Health Care Divided

Health Care Divided

Race and Healing a Nation

David Barton Smith

Ann Arbor

THE UNIVERSITY OF MICHIGAN PRESS

Research for this book was conducted with the support of a
Robert Wood Johnson Health Policy Research Investigator
Award Grant, Number 026426(IHP).

A CIP catalog record for this book is available from the British Library.

Library of Congress Cataloging-in-Publication Data

Smith, David Barton.
    Health care divided : race and healing a nation / David Barton
Smith.
        p.   cm.
    Includes bibliographical references and index.
    ISBN 0-472-10991-X (cloth : alk. paper)
    1. Discrimination in medical care—United States.   2.
Afro-Americans—Medical care.   I. Title.
RA448.5.N4   S63   1998
362.1'089'96073—dc21   98-40200
                                                       CIP

For my children, Alex, Barton, and Kara,
for my grandchildren, Jethro and Shannon,
and for their vision of a better world.

Preface

Telling the story of our racially divided health care system is difficult. Most readers bring their own baggage of strongly held opinions, anger, and resentments. Even if they are open enough to listen, most would prefer a story with clear-cut heroes and villains and a reassuring ending that makes them feel comfortable. The real story is more complicated and troubling.

I, too, have my opinions, and it would be false to claim to be providing an objective account. The telling of any story involves more than just a compilation of chronological events; it means imposing order on those events and making choices about what to include and exclude. Most of those choices are unconscious, reflecting the storyteller's own biases, experiences, and interests. The story told in this book reflects my own background in teaching and researching the organization of health services. I was drawn to it by a fascination with what it could tell me about how health care organizations work. People joke about going to a university hospital and being horrified when the academic physicians there show great interest in, rather than the usual boredom with, their complaints. They fear that the doctors suspect some really interesting—but fatal—pathology. With some embarrassment, I admit to a similar fascination with the problem of race and the organization of health care in America.

I view the story of our divided health care system through the experiences of the organizations that shaped, and were in turn shaped by, events. I look for the interconnectedness between those organizations and events, and how organizations adapted or were replaced by others better able to cope with the changes in their environment.[1] The story is guided by a recognition of the complexity of how organizations work. The organization of health care resembles a nested series of Chinese boxes,[2] each with its own rules and dynamics, and within each box is another one. I will try to look inside each of those boxes. The outermost box is national history and culture; nested inside that is national political and organizational dynamics; the next level down is state and local community dynamics; and inside that box is the local health professional community and their organizations. Each of these boxes or environments is shaped by individuals and the organizations of which they are members. Individuals and organizations exert influences on their environment and thus play a key role in choosing over time the environment or box in which they live. This book is, in essence, a case study of those choices.

As much as possible I have let the participants speak in their own words, either through interviews or from the written record. Just as in any case study, I have quoted extensively from these sources and supplied many numbers that help tell the more objective side of the story. I have tried to leave most of the interpretation in the hands of the reader.

The first part of the book describes in five chapters the choices that produced the health care civil rights struggle. The first chapter presents the background and evolution of our divided health care system. The second describes the early battles to integrate hospitals at the national policy level. Chapter 3 focuses on the battles in North Carolina, where the key legal precedents were set. Chapter 4 tells of the remarkable transformation that took place through the enforcement of the 1964 Civil Rights legislation in the implementation of the Medicare program. The final chapter of this section brings the story up to the present, describing the decline and dissipation of attention to civil rights issues in health.

The second part presents the legacy of a divided health care system produced by those early choices. It includes three chapters. The first assesses the accomplishments and uncompleted agenda of the civil rights movement as it pertains to health care. In spite of dramatic changes and the elimination of most financial barriers, racial differences persist in the life opportunities of those who are now being born and those who are growing old. These differences are explored in chapter 7, which looks at the impact on the provision of services to the elderly, while chapter 8 examines the lingering impact of this legacy on maternal and infant care. The final chapter deals with the choices remaining to us. It summarizes the lessons of the story and suggests some alternative organizational strategies for dealing with the continuing legacy of a divided health care system and the uncompleted healing of a nation.

In telling this story, I am indebted to the help of many individuals and organizations. Solomon Axelrod, Benjamin Darsky, Avedis Donnabedian, and Charles Metzner of the Bureau of Public Health Economics began my preparation more than thirty years ago in the Medical Care Organization doctoral program at the University of Michigan. Anne Torregrossa, Philip Tannenbaum, and Mike Campbell of the Pennsylvania Health Law Project sowed the seeds for this particular project over ten years ago when they persuaded me to look at some numbers related to racial access to nursing homes in Pennsylvania. Gordon Bonnyman and the Poverty & Race Research Action Council later encouraged me through their interests in using some of the conclusions from that early effort to challenge the federal failure to collect data to adequately monitor civil rights compliance.

No story this ambitious would have been possible to tell without the encouragement of the Fox School of Business and Management at Temple University and the Robert Wood Johnson Foundation. Temple provided a study leave during the early phases and subsequent flexibility in meeting my teaching and administrative obligations that made the field work part for the project feasible. The Robert Wood Johnson Foundation through a Health Policy Research Investigator Award provided the precious additional time, access to data resources and travel funds to pursue leads. Colleagues connected with Temple and with the Robert Wood Johnson Health Policy Research Investigator Program provided much intellectual stimulation and encouragement for this effort. At Temple, these included Morris Vogel, who first got me excited about medical history, David Webb and Scott Snyder of Temple's Social Science Data Library who helped translate my curiosity into numbers and colleagues in the Healthcare Management Program Bill Aaronson, Chuck Hall, Tom Getzen, and Jackie Zinn who read various pieces of the manuscript and provided suggestions and encouragement. I am also indebted to Sally Villar, the Program's Administrative Assistant, who handled much of the project's correspondence and graciously held the program together, giving me time to devote to this effort. Many students in the graduate program in Healthcare Management also read various drafts and, in some cases, helped supply from their own family histories stories that ended up being included in the book. My interactions with many of the people involved in the Robert Wood Johnson Health Policy Investigator program also found their way into the pages of this book. Those whose influence I can most easily identify include, Ruth Faden, Mark Peterson, G. Madison Powers, Mark Rodwin, David Williams, and Rodrick Wallace as well as the contagious excitement of Sol Levine who directed the program for the Foundation for my first two years as an investigator before his death.

Material written by the author and previously appearing in the *American Journal of Public Health, Hospital and Health Services Administration,* and the *Journal of Health Politics, Policy and Law* has been adapted and incorporated in this book. I gratefully acknowledge the permissions of these journals.

In the actual conduct of the research itself, I am indebted to many individuals and organizations that provided assistance. Brahim Bookhart, research assistant for the first two years of the project, did all the unglamorous but essential and often overwhelming work pulling together references, and data with grace, humor and efficiency. Many organizations assisted in providing access to staff and resources. Marianne Lado at the NAACP Legal Defense Fund helped set up interviews and shared much useful information from her own files. Dennis Hyashi, Director of the Office for Civil Rights in DHHS and staff members of the Office were most gracious in sharing insights and information. Bob Konrad and other colleagues at the Cecil Sheps Center for Health Services Research at the University of North Carolina went out of their way to serve as hosts and facilitators during my trips to North Carolina. In Greensboro, North Carolina, I am especially indebted to Dr. George Simkins, Dennis Barry, and Dr. Robert L. Phillips for their assistance and access to their records. The list could go on and includes more than one hundred individuals who assisted through interviews and access to documents and information. They unselfishly gave of themselves and have challenged me to try to the best of my abilities to be worthy of their trust.

As this book goes to press, I am struck by all the important parts of the story that I have left untold or incomplete. The stories of many cities, institutions, and individuals need more complete telling. In particular, I was impressed by some comments in reviewing the final version by Robert Ball, Commissioner of Social Security at the time of the passage of Medicare. He saw the need to tell more of the story of the local Social Security staff's role in the initial certification of facilities for participation in Medicare and that the bulk of the effort to integrate the hospitals in the South was accomplished by federal employees who were local southerners. I hope that such gaps, as well as those of which I am not now aware, will motivate others to fill them. At the same time, I am encouraged that the final chapter in the larger story may have begun to be written. In a significant departure from its predecessor, *Healthy People 2000,* the draft of *Healthy People 2010* has set as a key national goal the elimination of racial and ethnic health disparities. Efforts are also underway to include similar goals in the monitoring of standards in Medicaid and Medicare managed-care plans. This reflects a growing consensus that it is no longer morally or socially acceptable either to remain silent on the persistent disparities or to set different health goals for different racial, ethnic, or income groups. The public sanctioning of the unequal allocation among Americans of good health care and health, with all the opportunities it confers, is no longer acceptable.

For whatever clarity and precision I have been able to achieve on such a complex topic, I am indebted to those who shaped the writing. Bruce MacLeod and Florence Ann Roberts expertly reviewed and edited early drafts of the chapters. Rebecca McDermott and Perry Pearson at the University of Michigan Press helped fine tune and finalize the manuscript for publication. A special note of affection and appreciation is due my wife, Joan Apt, who, in this process, not only put up with my self-absorption and absent-mindedness but reviewed and offered helpful suggestions on all of its many drafts. Finally, a most affectionate debt is due my parents, Nancy Woollcott and Henry Clay Smith, whose storytelling gifts and unshakable belief in the unlimited capabilities of their children gave me the courage to plunge into these cold and turbulent waters.

Contents

PART 1

Health Care's Civil Rights Struggle

CHAPTER 1

Race and Health Care in the United States

The minimum categories for data on race and ethnicity for Federal statistics, program administrative reporting, and civil rights compliance reporting are defined as follows:

American Indian or Alaskan Native. A person having origins in any of the original peoples of North and South America (including Central America), and who maintains tribal affiliation or community attachment.

Asian. A person having origins in any of the original peoples of the Far East, Southeast Asia, or the Indian subcontinent including, for example, Cambodia, China, India, Japan, Korea, Malaysia, Pakistan, the Philippine Islands, Thailand and Vietnam.

Black or African American. A person having origins in any of the black groups of Africa. Terms such as "Haitian" or "Negro" can be used in addition to "Black" or "African American."

Hispanic or Latino. A person of Cuban, Mexican, Puerto Rican, South or Central American, or other Spanish culture or origin, regardless of race. The term "Spanish origin" can be used in addition to "Hispanic" or "Latino."

Native Hawaiian or Other Pacific Islander. A person having origins in any of the original peoples of Hawaii, Guam, Samoa or other Pacific islands.

White. A person having origins in any of the original peoples of Europe, the Middle East or North Africa.

Respondents shall be offered the option of selecting one or more racial designations. Recommended forms for the instruction accompanying the multiple response question are "Mark one or more" and "Select one or more."[1]

Thus read the Office of Management and Budget's revised federal standards for classifying race. Nobody liked the earlier version of federal standards, known as *Directive 15,* and the OMB's minor revisions, announced in October 1997, do little to heighten enthusiasm. Medical and health services researchers, black separatists, liberal guardians of political correctness, polished spokespersons for the conservative think tanks, and rabid white supremacists all hate them. The proud, self-identified ethnic groups subsumed under these categories do as well. Such categories make no sense as either biological or cultural groupings; nor does race as a whole. Most of those lumped into these categories share neither a common language nor a common history, and some feel strong prejudices against ethnic groups whose OMB category they share.

More than twenty years ago, *Directive 15* established the way racial data would be collected by all agencies of the federal government. The review that led to its revision lasted more than four years and involved more than thirty federal agencies, four congressional hearings, and extensive survey research. Yet it produced only minor tinkering with racial classifications that will, at least through the year 2000 census, racially define the United States population. One of the previous OMB categories was divided into two—Asians will now be distinguished from Native Hawaiian and other Pacific Islanders. In addition, individuals will now be able to check more than one box to identify themselves racially. The survey research suggested that only about 1 or 2 percent of the American population will choose this option.

Why not just stop collecting and using such information? Isn't it "un-American"? Eliminating the collection of data by race would, for all practical purposes, negate all affirmative-action programs, the Civil Rights Act, the Voting Rights Act, the Fair Housing Act, and other related legislation. Does discrimination grow or disappear without any way to assess it? Why classify people at all and, particularly, by such artificial categories? Why does race matter?

This book explores these questions for health services in the United States. Race continues to matter. Its influence has been so permanent and pervasive that it becomes an almost unrecognized part of the background of our culture. The Constitution of the United States, after all, used three of the recently announced six basic OMB racial and ethnic categories to allocate congressional representation to states according to their population (each white was counted as one person; black slaves counted as three-fifths of a person; and Indians were not counted at all). Friction over slavery among the framers of the Constitution contributed to our decentralized form of government. Some have argued that it was racial divisions that influenced the development of a welfare and indigent health care system that involves rituals of degradation in local means-tested programs, rather than a system of social entitlement like those typical in other developed countries.[2]

This book tells the story of how race has cast a pervasive shadow over the development and organization of health care in the United States. That influence, in part, is reflected in the lack of a national health insurance program. It has shaped how health care organizations are owned and governed. Race is reflected in the cost of health care in the United States, the highest in the world, and in the health status of its population, among the worst of developed nations. Health care expenditures in the United States in 1995 accounted for 13.6 percent of gross domestic product, or $3,219 per person. The United States is a lonely outlier whose per capita expenditures and percentage of gross domestic product devoted to health care are far above those of other developed nations. Yet, it ranks twenty-fifth among these countries in infant mortality, twenty-third in male life expectancy, and nineteenth in female life expectancy.[3] Race remains a thinly concealed influence on the debate over health care reform. It affects concerns over centralized control by a federal bureaucracy and the need for "market" solutions that more narrowly define health plan and provider responsibilities. Health care, however, is more than just a collection of goods and services fragmented by racial divisions. Health care is organized, and that organization sends powerful symbolic messages that help define our national identity. The story told in this book is about a divided nation, a divided health care system, and the uncompleted journey to heal both.

Race

Discussions about race are always awkward. Race is not a scientifically defensible biological or genetic classification scheme.[4] There is more variability within than between racial categories on any characteristic that should matter in shaping life chances. Race should not predict morbidity, mortality, or occupational success. Nor is it a classification scheme that defines distinctive cultural subgroups, despite the current wave of interest in "cultural diversity" training. There are as many cultural and class differences within racial categories as there are between them. Race does not fit the conventional American "melting pot" theories that predict the acculturation and intergenerational upward mobility of immigrant populations. Nuances aside, African Americans and white Americans share the same language, root for the same professional sports teams, enjoy most of the same popular music, and watch most of the same soaps. African Americans can trace their roots in the United States back much further than most white Americans can.

What makes race difficult to talk about is that it deals with resources and power. It has served as America's version of a caste system, while racism has been the ideology that justified it. The attributed cultural and genetic differences between the races have been used to justify slavery, Jim

Crow laws, and differences in life chances in a world where the "Whites Only" signs have been removed. Race remains the "American dilemma," as Swedish economist Gunnar Myrdal observed more than half a century ago. On the one hand, Americans value equality of opportunity. On the other hand, race continues to limit the equality of opportunity. It is one thing to make the visible symbols of Jim Crow disappear in order to embrace the rhetoric of equal opportunity. It has proved far more difficult to make the real differences in life chances disappear. That involves reallocating goods and power and effecting real change within institutions. However necessary, that is a much more difficult change to bring about.

The solution that we seem to have drifted into is not to talk about race, and particularly, not to talk about the racial separation that assures unequal access to resources. As one group of researchers recently observed, we have done a good job of that: "During the 1970s and 1980s a word disappeared from the American vocabulary,"[5] they write. The word is *segregation.* The word was not a part of the vocabulary of politicians, private foundations, government officials, journalists, academicians, or business executives in their discussion of the nation's social problems. Current health care reform proposals that express the desire to assure universal access and an end to a tiered system of care do not mention it. In no area has the silence been as complete as in health care. We compile statistics on segregation in housing, schools, and employment. No such information has ever been systematically collected on health care. Title VI of the Civil Rights Act of 1964 specifically prohibits the use of federal financial assistance for any activity or program that denies benefits or excludes participation based on race, color, or national origin. Yet, more than thirty years after the passage of Medicare and Medicaid, which made the federal government the dominant source of funds, this information void continues. Far more federal dollars flow into health care than into housing, schools, and employment. Far more federal dollars flow into collecting data about health and health care than into data about education and housing. Yet no one reports information on segregation in health care. We have done a good job of making the word disappear, but the problem remains. It is what Philip Slater in *The Pursuit of Loneliness* described as the "toilet assumption," the

> notion that unwanted matter, unwanted difficulties, unwanted complexities and obstacles will disappear if they are removed from our immediate field of vision. . . . when these discarded problems rise to the surface again as a riot, a protest, an exposé in the mass media we react as if a sewer had backed up. We are shocked, disgusted and angered and immediately call for the emergency plumber (the special

commission, the crash program) to insure that the problem is once again removed from consciousness.[6]

It is time to take a harder look at the plumbing.

Health Care

Health care is a perfect place to start looking at that plumbing. Most acknowledge that health care has always been something more than just another good or service bought or sold in the marketplace.[7] Because health care directly influences not just lifestyle, but life itself, health care is different. As such, it provides both an ideal window for observing the effects of race and, perhaps, the best place to begin to minimize them. There are three aspects of health care that make it distinctly different from most other goods and services.

First, health care, from a political perspective, serves as a *mechanism of social control,* which contributes to social stability. Health care is a part of the way any society, community, or large organization tries to maintain itself as an effective collective unit. For example, health care helps organizations deal with members who no longer do what is normally expected of them, encouraging them to be admitted to a hospital for cardiac bypass surgery or to an outpatient drug treatment program. Knowing that they will be taken care of if they get sick, in turn, strengthens individuals' identification with and commitment to an organization. Families, churches, schools, and the criminal-justice system, as well as health care, all play a role in assuring a necessary degree of social cohesion in a community. Health centers are constructed amid the charred ruins of urban riots in an effort to build social cohesion where it is absent. Health care reform efforts in nations take place after wars in acknowledgment of the social cohesion and individual sacrifices necessary to bring the war to a successful conclusion.

As a result, reducing the investment in health care sometimes does not save money. Reductions in health care may simply shift the costs of dealing with social problems to other institutions that are concerned with social control. For example, the admission rate to inpatient drug and alcohol treatment programs dropped by 22 percent, or more than five thousand admissions, in Philadelphia between 1980 and 1992, while the incarceration rate in state prisons increased by more than 233 percent, from 2,790 to 10,856 inmates. In constant dollars, the jail expenditures for prisoners from Philadelphia have increased from $42 million to $163 million, and the average expenditures per inmate per year have been estimated at more than fifteen thousand dollars. Most of these incarcerations were drug related.[8] A similar situation exists with the decline in state-supported inpatient psychiatric care, lack of adequate transitional assisted-living arrangements, the corresponding growth of homelessness, and the growing cost of temporary shelters to house this population. Squeeze the investment in one place, and it expands in another.

Second, health care, from an economic perspective, is in part a *public good.* That is, the public in general benefits, and benefits can't be restricted simply to the person receiving services. Much of the effort earlier in this century to provide health services to blacks was driven more by a concern for protecting whites from TB and other infectious diseases than for protecting the health of blacks.[9] More recently, one analysis has suggested that so-called inner-city markers such as AIDS, tuberculosis, and low birth weight diffuse rapidly across suburban commuting fields, creating the potential for enveloping entire regions in "synergisms of plagues."[10] Such analysis makes a strong argument for regional efforts and the pooling of the resources of suburban counties to combat inner-city problems.

The boundaries between public and private goods in health care are fuzzy. For example, death rates from asthma have increased dramatically in Philadelphia over the past twenty years, particularly for young people, blacks, and those living in low-income neighborhoods.[11] Allowing a child to die in the streets from an acute asthma attack just because her family cannot pay for admission to a hospital is unacceptable to all of us. We are quite clear on this, even making it illegal to deny such care. Is such care a public good? Asthma is not an infectious illness, but we will all pay the cost of that hospitalization, whether it be in the form of a tax increase, higher hospitalization insurance costs, or subtle degradation in the hospital care that we as individuals receive that results from underfunding.

When presented with the bill for these costs, people usually say, "Yeah, it's sort of a public good, and we should pay for it." Yet who is the "we?" Should that "we" be the extended family, friends, the hospital, the local community, the state, or the country as a whole? This is what economists call the "free rider" problem, and most of the debate about health care financing revolves around it. That is, we all benefit, at least psychically, from knowing that care is provided to asthmatic children, whether we chip in to pay or not. Public programs reduce the payments recipients make to providers, thus shifting more of the cost for indigent patients onto the providers. The providers then raise the fees to their private patients, thereby shifting the burden onto private insurers. Private insurers, in turn, shift costs onto the employee benefit plans, which shift them onto the employees, which in turn increases the pressure on public programs, and so the vicious cycle continues. The cynics might say that management and managed care mean taking the monkey off your back and putting it on someone else, but that monkey, eventually, comes around again.

For the less cynical, well-managed care would mean finding the most cost-effective way to address a problem defined as a public responsibility. For example, most asthma admissions could be prevented with adequate primary care. Is such primary care a public good? It would be a cheaper way of managing asthma.[12] It is far less costly than permitting frequent crises that require hospital admissions. The rise in rates of admissions for, and deaths from, asthma, however, may not be related to any sharp decline in indigent access to primary care. Some research suggests that the major cause is crowded, substandard housing, in particular, the dust of cockroaches.[13] We have come full circle again.

Health care is more than just a peculiar struggle over who gets what kind of care and who gets stuck with the bill. As the preceding discussion suggests, health care is an *ethical and moral matter.* Lack of access to adequate health care can restrict an individual's normal range of opportunities and raises basic issues of fairness and social justice.[14] Health care and the way we organize public health services has a profound effect on people's well-being and opportunities. Health care can provide the information we need to plan our lives in the face of illness, prevent premature death, alleviate pain, and restore function. As a culture we profess a moral commitment to equality of opportunity. Access to health care often has a more immediate impact on opportunities than access to the ballot, education, housing, and jobs.

Health care, in summary, serves as (1) a mechanism of social control, (2) a public economic good, and (3) an ethical and moral touchstone. These three characteristics distinguish it from other goods and services. The tensions created by these three distinctive characteristics have shaped the development of health services in the United States, as they have in other countries. In the United States, however, they were shaped through the filter of race.

Health Care Divided: Race and the Development of Health Care in the United States

My father's family came from Georgia, where they owned a farm. The story goes that in the 1930s a neighboring white plantation owner wanted the land, but my granddad refused to sell it. I guess the plantation owner got angry, and the Klan came the next night, grabbed two of my grandmother's brothers, and lynched them. My grandfa-

ther returned, killed the plantation owner, and escaped. My grandmom and her kids had to escape also to avoid retaliation. They ended
up in Greenville, South Carolina, and my grandmom took in washing. She never saw her husband again, but they never caught him
either. He ended up in the Winston-Salem area living under an
assumed name. Every once in a while she'd get word passed along
about him. There was an underground thing; an understanding that
you helped other blacks who had got in trouble. That's how my
grandmother was able to move to Greenville.

I grew up on a farm outside Greenville. There was a thing about
going to town on Saturdays. We'd all walk three miles to town. In
Walgreen's or Woolworth's we'd see something different. There were
"white" and "colored" water fountains. I wanted to see what the
white water tasted like. You'd get there and one of the other kids was
always daring you. One day I got up enough nerve to dip my head
down and squirted it up. Got in a lot trouble for that. My parents
didn't want any trouble.

When I was growing up, Dr. Bailey on Main Street in Greenville
was the family physician. There was a separate waiting room for
blacks, and you had to wait till all the white patients had been seen
before he'd see the blacks. As long as the white patients kept coming
in, you kept being pushed further and further back. Later, when a
black physician set up practice in Greenville, blacks flocked to him. I
got a bad virus when I was a little kid and was admitted to the hospital. I got a private room on a white floor. My aunt did washing for a
white physician, and that gave me special pull. I felt extra special. I
remember when I was a teen I had to help my grandmom go for care
at Greenville General. She had cancer. We had to wait in a horrible
small room for black patients in the basement. We'd get there at 9:00,
and we often didn't return until 5:30. The local mortician provided
the transportation to the hospital. The understanding was that the
transportation was free, but he would get the body. It wasn't a bad
experience. It was the way it was.[15]

"The way it was," the underlying caste divisions in American society
shaped the institutions that developed to care for the health needs, patient
expectations, and the very purposes of the services provided. It also shaped
outcomes. A research memorandum prepared as a part of the Carnegie
Foundation–supported study that would produce Myrdal's watershed
book, *The American Dilemma,* concluded that if black death rates in 1930
were made equivalent to white death rates, 70 percent of the black deaths
would have been eliminated.[16] That same memorandum concluded,

The economic problem of providing medical facilities for Negroes is complicated by racial discrimination. Color restricts the Negro's access to many medical facilities even when he is able to pay for the services rendered. Negro physicians are admitted to some hospitals operated by white persons but the more usual situation is to bar them entirely.[17]

Segregated systems of care that developed in slavery were perpetuated in the post-Reconstruction period. The underlying assumptions of scientific medicine and the mechanisms developed for financing health services helped reinforce these divisions. Thus, the transformation of medicine in the twentieth century heightened both racial segregation and inequalities.

Antebellum Health Care

Medical care in the United States before the Civil War was limited and unorganized. The country was largely rural, populated by farmers and independent craftspersons. There was no standing army, and there were few large employers. Medical care, except for a few institutions established for the destitute by local governments and philanthropists in the larger cities, was provided by independent, fee-for-service practitioners. They took diverse, sometimes conflicting approaches to disease and applied treatments that were often ineffectual or even harmful. Many were part-time practitioners whose practice income was not sufficient for a livelihood. With the mix of altruism and self-interest that is always present among professionals, local groups of physicians began to organize. Physicians in a New Jersey medical society, for example, as early as 1786 established a fee schedule that "shall be deemed the general rule of charging by the members of the Society and so far binding that in no instance [shall a member] exceed it and further, the Society will deem it highly dishonorable in any member to make a different charge with a view to injure a neighboring practitioner who is also a member."[18] In effect, discount fee competition among physicians was stifled by local medical societies until the recent emergence of managed care.

The only instances of organized medical services comparable to current managed-care plans were found on the plantations and directed toward slaves. Plantation owners were the only group of large employers before the Civil War. They were also the only employers that had a direct financial interest in protecting the health of their employees. In 1860 the estimated four million slaves in the United States were valued at more than two billion dollars.[19] Slaves sometimes received better health care than poor southern whites or northern laborers. Every major plantation had a hospital of some kind, and some were well equipped by the standards of the day. An older black woman was typically placed in charge. Some of these black attendants were considered so knowledgeable that whites consulted them. Occasionally, white physicians sought to prevent such competition. Courts in Tennessee, for example, ruled that slaves could not practice medicine. In the larger towns of the south, such as New Orleans, Savannah, and Montgomery, private physicians organized hospitals for slaves. Natchez, Mississippi, had several slave hospitals, including a two-story building next to the slave market known as the Mississippi State Hospital and the Homeopathic Infirmary for Slaves. The infirmary provided care for one dollar a day. Several hospitals in New Orleans provided separate wards for slaves. Alternatively, plantation owners sometimes arranged for physicians to care for slaves on an annual retainer. Those arrangements with health care facilities served as the first form of employer-based health insurance in this country, and those contracts between the plantation owners and physicians for overseeing the care of slaves represented the first forms of managed care.

Post-Reconstruction Health Care

The plantation system of medical care ended with emancipation. Massive dislocation and migration to southern urban centers began to take place. The federal government established the Freedmen's Bureau to help the emancipated slaves. Its medical department set up more than ninety hospitals and dispensaries in the South but closed all except one by 1868. Only Freedmen's Hospital (Howard University Medical Center) survived. Whose responsibility would black health care be now? Blacks were mostly excluded from existing health and social-service organizations. Orphanages, private charitable hospitals, local almshouses, and state facilities, with rare exceptions, served only whites. Local municipalities reluctantly began to develop segregated services for blacks, largely in response to pressures from local black populations exercised through the ballot. Some private hospitals in the larger northern cities provided care in segregated services for blacks. They tended to be less exclusionary, but the bulk of the black population remained concentrated in the South. As another method of providing care, local municipalities and states in the nineteenth century instituted lump-sum payments to municipal and some private hospitals to subsidize the care of the indigent, which included segregated services for the poor. (That approach is now being reinvented. In order to control escalating costs, most state Medical Assistance programs have adopted regional capitation approaches.)

An implicit division of labor emerged between public and voluntary hospitals in cities and towns large enough to accommodate both types of facilities. Both types of nineteenth-century hospitals had been asylums or refuges for the destitute who lacked housing or the means to pay for private nursing and physicians in their home. The voluntary hospitals, however, created through the donations of local community members and philanthropists as private charities, defined their mission in more narrow, moralistic terms. They saw their role as providing care to the "deserving poor," not as a service to all people in the community. It was the role of governments, not voluntary hospitals, to provide for the "undeserving." Government hospitals should provide the shelter and basic services to the unworthy, impoverished social failures, as well as the chronically ill whom charitable hospitals were not prepared to admit.[20] Being a "socially worthy" impoverished patient meant being morally respectable and suitably deferential. Those whose need for care resulted from alcohol or drug abuse or sexual indiscretions were not deserving of such charity. Being a member of the right racial, ethnic, or religious group also helped. Board members of voluntary hospitals often personally participated in admission decisions. Both the public and voluntary hospitals served to police and control individual behavior. The voluntary hospitals supported the socially worthy, and public hospitals controlled those who were not. This meant that blacks were mostly relegated to the use of public institutions. Blacks, nevertheless, were increasingly able to exercise influence over those public institutions and the care they provided through their growing political influence in local elections.

Toward the end of the nineteenth century, however, both the public and voluntary hospitals were becoming more important to medicine. Asepsis, anesthesia, and other surgical advances were transforming these institutions into workshops essential to the practice of medicine. Increasingly, middle- and upper-class patients would receive and pay for care in these facilities. Some voluntary charitable hospitals felt uncomfortable with that shift. The board of one Philadelphia hospital for a decade debated the appropriateness of accepting paying patients, before acquiescing to an experiment with six private rooms in 1899.[21] The shift of private medical practice to hospital settings spread quickly; correspondingly, effective control of the institutions shifted from their boards and charitable benefactors to the hospitals' medical staff.[22]

The Social Transformation of American Medicine

The transformation of medicine at the turn of the century coincided with the failure of Reconstruction and the passage of Jim Crow laws by states across the South. Until the last decade of the nineteenth century, the divisions between the races had been more fluid. While there was informal segregation, as there is today, little had been prescribed by state laws.[23] The climate hardened in the 1890s. The *Plessy v. Ferguson* Supreme Court decision in 1896 ruled that a Louisiana state law segregating railroad passenger cars did not violate the Fourteenth Amendment guarantee of equal protection. Modern medicine and the organization of health services in the United States were a particularly bitter part of the harvest of the seeds sown by *Plessy v. Ferguson.* The subsequent wave of Jim Crow legislation solidified a caste system that most whites and blacks seemed either to endorse or dare not to defy. The modern U.S. health care system was constructed according to those blueprints restricting the opportunities available to blacks, shaping the physical design of facilities and even influencing the nature of scientific inquiry.

Much of the care provided in increasingly segregated black communities was provided by black physicians. For those practitioners and the communities they served, the social transformation they experienced was traumatic. The net impact was to (1) restrict the supply of black physicians, (2) limit the ability of black communities to control the hospitals that served them, and (3) exclude black physicians from hospital practice.

Restriction of Entry into the Profession

Between 1900 and 1920, reforms in medical education and a tightening of medical licensure restricted opportunities for blacks to enter the profession. In the beginning of the century the United States had the highest ratio of physicians to population in the world. The practice of medicine included a chaotic, warring assortment of cults trained by schools with stark differences in rigor and resources. By 1920, reforms in medical education had changed medicine into an occupation restricted to a professional elite. Four-year university training programs modeled on the one at Johns Hopkins became the standard. The strongest schools were generously supported by private philanthropies such as the Rockefeller and Carnegie foundations. The foundations were attracted to the new concept of scientific medicine, just as their benefactors had embraced new concepts in industry during their early careers. Scientific medicine gave the illusion of elevating the profession above political, class, and racial conflicts. Medicine became largely an upper-class, white, male profession. In 1900 seven medical schools were training blacks, not including several proprietary schools in Washington, D.C., which provided evening programs, or "sundown" medical schools, largely for those who had full-time day jobs as federal employees. Jobs in the federal government were among the few nonmenial ones available to black Americans at the turn of the century, and many became trained as physicians in evening programs.[24] By 1920, however, only two medical schools for blacks survived the reform efforts, Howard and Meharry. They remained the almost exclusive sources of the limited supply of black physicians until the 1960s.

The transformation in medical education had been encouraged by a report produced by Abraham Flexner in 1910. The Flexner report had been supported by the Carnegie Foundation and helped bolster the efforts of the AMA's Council on Medical Education to restrict eligibility for state licensure to physicians graduating from approved medical schools. Flexner, who later served on the board of Howard University, acknowledged the importance of providing adequate medical education to blacks in a racially divided health system.

> The medical care of the Negro race will never be wholly left to Negro physicians. Nevertheless, if the Negro can be brought to feel a sharp responsibility for the physical integrity of his people, the outlook for their mental and moral improvement will be distinctly brightened. The practice of the Negro doctor will be limited to his own race, which in turn will be cared for better by good Negro physicians than by poor white ones. But the physical well-being of the Negro is not only of moment to the Negro himself. Ten million of them live in close contact with sixty million whites. Not only does the Negro himself suffer from hookworm and tuberculosis; he communicates them to his white neighbors, precisely as the ignorant and unfortunate white contaminates him. Self-protection not less than humanity offers weighty counsel in this matter; self-interest seconds philanthropy. The Negro must be educated not only for his sake, but for ours. He is, as far as human eye can see, a permanent factor in the nation. He has his rights and due and value as an individual; but he has, besides, the tremendous importance that belongs to a potential source of infection and contagion.
>
> The pioneer work in educating the race to know and practice fundamental hygienic principles must be done largely by the Negro doctor and the Negro nurse. It is important they both be sensibly and effectively trained at the level at which their services are now important. The Negro is perhaps more easily "taken in" than the white; and as his means of extricating himself from a blunder are limited, it is all the more cruel to abuse his ignorance through any sort of pretense. A well-taught Negro sanitarian will be immensely useful; an essentially untrained Negro wearing an M.D. degree is dangerous.[25]

Flexner clearly saw the place of black physicians in the natural order of things. Their practice would be limited to blacks. They could be useful in preventing the spread of TB and other infections to white populations, and, thus, their education should focus on the principles of hygiene rather than the techniques of surgery. Germs may not have a color line, but medical practice should.[26]

The Transformation of the Hospital and the Consolidation of Racial Divisions

Reforms in medical education and the credentialing of practitioners led to similar changes in hospitals, further exacerbating racial inequities. Hospitals at the turn of the century represented a diverse assortment of private sanitoriums run by individual physicians, county and municipal facilities evolving out of eighteenth- and nineteenth-century's poorhouses, and privately endowed philanthropic institutions. These facilities now became increasingly important to the practice of medicine and essential to surgical practice. Medical staffs, bodies organized by the independent practitioners who used a hospital for their patients, quickly wrestled effective control of hospitals from their boards. The American College of Surgeons played a key role in this shift. By 1920 it had launched an ambitious effort to standardize hospitals through a voluntary certification program. Since medical records were important in evaluating the eligibility of surgeons for membership in the College, they became an important focus of the College's standardization and certification efforts. More important, certification required that medical staffs be organized and exert control over medical practice in the hospital. Medical staffs now became much more than a loose collection of practitioners who volunteered some of their time to care for patients who could not afford to be cared for by private practitioners in their homes. They now decided who would be accepted as staff members and what kinds of procedures they would be permitted to perform; they monitored the quality of care provided; and they disciplined their members. The authority of the staff to accept or deny membership was absolute. Physicians from many ethnic groups were excluded from medical staffs in institutions that operated essentially as private clubs. The only recourse for these physicians was to organize support within their own ethnic communities to build their own hospitals. Hospitals were founded not just by Jewish and Catholic religious communities, but also by Russian Jews and German Jews, Irish Catholics and Italian Catholics.

Part of the response by black physicians, similar to that of other excluded groups, was to build their own hospitals. Provident Medical Center and training school, the first black-owned and controlled facility, was established in Chicago in 1891. More would follow. Most would be created with a certain tension and ambivalence. The Frederick Douglass Memorial Hospital and Training School, opened in Philadelphia in 1895, was no exception. Nathan Mossell, a founder and a black University of Pennsylvania Medical School graduate, would later reflect that Douglass "means extravagance, inefficiency, duplication of effort, and is undemocratic in that it establishes a caste."[27] Some white leaders were concerned that it was an unnecessary addition to the already crowded list of charitable institutions in the city. The *Weekly Tribune,* a black paper, viewed it as surrender, arguing that it was the "quintessence of foolishness to continually prate about breaking down color barriers and then go on rearing them ourselves."[28] By 1910, however, one hundred such institutions dotted the American landscape.[29]

The fear among black medical leaders was that the American College of Surgeons standardization effort could eventually result in the elimination of black hospitals and even the death of the black medical profession. These leaders had formed their own organization, the National Medical Association (NMA), in 1895 in response to their exclusion from AMA-affiliated local medical societies. At the NMA's annual meeting in 1923 the organization established its own hospital association and standardization effort, the National Hospital Association.[30] Corresponding efforts were initiated to support and strengthen medical and nursing training, medical societies, and journals, all established to assure survival. The NMA also sought the help of private white philanthropies to build and improve black hospitals. The Julius Rosenwald Fund, with the assistance of the Duke Endowment, had helped fourteen such projects in the Carolinas by the end of 1930.[31]

The story of the formation and expansion of Lincoln Hospital, a black institution in Durham, North Carolina, illustrates the complex interplay between white philanthropy, black communities, and the struggle of black physicians to avoid exclusion from hospital medicine. Evolving out of the earlier benevolent association organized by freed slaves after the Civil War, North Carolina Mutual in Durham had grown to be the largest black-owned business in the United States. The two founders of the company were Dr. Moore, Durham's first black physician, and John Merrit, an enterprising barber who operated about five shops in Durham. Dr. Moore helped to found Lincoln Hospital at the turn of the century. In 1895 a local white benefactor had provided fifty thousand dollars in his will for the construction of a hospital in Durham, stipulating that it serve white patients only. About 25 percent of the population of Durham was black. In response, Dr. Moore in 1902 pressed the Duke family for ten thousand dollars to build Lincoln Hospital, a sixteen-bed cottage hospital.

In 1924 the Duke family matched $75,000 raised in the black community to build a more substantial one-hundred-bed facility.[32] It would grow to become an important center of training for black physicians. For example, Charles Watts, a black surgeon and the first in North Carolina to become a member of the American College of Surgeons, began his practice at Lincoln in 1950. In the 1950s a black surgeon wishing to be in private practice had few other options.

In the absence of any white philanthropic support, some efforts to build black hospitals exhibited remarkable ingenuity in tapping into black resources. The work of Dorothy Ferebee and her sorority sisters is a particularly compelling example. Ferebee, the first black female graduate of Tufts Medical School in 1924, served on the faculty of Howard University's Medical School.[33] She organized her Alpha Kappa Alpha sorority sisters in volunteering to help blacks in the Mississippi Delta. A community organizer arriving in Mound Bayou in 1967 to organize the recently federally funded Tufts rural health center demonstration project was in awe of what had been accomplished with so little.

Beginning in 1934, Dr. Ferebee had recruited sisters from her national black sorority, Alpha Kappa Alpha, to join her as volunteers in Mississippi. They established contacts in Mound Bayou through a network of churches. Dr. Ferebee's volunteers set up seven clinics on plantations, did immunizations, nutrition counseling, and so forth. They also worked with a local fraternal order, the Knights and Daughters of Tabor. Black benevolent groups like the Knights had sprung up all over the South after the Civil War.

In my own family, we belonged to a similar order that looked after members facing crises. My grandfather and great-grandfather were active in such organizations. They saw it as an extension of their social responsibility. As a member, you were assured of a burial with dignity. If you became ill, someone was there to assist you and your family. The community has to come together on some things. In my family, this meant helping to maintain the community well and burial ground and to help people who became ill. Many were subsistence farmers, and others would go in and make sure that they got their crops in for that year. They assigned responsibility. My father, who was doing fairly well, contributed two pigs a year to the community larder. The community owned these resources, which could carry a couple of families who were in trouble with food for the year. Almost everybody back in the 1930s and 1940s were members. It included the schoolteachers, preachers, plus tenant farmers and sharecroppers on the plantations. It was organized in such a way so that the collector would see them every month and collect the nickel for the insurance system. It was a powerful communication system.

I think Dorothy Ferebee understood all this. She talked to the Knights and Daughters of Tabor about expanding their mission to health. That was the beginning of a real presence of health. This black woman of some prominence went into Mississippi when most black people would not do that and convinced the local fraternal order to build a hospital. The bottom line is that in 1941 in what was the second or third poorest county in America, the fraternal order built with their own resources what was then a modern forty-two-bed hospital for black people. It was beyond doubt the best hospital for black people in Mississippi at that time, Taborian Hospital.[34]

Sometimes black hospitals also represented a defiant response to a racial incident in the absence of any outside help. Most of the thirty thousand blacks in 1940 in south Florida's Broward County had come to the area to work in the fields or in the construction of roads and railroads. Dr. Von Delaney Mizell, Broward's second black physician, returned home to Broward to practice medicine in 1937. By default, he became a leader in many civil rights struggles and founded the local chapter of the NAACP. Blacks then were routinely arrested on the streets of Ft. Lauderdale for vagrancy. If they could not pay stiff fines, they were put on work gangs to help harvest crops.[35] In 1940, a young black man, John McBride, was shot in the abdomen by a gang of white youths bent on more aggressively policing the streets. South Florida's two black hospitals, the only ones that would accept black patients, were in Miami and West Palm Beach. McBride was denied admission to the two local hospitals, one municipally operated, the other private, and he died without hospital care. His death galvanized the African American community, under the leadership of Dr. Mizell. They responded by raising funds in the community to create Provident Hospital, a modest thirty-five-bed cottage hospital.

Some efforts in the black community, similar to other physician-established proprietary facilities, were more entrepreneurial than communal ventures. They reflected class, racial divisions, and the informal understandings that took place in racially divided communities. Just like other physician-owned hospitals, they were often lax in their control of surgical practices. A black surgeon recalled his pre-medical-school experiences in 1940 working at his uncle's hospital in Detroit.

He wanted me to sleep in the hospital, keep people from stealing from the refrigerator at night, and be the night watchman. I did that from

February to the following fall. The system of indigent care in Wayne County then was that entrepreneurs were encouraged to open hospitals, and the county would furnish indigent patients and pay for them. They did that rather than build an indigent hospital. Receiving Hospital was the indigent hospital, but it was nowhere near large enough to take care of the indigent. What they really did was take care of the white indigents at Receiving and allow the black physicians to open their own hospitals to take care of the blacks. There were about ten fifteen to one-hundred-bed or so hospitals like this. It was a terrible system. They couldn't maintain standards. They allowed private physicians to bring in patients for anything. We could see who was competent. One fellow was a very dapper and fashionable fellow who liked to take out tonsils. That was still in then, when we thought every child should have his tonsils out. Whenever he did several tonsillectomies in the morning, we kept the room warm because we knew they would be back that night to stop the bleeding.[36]

Some progress, however, had been made by black physicians in gaining privileges and integrating the medical staffs of public hospitals in some northern cities after World War I. These hospitals were caring for an increasing number of black patients in neighborhoods that were becoming predominantly black. The appointment of Dr. Lewis T. Wright to the low-ranking position of clinical assistant visiting surgeon at Harlem Hospital in 1919 was a first major breakthrough. A cum laude graduate of Harvard Medical School and a Purple Heart–decorated World War I veteran, he would later become the director of the hospital's surgical department and chairman of the board of the NAACP. His appointment resulted in the transfer of the hospital's white superintendent and, subsequently, a wave of resignations of white medical staff members.

Harlem, with its attractive brownstone neighborhoods, had become a magnet in the 1920s, a national epicenter of the black business, professional, and intellectual elite. It was the period of the Harlem Renaissance, and many of Harlem's residents were prolific contributors to literature, music, and the arts. It was also a sophisticated, politically well organized community with growing political power.

Harlem Hospital was a public hospital, and thus it was not completely insulated from local political pressure. Its all-white medical staff had served a growing black community that increasingly resented what they perceived as the racially prejudiced treatment that they were receiving. Under the leadership of the North Harlem Medical Society, with support from the NAACP, a recently appointed black civil-service commissioner, and pressure from a Harlem newspaper, more black physicians were appointed to the staff, slots were opened for interns through competitive examinations, black nurses were hired, and a nursing school was established. The hospital's unusually gifted group of physicians served as the center for the debate over the future of black health care. Harlem Hospital served as a model, and by the 1930s six other nonsegregated municipal hospitals followed, appointed blacks to their medical staffs: Bellevue in New York, Cook County in Chicago, Detroit Receiving, Boston City, and Cleveland City.[37]

Yet, for the most part, black physicians were squeezed out of hospital-based practice at other historically white-controlled institutions. Most black hospitals available to them did not have the staff and equipment to support the rapidly changing state of medical practice. In many communities, such as Atlanta, black physicians were restricted to the hospital for the indigent and had to refer private paying patients elsewhere to white physicians with staff privileges at voluntary hospitals with segregated accommodations for black patients.

The black physicians faced an elaborate catch-22. Many institutions available to black physicians did not meet necessary standards and were inadequate sites for training new physicians. Medical licensure required graduation from an approved medical school, specialty credentials required successful completion of an approved residency program, and staff appointments required a physician to be a member in good standing in the local medical society. Black physicians were excluded from all three.

Blacks struggled to deal with these exclusions by forming their own medical societies, journals, hospitals, and credentialing programs. In doing so, they faced a divisive contradiction. If successful, they would legitimize the "separate but equal" argument for segregation. If unsuccessful, they would serve as proof of inherent inequality. It was a lose-lose proposition for black physicians and a win-win proposition for those who embraced the status quo of inequality. Yet, a segregated medical world was better than the alternative: none at all.

Scientific Medicine's Reinforcement of the Racial Divide

Meanwhile, the mainstream of medical science and medical care marched onward. Medical science, however, did not take place in a social vacuum. It was heavily influenced by attitudes about race, morality, and the politics of segregation.

Race was routinely defined as both a behavioral and a biological risk factor. The view at least of many southern white physicians writing before the turn of the century was that emancipation had increased the death rates of blacks. This, they felt, proved both the value of slavery and the incapacity of blacks to take care of themselves. They believed that blacks' inferior constitution, natural tendencies toward sexual promiscuity, drug and alcohol abuse, and lack of personal hygiene would, in Darwinian fashion, solve the race problem through extinction.[38] Medical discourse blended naturally into racist diatribes on miscegenation. A commentary on a paper on the prevalence of high TB rates among blacks presented at the Tennessee State Medical Association meetings in 1907 reflects this mixture of attitudes.

It is principally the yellow Negro that shows the enormous death-rate from tuberculosis today. In all cases, wherever we find a hybrid race, we find a race which has not the stamina, physical, moral or mental, of either of the races in the mixture. Then, again, we must remember that in the hybridization, as a rule, we add a vicious tendency to what might be expressed as the lowest strata of the upper race, mixed with the vicious tendency of the lower race. That carries with it to begin with a poor hereditary foundation, one lacking in natural resistant qualities. Again, we are in the attitude in regard to the Negro question of attempting to force in one or two generations a civilization upon an inferior race which it has taken the Caucasian race centuries to attain. He staggers under the burden and falls, as you would naturally expect, even though you had no data on which to base your judgement. Then, his other vices add to the list of predisposing causes. Syphilis is almost universal among Negroes in cities, so that in our dispensary work we do not say, "Have you got syphilis?" but say to them, "When did you get it?" (Laughter.) We take it for granted that he has got it just the same in most cases. That helps to lay the foundation for Tuberculosis.

Again, in the antebellum days the Negro got a drink now and then, when it was good for him possibly. Now, he gets a drink every time he gets paid off, and in between if he can. As has been said by one of the French writers, alcoholism makes a bed for tuberculosis. You gentlemen, who are familiar with the conditions in the larger cities know to what extent addiction to drugs, especially cocaine has reached among Negroes. Besides that, you also know the extent to which abortion is practiced among Negro women. These things in the older days were not known, and yet every one of the factors I have mentioned is of stupendous moment as a predisposing cause in any infectious disease. Possibly no one cause mentioned would of itself suffice to insure contracting of the disease, but taken collectively they leave an outlook for the race which is hopeless, if help from without is not forthcoming.[39]

Gradually, however, the pessimistic view that the poor health of blacks would lead to extinction gave way to acknowledgment that it was a problem. Often, this was defined not so much as a problem for blacks but as a problem for whites.

> I feel that not only is the Negro mortality of the Southern city increased by these diseases from the lack of preventive measures amongst this people, but that the white mortality and morbidity is raised by these same causes, through their prevalence in the other race. To quote from another paper on this subject: "These Negro citizens among whom we find such an undue prevalence of diarrheal diseases, tuberculosis and venereal infections, who live under the worst of sanitary conditions, through circumstances, racial inferiority or our neglect, mingle with us in a hundred intimate ways, in our stores and factories, our kitchens and nurseries. They kneed our bread and rock our babies to sleep in their arms, dress them, fondle them and kiss them; can anyone doubt that we may not escape close exposure? The missed and carrier cases of typhoid and other intestinal diseases that wait upon our tables must exact their toll nor is this lessened by any habits of personal cleanliness discernable."[40]

Black physicians did not take kindly to this new genre in the medical literature that defined blacks simply as vectors of disease, "[l]ike the fly, the mosquito, the rats, and mice, an arch-carrier of disease to white people."[41] Yet, black hospitals were not averse to using such racial fears to raise funds in the white community. When the oldest black-controlled hospital in the country, Provident Hospital in Chicago, began a fund drive in 1929 to raise funds for black medical education at the hospital, the slogan was "Germs Have No Color Line." This reminded potential white donors of their own self-interest in providing support.[42]

The discovery of the sickle-cell trait in 1910 in blacks illustrates the peculiar way that medical knowledge blended with ideologies about race. Sickle cell became quickly defined as a genetic marker of "Negro blood." Those with the trait who denied any such heritage were suspected of lying out of shame or guilt. The spread of this trait into an apparently white person was twisted to provide proof of the dangers of race mixing or miscegenation. One physician in 1943 went so far as to declare it a national health problem. He argued that intermarriage between Negroes and whites directly endangered the white race by transmission of the sickling trait and that such intermarriage should be prohibited by federal law. Similar ideas in less strident terms found their way into an editorial in the *Journal of the American Medical Association* in 1947. Another physician used the "Negro blood" theory to argue that it suggested a more general physical inferiority and that blacks should not be inducted into the armed services in World War II.[43]

The Use of Blacks in Teaching and Research

Medicine's most troubling legacy has been the use of blacks as clinical material in teaching and research. That legacy has produced a schizo-phrenic political marriage of convenience between medical schools and teaching hospitals and state and municipal financing of indigent care. On the one hand, teaching hospitals have complained about the paucity of indigent care payments, while, on the other hand, their medical chiefs have worried periodically during the ebb and flow of indigent care financing that individual patient payments might be too high, thus encouraging competition with private-practice physicians and the erosion of the num-bers they need to accredit residency programs. Reflecting on his experi-ences, Aubre Maynard, one of the surgeons who successfully challenged racial exclusion in making staff appointments at Harlem Hospital in 1926, observed,

> As the helpless slave, as the impoverished freedman following eman-cipation, as the indigent ghetto resident of today, the share-cropper or dirt farmer of the South, the Negro has always been appropriated as choice "clinical material" by the medical profession. In the mind of the unregenerate racist, who, unfortunately, has always been repre-sented in the profession, the Negro was always next in line beyond the experimental animal. Without option in the peculiar situation, he has contributed to the training of generations of surgeons, his fate subject to the quality of their skill, and the integrity of their character. He has sometimes benefited from their efforts, but he has also occupied the role of victim and expendable guinea pig.[44]

Such fears about being used in experiments and as teaching material are well embedded in the concerns many blacks have with medical encoun-ters even today. They reflect a troubling history. In the antebellum period slaves were sometimes used to test experimental surgical procedures.[45]

The "teaching material" of northern white medical schools and urban hospitals became increasingly African American after World War I, coin-cident with the great migration from the South to northern cities. That migration had been preceded by the shipment of southern Negro corpses concealed in the barrels labeled "turpentine" to northern medical schools for teaching and anatomical research that began after the Civil War. A survey of such practices in 1933 showed that for years most southern medical schools had taught their students fundamentals of human anatomy on African American cadavers. Reflecting on this practice, Howard University professor of anatomy and editor of the *Journal of the National Medical Association,* W. Montague Cobb, was struck by the irony that such acknowledged physical equality of the races was restricted only to corpses.[46]

The Tuskegee syphilis experiment, which involved following the natural course of syphilis over a thirty-year period in 399 black males, is the most commonly cited example of such abuses. It was the longest experiment in withholding treatment from human subjects in medical history, lasting from 1932 to 1972. The health professionals involved in the project clung to three assumptions that vividly illustrate the powerful hold of the racial legacy on judgment. These assumptions still exert a powerful hold on the organization of services and on treatment decisions. Today, however, they exist in more subtle forms.

1. *The disease affected blacks differently than whites and thus was a legitimate focus of research.* While such ideas did not square well with the bulk of the medical evidence even at the time the study began in 1932, it continued to serve as the justification for a black-only study of the withdrawal of treatment.

2. *Since the subjects had no access to medical care, whatever was provided was better than what they would have received without the project.* The subjects were "uncontaminated" by any form of treatment and thus more useful from a research perspective. They posed no ethical dilemma, at least from the perspective of the researchers, since they were not withholding something the subjects would have received in the absence of the experiment. When the project began, few of the subjects had ever seen a physician. Rural blacks in Alabama did not go to physicians. Thus, whatever care was provided to them, project directors argued, was better than what they would have received without participating in the project. (Through various public-health programs and eventually through the passage of Medicare and Medicaid, the availability of medical care for these subjects changed dramatically over the lifetime of the project.)

3. *The subjects were poorly educated, poorly motivated, and the course of treatment was too demanding and complicated to assure the compliance necessary for success.* The treatment became less difficult and problematic with the introduction of antibiotics after World War II. Educational levels of the subjects and their families proba-

bly also increased. Yet, the assumption that these rural Alabama black males were not good patients or good risks for treatment persisted.

Most remarkable, however, is how pervasive and well entrenched were the basic assumptions that permitted the study.[47] It was not a secret experiment conducted by rogue researchers. Outside professionals regularly reviewed the project's protocols. More than a dozen publications were generated by the project and were widely read. Active participants included the Milbank Memorial Fund, the Rosenwald Fund, the United States Public Health Service, state and county public-health officials, and members of the local white medical society. It also used the facilities and had the full support of the Tuskegee Institute, the proud creation of Booker T. Washington's efforts to assure self-sufficiency for blacks. Even after integration had taken place and the county medical society had become a predominantly black body in the late 1960s, the project continued to receive full support, including the referral of patients to the project's control group, which was not supposed to receive treatment for syphilis. Much of the more progressive, liberal wing of medicine and public health during this period was involved in the project.[48]

The Tuskegee syphilis project, the legacy of a divided health care system, continued with a life of its own. No one, black or white, questioned it for forty years. A faculty member at Howard's medical school reflected,

I have thought about it many times and have asked myself how in the hell I knew about it and I thought it was perfectly all right to do this experiment. I remember reviewing an article in *Public Health Reports* in the early 1950s, and I said, "This is interesting." I have asked myself many times why I didn't raise that ethical point. I didn't, and nobody else did either.[49]

The Tuskegee study and the myths surrounding it continue to resonate in black low-income neighborhoods. The distrust of medical providers reflects an historical legacy of which the Tuskegee study is but a small part.[50] That distrust has undermined many outreach efforts of health care providers, including childhood immunization drives, flu vaccinations for seniors, and AIDS education projects. For example, a federal pilot study of the prevalence of AIDS in the District of Columbia had to be scrapped in 1988. Many local people accused the project of using Washington's black community as a "guinea pig" in a study that would stigmatize the city and minority communities.[51]

The assumptions that served as the justification for the Tuskegee study remain in evidence among those providing health services to this population. They appear to be reflected in substantial differences in rates of use of many more complex medical procedures. Blacks have lower rates of use of kidney transplants, coronary bypass surgery, and many other procedures, even where no differences in insurance or the ability to pay exist.

The assumptions were embedded in the training of physicians. The larger public hospitals in the United States persisted as the premier training centers up until the 1960s as well as the almost exclusive source of care for a growing urban black population. A physician reflected on his experience as an intern at Cook County Hospital in Chicago in the late 1940s.

> On the medical side it was a premier training place. I got there just after World War II, and it was still riding on its prewar reputation as a training center. It was a very sought-after site. Yet the patient loads were ridiculous, you had limited support. and your training came largely from the resident and by the seat of your pants. I think it trained a lot of people very well, but at what cost, one wonders.
>
> The place had a battle mentality. It was not a place for liberals. At County you either had a very conservative right-wing view that the people you were seeing were getting their just rewards for their substance abuse, fornication, and that this was God's will, or you would see it more as the congealed oppression and the end product of lousy housing, poor education, poverty, and ignorance. The group was divided up that way because doctors tend to come from conservative origins, but the County could make you pretty radical. Much as you'd like to think that the good doctors were the bleeding hearts and the bad doctors were the reactionaries, it wasn't so. You were judged by your colleagues on how well your patients did, and your attitude didn't matter. But some were pretty terrible people who I'd have huge shouting matches about their racism. They could justify their attitudes. They'd see the pregnant woman who was shooting up, but how do you interpret the experience that she has had? Is she violating God's law or is she a victim of capitalist oppression? Which? Both! God's a capitalist.[52]

The view of the more conservative public-hospital-trained physicians and the underlying assumptions that sustained the Tuskegee study prevailed in the development of health insurance in this country.

Race and the Soul of Insurance

As medicine developed into something that could make a difference in people's lives, a parallel struggle took place over how to pay for it. It has been, in essence, "a struggle for the soul of insurance."[53] It has also been a struggle over the national soul. Should medical care be provided based on need rather than the ability to pay? Should one pay only for the medical services one receives, or should one also pay a share of the excess expenses of others? In other words, should the logic of the market and actuarial forecasts be substituted for the logic of solidarity? The logic of solidarity dictates, just as the early black fraternal orders recognized, the social importance of protecting all members of the community and spreading the costs equitably. The answer in the United States, unlike any other developed country that has embraced the logic of solidarity through some form of universal health insurance, is, "It depends." Race has played a role in shaping that answer.

Just as in other countries, insurance started in the nineteenth century as a way for groups that shared a common bond to care for the misfortunes faced by their members. The black benevolent societies created by freed slaves after the Civil War were an impressive example of such efforts. Other mutual-aid societies were formed by guilds, craft unions, and churches. All these groups, the precursors of modern forms of health insurance, valued group solidarity. Many helped to cover the costs of illness among their members. One way that such mutual-aid societies helped their members was through arrangements negotiated with a local physician. They would typically negotiate an annual fee per member with the physician. Such "lodge practice of medicine," an early form of managed care, was fought by local medical societies.[54] The ability of medical staffs to exclude physicians involved in such lodge practices from hospital staffs eventually discouraged such practices.

In other developed countries such arrangements naturally evolved into universal-entitlement programs for health care, covering the entire population. In part because of race, that evolution never took place in the United States. Insurance, as it developed in the United States, was divided along racial lines. Accepting the conventional wisdom of medical practitioners at the turn of the century, most life insurance companies would not write insurance policies for blacks. Uninsurable risks for one life insurance company in 1930 included "Negroes, Chinese, Japanese, Mexicans and more than one-fourth blood Indians."[55] Enterprising blacks in Durham, Atlanta, and elsewhere created their own life insurance companies, and some became the first black millionaires. They took advantage of the niche offered by these racial exclusions, building on the strong tradition of black benevolent societies.

Many groups in the United States resisted the expansion of the idea of the mutual-benefit societies to the whole population. Divisions similar to those that had existed between the roles of private voluntary hospitals and public hospitals emerged in the financing of health care. Public programs were for blacks; private ones for whites. The Committee on the Cost of Medical Care, whose comprehensive pathbreaking research efforts in the 1930s set the direction of the financing of health care for the rest of the century, even excluded blacks from their survey of nine thousand households used to estimate patterns of expenditure and use of health services. They concluded that "the procedure adopted could not procure satisfactory information from Negro families."[56] Trade unions resisted efforts during World War I to expand coverage through public health insurance programs. They saw such programs as threats to their own influence and control, preferring to negotiate their own arrangements directly through the workplace. Organized medicine and the emerging voluntary hospital system preferred the development of voluntary insurance programs, thus assuring greater influence and control for themselves. The consequence was a sharp division along racial lines between those dependent on the public system and those whose employment offered benefits or who could afford private care in the voluntary system. The self-interests of labor unions, physicians, and hospitals against such national comprehensive plans was not that different from those in other developed countries where such comprehensive plans were enacted. What were different were the racial divisions that made more universal approaches less attractive to the white majority.

The voluntary health insurance system developed as a defense against public or government-run programs that would also be more racially integrated. Rufus Rorem, a key staff member of the Committee on the Cost of Medical Care, was the chief architect and advocate of the Blue Cross voluntary hospital insurance system. In 1938 he predicted that "voluntary hospital care insurance may postpone indefinitely the need for nationwide compulsory health insurance."[57] Many early practices of the voluntary hospital insurance plans were modeled after those of the benevolent societies. Some of these early Blue Cross hospital insurance plans relied on volunteers to collect monthly premiums, just as the benevolent societies had of their members. They also were firmly committed to something called "community rating." That is, all members of the plan would pay the same rate, and that rate would be based on the average hospital cost per member. Just as in the early benevolent societies, each member took on responsibility for a fair share of the misfortunes of other members. This romanticized ideology was the trump card in defeating national health insurance in the 1940s. The "community" in "community rating" excluded a large portion of the population. Coverage privately found through employment also insulated such programs from the political power of blacks to affect change.

The early racial divisions between publicly financed and privately financed health programs propelled further divisions and fragmentation. Community rating was an alien notion to commercial life insurance, which could not resist the lure of the rapidly expanding market for employer-based health insurance after World War II. Their version of fairness was quite different and based on actuarial calculations. Each person's premium should be based on their own estimated risk, rather than the sharing and pooling of risks across all community members. In reality, the underwriting process took on moral tones, similar to the idea of the "deserving poor" found in nineteenth-century voluntary hospitals. The moral tones adopted in the underwriting of life insurance were eventually applied to health insurance. One simply separated out the "good risks" and resigned others to the purgatory of the uninsured. According to the commercial insurance companies, "there were only two classes of people in the world: one entitled to all the privileges and benefits of life insurance and the other entitled to nothing."[58] The same principles of underwriting were applied eventually to health care through experience rating of groups.

What then, is the ethic that should govern health care? Who are we, and what are we responsible for? What is the "soul of insurance?" In small homogenous societies and communities with shared values people are willing, as the black benevolent societies were, to give whatever limited pooled resources are available to the most needy. In a large racially divided community, no one wants to put much in the common pool. People's willingness to contribute is guided by their calculation of the payback for themselves and their immediate families. Perhaps the most that can be hoped for is a contribution to a floor of basic needs we are unwilling to see others fall below. We do not want to see children die on the streets from asthma attacks because hospitals refuse to admit them.

The legacy of racial segregation and the caste structure of American society is one we are yet to free ourselves from. It is a legacy that divides the world of private insurance from the world of public responsibilities. Ultimately the story of the civil rights struggle and the struggle to assure a decent level of basic health and health care were essentially the same.

That viewpoint was expressed by Dr. Louis T. Wright, the black physician who had integrated Harlem Hospital's medical staff in the

1920s, when he spoke out at a hearing on national health insurance in 1938.

It is hoped at this time that the American people will begin to realize that the health of the American Negro is not a separate racial problem to be met by separate segregated set ups or dealt with on a dual standard basis, but that it is an American problem that should be adequately and equitably handled by the identical agencies and met with identical methods as the health of the remainder of the population.[59]

Unfortunately, his advice was not followed. Yet a small but growing group of physicians, nurses, and kindred spirits had begun to speak out for the racial integration of health services. Their story begins in the next chapter.

CHAPTER 2

Attending the Birth of the Struggle

Only black docs used to come into black communities to take care of blacks. Meharry and Howard docs went back to the communities from which they came. My dad and uncle were GPs. Sometimes they just got paid in staples. My first memory of medical practice was going with dad to deliver a baby in someone's home. He took me to help him stay awake. My sister and I were born at home. The hospital would not accept black patients. We had a birthing room in my house. My brother was born with CP because he was too big and needed to have a C-section. Although my mother was a wife of a physician, she could not be admitted to the hospital. He was born vaginally and had a bleed in his brain and CP because of it in 1956. My uncle went to Leonard, one of the black medical schools that closed. When my dad finished at Meharry, he joined the practice. He would go out to the farms and provide care for the sharecroppers. He worked twelve hours a day, six days a week. The trust that people had for them was great. They grew up in the community. No one ever went to white doctors. They didn't trust them, didn't think they cared, and most felt they couldn't afford them, even if they had accepted them as patients. We had two black pharmacists, two docs, and two dentists, all in the block where my dad practiced. Literally, it was like a community health center before the term was invented. Even though they didn't have the access to hospital care, few kids didn't get immunized. Now it's different. Medicine is more of a business.[1]

Black physicians and other health professionals not only helped deliver the babies in their communities; they also assisted at the birth of the civil rights struggle in the United States. Without their help the civil rights struggle would have been stillborn. World War II signaled the beginning of active labor. There was a new aggressiveness, an increasing restlessness among black health professionals with a racially divided world and the constraints it imposed. A growing minority pushed for real integration rather than separate development. Black professional societies and communities, however, were often bitterly divided by this shift.

The Separate and Unequal Compromise

Two events following within a year of the founding of the National Medical Association in 1895 profoundly shaped the environment faced by this professional association for the next half-century. Booker T. Washington delivered his famous "Atlanta Compromise" speech in the Cotton Pavilion a month after the NMA was founded on the same stage. Washington's compromise, widely embraced by both whites and blacks, seemed to boil down to this: Blacks would accept restrictions on voting rights and make no further demands for social equality, and, in exchange, the South's white rulers would accept gradual economic self-improvement for blacks and would rein in the more violence prone racists.[2] The *Plessy v. Ferguson* decision followed a few months later, putting the Supreme Court's stamp of approval on "separate but equal" actions by state and local governments. A wave of Jim Crow legislation followed, cementing a segregated new social order.

The charter of the NMA resonated with Booker T. Washington's message of racial solidarity and self-help. State and local groups such as the Medical-Chirugical Society of the District of Columbia, the Lone Star State Medical Association of Texas, and the Old North State Medical Society of North Carolina had grown up in response to exclusion from other local medical societies. As did their white counterparts, the National Medical Association and its constituent medical societies reflected the conservative, practical bent of the practitioners who made up their membership. They were interested in the expanding opportunities to learn, practice, and earn an income. In the starkly segregated society of pre–World War II America, that meant developing, controlling, enhancing, and defending black hospitals.[3]

Growing Division in the Ranks

Increasingly, however, dissension grew in the ranks of black medical professionals. Another organization competed for the loyalties of black physicians and dentists, the National Association for the Advancement of Colored People (NAACP). It was formed in 1909 by black and white intellectuals and activists who were united in their opposition to Booker T. Washington's "accommodationist" position. By 1920 membership had grown to ninety thousand, half of it in the South, and the NAACP had begun to attack discrimination in the electoral process in the courts. Much of the leadership locally and nationally was made up of black physicians and dentists. Only a minority of black physicians and dentists actively participated in the NAACP, but by the force of their personalities and medical credentials they had influence well beyond their numbers. For example, Dr. Louis T. Wright, who had the distinction of being the first black physician to be named to the staff of Harlem Hospital and the second to be admitted into the American College of Surgeons, served as chairman of the NAACP board of trustees from 1935 until his death in 1952.

In 1930 the black medical community in New York City was split by open warfare, with the Rosenwald Fund caught in the cross fire. At the time, staff privileges at Harlem Hospital for black physicians were critical to their practices. Other than three marginal private black hospitals or sanitariums, it was the only hospital in New York City where black physicians could get hospital privileges. A reorganization of the medical staff at Harlem, engineered by a contingent of physicians supported by Dr. Louis Wright, the first to break the color barrier at the hospital, had stirred divisions. Wright's refusal to appoint some prominent black physicians whom he considered incompetent split the North Harlem Medical Society. The dissident group, led by Dr. Peter Marshall Murray, took control of the North Harlem Medical Society. Wright's group responded by resigning and forming its own association, the Manhattan Medical Society.[4]

Dr. Aubre Maynard, one of Wright's equally blunt surgical colleagues, later observed of the Murray contingent,

> . . . the vast majority of black physicians were from Howard and Meharry, Negro schools. Conditioned in their personal and professional lives to separatism, it is understandable that many eschewed professional contact with whites as did some whites with them. Psychologically, they were unready for the issues that were involved, particularly the basic one of racial integration with equal opportunity but open competition in the arena of medicine. For them it was still preferable to be at a Negro hospital, which assured them of acceptance with greater comfort, even special considerations, which, on pragmatic and empathetic grounds, would probably be less stringent in its demands for dedication, performance and competence.[5]

W. E. B. Du Bois, editor of the NAACP's *Crisis* magazine throughout most of this period, was the most influential spokesperson for integrationists and an intractable adversary to Booker T. Washington's approach. He supported Wright's position, observing that "to fill Harlem Hospital with such dead weight was to play directly into the hand of every 'Nigger hater' in the land, and 'prove' the inability of the Negro physician to measure up to modern exacting standards."[6]

The Murray faction, excluded from municipal political support, sought the assistance of private philanthropy to establish a black hospital in New York. The Julius Rosenwald Fund, established by the head of the Sears Roebuck empire in Chicago, announced its intention of making a "survey of black physicians in New York." The unstated purpose, at least from the view of the Wright group, was to establish a Negro private hospital. The Rosenwald group met with both factions, receiving angry denunciations from the Wright group and support for the study from the Murray group. It was, however, a letter from Ferdinand Morton, a member of the Municipal Civil Service Commission and an influential Harlem Democratic leader that probably killed the project.

> Mr. Rosenwald's projects on behalf of the Negro, while doubtless well intended, have perhaps done us more harm than good. The Negro does not need philanthropy; all he asks is a square deal at the hands of the state and he will be able to take care of himself. It is not bounty that we want, but simple justice.
>
> Certainly, in this section of the country, we do not need Mr. Rosenwald. In communities such as ours, where the Negro enjoys in full measure his civic and political rights and equality of opportunity at the hands of the state; he is well able to take care of himself. He is in no sense a "problem" and does not need to be "surveyed" nor "analyzed." We are American citizens, a little handicapped perhaps by reason of our color, but we are able to fight our own battle.
>
> If Mr. Rosenwald's interest in colored Americans is sincere, it would be a fine thing for him to prove it by extending to colored men and women, in his vast business organization, equality of opportunity in employment and promotion, a thing which he does not now do. He has made millions of dollars by the sale of merchandise to colored farmers in the South and, instead of offering us bounty in the form of colored hospitals where they are not needed, he should do that which we are entitled by right, equality of opportunity.[7]

A letter from Wright to the president of the Rosenwald Fund, expressing similar sentiments, put the final nail in the coffin. The president of the foundation announced that it would not continue with its proposed study since there was not unanimity of support in the black community. A defiant line in the sand had been drawn. The tide would slowly turn toward the integrationist position.

The dream of a separate high-quality hospital system for blacks was slow to die. In 1934 Reverend Amos H. Carnegie announced the formation of the National Negro Hospital Fund.[8] The stated plan was to raise $150 million and build seventy-five hospitals across the country, in every city with more than ten thousand blacks. The first one would be built in Harlem. Dr. John A Kenney, former private physician of Booker T. Washington and editor of the *Journal of the National Medical Association*, was among the people named to the board. The plan to raise the funds involved solicitation of weekly contributions from every black person in the country, a vision of the older black benevolent societies on a grand scale. Carnegie's effort irritated both the accommodationist and the integrationist factions. For the integrationist it was capitulation; for the accommodationists, it belittled their efforts. When asked for comment on Carnegie's plan, E. B. Perry, president of the National Hospital Association, found it hard to contain his irritation.

> In the first place Carnegie is making a racket out of the hospital situation as concerns our race. You will pardon personal references in this communication. He has no organization, his plan is not possible to realize, for instance, a penny a week from twelve million Negroes, to be collected in various churches—He couldn't find the personnel; even if he had the hospitals. There are twenty "A" class Negro hospitals, satisfying the requirements of Surgeons. There are 110 hospitals registered by the American Hospital Association as being able, not always as adequate as desirable, for care of Negro patients.[9]

Dr. Harry Barnes, president of the National Medical Association, was even less diplomatic.

> It is impossible for me to discuss Rev. Carnegie's article. A careful study of his proposition would convince one that he is insane or trying to make a living from an appeal for a great human need. I think it is the latter, and the more his proposition is discussed, the more publicity he will get and the more money he will make. . . . The very reason that we are acquainted with these matters and have been working on them, enables us to see at once how impossible his plan is of accomplishment.[10]

Rev. Carnegie continued to make his appeals. The hospital in Harlem was never built, but in 1951 he appealed in an article published in *Modern Hospitals* for contributions from blacks (now a dollar a year, not a penny a week) for help in building a black hospital in Washington, D.C. He offered a site and the possibility of matching funds through proposed federal legislation.

> So now it is up to us! Do we want a to see a first-class, 200 bed hospital, second-to-none in the country, established in Washington to be owned and controlled by us in which we shall demonstrate the practice of democracy and Christianity? Do we want to experience the thrill of having a hospital of our own in which our people will always find welcome and where the most modern service can be rendered to the sick? If we do, then it is up to us to take hold of this simple plan and put it over the top in a big way and in the shortest time possible.[11]

Among the black leadership in Washington, the appeal fell on deaf ears. The integrationists were in ascendancy. In the same year that this appeal was published, W. Montague Cobb reflected on the dilemmas of the two approaches to health care for blacks in a speech at Tuskegee—the institution Booker T. Washington founded—shortly after assuming a role almost identical to that of Du Bois, as the forceful integrationist editor for the *Journal of the National Medical Association.* He tried to pull the two antagonistic strands back together.

> For nearly fifty years the retarded health status of our Negro population has been common knowledge and the object of sporadic corrective effort. In the early part of the century no one seemed to take the view that this problem could be practically addressed except in separate treatment apart from that of the general health problems. The first scientific approach to the problem came in the publication of an objective monograph, *The Health and Physique of the Negro American* published by Dr. W. E. B. Du Bois in 1906. This was a remarkable document for its time and was Du Bois' sole sojourn into the health field. The Negro public, however, both professional and lay, was not prepared to appreciate the significance of such a comprehensive report and the limited white public to whose attention it came was essentially hostile to the logical scientific approach indicated by the data presented. Hence, tangible results were few. The appearance of this work was, in effect, a long forward pass heaved the length of the field, for which there was no receiver.
>
> By contrast, a program with mass appeal initiated by Booker T. Washington at his institution Tuskegee Institute in 1915 received general approval. In that year he established what came to be known as

the National Negro Health Movement. . . . Howard University, the National Medical Association and the national Negro Insurance Association joined with the Tuskegee Institute as co-sponsors.[12]

Cobb then went on, diplomatically, to clearly align the future of Negro medical organizations with Du Bois and the NAACP integrationist vision.

Independent Practitioners Transformed into Civil Rights Activists

In the rising groundswell of opposition to racial discrimination, physicians and dentists played a key role. The nursing-home patient, the hospital patient, the patient waiting to see a physician rarely complains. He or she feels vulnerable and, rightly or wrongly, fears that such complaints will worsen the care he or she receives. Patients don't complain; doctors complain. A private-practice physician can complain about what happens in a hospital or nursing home. A physician is hired by the patient to serve as their advocate in those settings. Thus, the livelihood of a general practitioner is not dependent on keeping the administrator or the nursing director happy; it's dependent on keeping patients and the families of patients happy. Few in starkly segregated communities felt as much freedom to speak out as advocates as did black physicians and dentists. They were insulated from the white medical care system and beyond the control of the dominant white community. In most communities, they and the black clergy were the only ones who could push without fear of losing their livelihood. True, black physicians occasionally needed the help of a white physician to look after a patient admitted to a hospital or referred to specialty care. They might, therefore, hesitate to appear too confrontational. Dentists, however, who had far less need for hospital services or referrals to specialists for their patients, were less constrained. Black physicians and dentists made up the backbone of local chapters of the NAACP.

Black physicians and dentists were scarce and much preferred by black community members. In essence, they had a lock on this market segment in whatever community they chose to set up their practice. As did their white counterparts, most gravitated to communities that (1) had a more affluent population who could afford to pay for their services, and (2) offered the amenities of a middle-class lifestyle. Black physicians and dentists setting up practices in such communities could earn a comfortable living and had positions of social prominence in the local black community. Their aspirations for themselves and their children were constrained more by Jim Crow practices of the South and their more informal equivalents in the North than by ability, education, or income. More than a generation before Martin Luther King assumed leadership of the Montgomery bus boycott and the formation of the Southern Christian Leadership Conference, some of these individuals and their families had already begun to push for change.

The Threat of Violence

In pushing against barriers, they walked a fine line between courage and foolhardiness. In spite of their seeming economic positions of security and status they enjoyed, the threat of a violent seething world lay close to the surface. Dr. T. R. M. Howard was a practitioner in Mound Bayou, Mississippi, in 1955 when Emett Till, a fourteen-year-old boy visiting from Chicago, was kidnapped and murdered nearby—for allegedly whistling at a white woman. Dr. Howard managed to hide two eyewitnesses to the slaying in his home and then transported them to court in Sumner, Mississippi, to testify in the trial. A cash price was apparently put on Dr. Howard's head for this action, and he was forced to leave Mississippi. Dr. Howard was president-elect of the National Medical Association at the time. His presidential message at the NMA meetings in Chicago in 1957 had a little more sting and stridency than was usual for such addresses.

> We have still got too many gradualists among us. Too many Negro doctors in this nation have not concerned themselves about this "all-out fight for first class citizenship for our people." We the Negro physicians of America are spending too much money on Cadillacs, yachts and mansions in this grave hour. . . . Wake up—Negro Physicians, it is later than we think: Most of us are so financially secure ourselves that we have forgotten that we are our "black brother's keeper." . . . Some timid men among us have tried to criticize the NMA, in the Imhotep National Conference on Hospital Integration. The criticisms were based on the fact that in this conference, we joined hands with the NAACP.[13]

Years later over drinks a friend congratulated Thurgood Marshall, Supreme Court justice and former NAACP lawyer, for his own bravery in going into racially charged places to represent blacks. Marshall responded with characteristic bluntness. "Cut the shit. . . . You forget just one little f——ing thing. I go into these places and I come out, on the fastest vehicle moving. The brave blacks are the ones who have to live there after I leave."[14] Many of them were doctors and dentists.

Focus on the Public Institutions

The target of all the early efforts at integration was public institutions. The black physicians paid taxes and voted. The Harlem Hospital battles were the prototype of such struggles. They were the first such efforts to translate the growing political power of blacks into influence over the policies of a public hospital serving a predominantly black community. The Harlem coalition, which included the North Harlem Medical Society, Urban League, and the NAACP, had secured from the city both a training program for black nurses and internships for black physicians in an agreement in 1925. Similar concessions were soon extracted from other public hospitals in New York, Chicago, St. Louis, Cleveland, Detroit, Kansas City, and Boston.[15] (In some cities in the South, such as Atlanta and Memphis, the need to woo black votes actually produced the construction of *public hospitals* for the *private* paying black patients of black physicians, who, because of policies of the voluntary hospitals, had been restricted to public hospitals for indigents.) The pressures from black physicians and dentists for hospital privileges continued to build. The NAACP and its local chapters tried to respond to complaints reflecting the growing assertiveness of these professionals in the 1940s.

In 1941, an exasperated Dr. Charles Prudhomme wrote the secretary of the NAACP for help. He had been denied the opportunity to receive training as a psychiatric resident at St. Elizabeth Hospital in Washington, D.C., a federal facility serving a predominantly black population. High civil-service test scores and letters from Senator Harry Truman and from Eleanor Roosevelt had been to no avail.[16]

In 1942 Thurgood Marshall, as counsel to the NAACP, was actively involved with local lawyers who were seeking to force Newark City Hospital to grant blacks medical-staff appointments or admissions to its nursing school. A local NAACP lawyer, anticipating the arguments surrounding subsequent struggles, observed to Marshall in a letter,

> I also have had the feeling that in some way we could bring in the fourteenth amendment, and have got out my old Anti lynching Bill correspondence. . . . Perhaps our chief difficulty grows out of the fact that the wall of discrimination has been so effectively applied over a period of years that very few Negroes have definitely tried to breach it and so we have difficulty finding individuals who can make a case of legal discrimination as applied to them personally.[17]

Others simply rebelled on their own in actions reminiscent of the Boston Tea Party and the Wild West. A physician from Paducah, Kentucky, wrote to one of the NAACP lawyers in New York on May 27, 1942,

Dear Prentice:

Here it goes again! . . . The situation is this. I do not believe that the occupational tax imposed on me is legal, since I am denied all hospital privileges. I cannot work on colored patients in the City Hospital. Since hospital facilities have a strong bearing on my occupation I do not feel I should pay the occupational tax under these circumstances. Judge Price has asked me to ask you to make out a brief and go on to argue my own case. He tells me I have the right to test the validity of the tax. I shall remain indebted to you forever.

Yours,

"Hoss"[18]

The ability to bring political and legal pressure to bear through the black vote made the public institutions the only realistic targets. The voluntary hospitals remained distant, impenetrable fortresses. That would soon change.

Nursing Breaks the Color Barriers

The first real breakthroughs, however, came in nursing. World War II changed circumstances dramatically for black nurses.[19] Earlier in the century nursing had been predominantly a cottage industry. After completing training, many nurses contracted directly with families for the care of the sick in their homes. With the development of the modern hospital and the growth in demand for its services, the bulk of employment of nurses shifted to hospital settings in the 1930s. Local nursing organizations or registries that had been organized to control private-duty nursing, much in the way local medical societies were organized to control practice activities of physicians, declined in influence.

Hospitals faced a growing need for graduate nurses; yet they were either unwilling or unable to increase the salaries to improve recruitment and retention. As a result, hospitals were constantly experimenting with ways to solve their nurse staffing shortages. In the 1940s, stimulated at first by the drain on the civilian labor force by the war effort, white hospitals increasingly began employing black nurses. As the editor of a national hospital trade publication noted in 1952, the motives of the hospitals in breaking down barriers to employment of black nurses were mostly self-serving, "a case of arriving at the right answer for the wrong reason."[20]

Hospital management generally stood firm in reacting to the protests of white employees to such moves. One Philadelphia administrator faced a threatened strike by white employees after he began employing blacks. "I told them to go ahead and strike if they wanted to and said, 'if you strike or quit, what I will probably do is put a Negro in your job.' [After that] there was absolutely no trouble."[21]

More serious challenges took place in integrating nursing staffs in some border states. For example, in 1951 St. Francis Hospital in Charleston, West Virginia, a hospital operated by a Catholic order, faced a walkout of some of its graduate nurses because the hospital refused to discharge three black nurses it had hired.[22] The protest was short lived. With the full support of the bishop of the Diocese of Wheeling, West Virginia, the hospital flew in graduate nurses from other hospitals operated by the order. Many local and out-of-town nurses offered their assistance if needed. In a formal statement the hospital said: "To uphold Christian principles of charity and justice, as well as the spirit of the United States Constitution, St. Francis will not dismiss any nurse or employee on account of race."[23] The local newspaper joined in support of the hospital, lecturing the striking nurses on the meaning of the Florence Nightingale oath. In the face of this united front, some of the medical-staff support for the striking nurses dissipated. One physician denied an earlier report that the physicians had voted in favor of dismissing the black staff members and said that the majority of physicians agreed that the argument did not concern them.

Such resistance to integration might have fared better were it not for the strong support for integration by the American Nurses' Association (ANA) leadership and most state nursing associations. Throughout the 1940s leaders of the National Association of Colored Graduate Nurses (NACGN) and the ANA had worked together, setting the stage for eventual consolidation. Whatever the motives of the leadership of the white nursing associations for including black nurses, the integration strengthened the position of their organization. Their total membership increased. The ANA had prevented the threat of separate negotiations between black nursing organizations and white hospitals. For example, in 1946 the ANA House of Delegates supported the exclusive use of state and district nursing associations as collective-bargaining agents for their members. The ANA, however, was careful to ensure that even in states where black nurses could not be members of the nursing associations, these associations could still represent them. During the same convention the ANA also endorsed a plan to admit into the ANA qualified black nurses denied membership in their state associations.[24] In 1949, state nursing associations in both North Carolina and Arkansas—states with extensively segregated health services—opened their doors to black nurses.

Organized nursing continued to actively support efforts toward the racial integration of nursing and hospitals. Many leaders of organized nursing, who had been nursing educators, were less concerned with issues of economic self-interest of the average nurse than with broader social issues such as integration.

In 1951, the 250 delegates to the NACGN convention voted unanimously to disband. Founded in 1908 to encourage the integration of blacks into the nursing profession, its members concluded that their activities were no longer necessary. The executive secretary of the association noted that "there were a few problems but Negro graduate nurses are now being widely employed in hospitals, public health agencies and the armed services."[25] Now, all nurses would join the ANA and the Nursing League of America. Coming well before medical-society integration and most other efforts at integration, it was an occasion of some note. The *New York Times* paid special attention to the event on its editorial page.

> It is not very often that an organization devoted to the welfare of a minority group in the community voluntarily disbands. . . . It has formally terminated its own existence because it feels that the time has passed for a separate organization to promote the interests of Negro nurses as such. In all but four laggard states and, ironically enough, the District of Columbia, Negro nurses are now welcomed into local chapters of the ANA; and there has been so much improvement in the treatment accorded Negro nurses in recent years that they are now considered well integrated into the profession as a whole.[26]

The combination of nursing shortages, forceful effort of hospitals and administrators acting in their own self-interest, and the strong support of most nursing-association leaders produced the rapid collapse of much employment discrimination of nurses in all but the Deep South. While doubts continued as to whether the move best served the interests of black nurses, the disbanding of the NACGN and its absorption into the ANA in 1951 was a logically inevitable step in a decade-long process.[27]

Walter White, executive secretary of the NAACP, attended the organization's final banquet at the Essex House in New York, with more than one thousand persons attending to celebrate its demise. He gave certificates to eleven individuals and twenty-one organizations to recognize the work they had done with the NACGN. He would comment later,

> For the first time in my life I have enjoyed a funeral, instead of being lugubrious the obituaries were gay and congratulatory. The quite lively corpse handed out thank you scrolls to individuals and organizations which had helped and cooperated with the late departed.

Stripping off its sable shroud, the corpse promptly marched into a new life of greater usefulness [through amalgamation with the American Nurses Association].[28]

The American College of Surgeons Changes Course

Meanwhile, black physicians and the NMA were just beginning a long and difficult legal struggle to get its members in the front door of the white voluntary hospitals. The credentialing of physicians represented a growing barrier. The American College of Surgeons (ACS) through its control of the hospital standardization program had become the country's most powerful hospital gatekeeper. The ACS defined the process by which physicians gained privileges at hospitals, and some of the growing hospital insurance plans in the 1940s had begun to use ACS hospital accreditation as a requirement for hospital contracts. A key to such accreditation was the control of physician appointments by an organized medical staff. Appointment to the medical staff required membership in good standing in the local AMA-affiliated medical society. The gap between the AMA and NMA, however, was a chasm. In 1938 the NMA created a "good will committee" to approach the AMA with three requests.[29]

1. Recognize membership in the NMA as sufficient qualification for AMA membership, thus circumventing the white-only local medical societies.
2. Eliminate the racial identification of black physicians who were AMA members in the AMA directory. (Black members were identified in the AMA directory with "Col." appearing after their name).
3. Support the admission of black physicians to staff privileges at tax-supported hospitals.

While the AMA initially suggested a compromise, replacing identification of black physicians with what they thought would be a less offensive box symbol, all racial identification was dropped in the 1940 AMA directory.[30] Nothing of substance ever happened to the other two requests. By 1945, it was increasingly clear according to NMA leaders that "full access to modern hospital facilities was the number one problem facing at least half of our doctors."[31]

The American College of Surgeons, founded in 1913, had been the sole body conferring specialist's status to general surgeons and surgical specialists until 1937. Dr. Daniel Hale Williams, a black and chief surgeon of Provident Hospital in Chicago, had been among the first inductees in

1913. Dr. Louis Wright followed as the second black to become an American College of Surgeons fellow in 1934. The consideration of his admission had apparently produced strong opposition and the tacit understanding that no additional black applicants would be considered.[32]

In April 1945, Dr. George Thorne, a black member of the surgical staffs at Sydenham and Lincoln Hospitals in New York City, had requested an application for membership from the College. He received a surprisingly frank and inept response in writing that stated, "Fellowship in the College is not conferred on members of the Negro race at the present time."[33] Dr. Thorne promptly shared the letter with the press, and the College suffered the predictable public maelstrom of indignation in silence. Behind the scenes, however, the wheels of change had begun to turn.

Dr. Henry Wisdom Cave, a surgical chief at Roosevelt Hospital in New York, now found himself cast in the unlikely role of a civil rights activist. A southerner born in Paducah, Kentucky, a regent of the American College of Surgeons, and a man of patrician bearing, he now faced the task of extricating the ACS from the public-relations debacle. Dr. Aubre Maynard, one of the black surgeons at Harlem, had approached Dr. Cave informally concerning membership prior to this flap and recalled his response vividly many years later.

> Dr. Maynard, I am to attend a meeting of the Regents of the College at Hot Springs, Virginia and I shall bring up the matter of the policy of the College in regard to Negroes. I shall say to them: "Gentlemen, if this is a social organization, then as a Southerner, I shall not push further for their admission to the College. On the other hand, if this is a professional and scientific organization, then I shall demand admission of qualified Negroes as the only fair thing to do."[34]

In May 1944, Dr. Cave had requested that the regents set up a committee to study the subject of the Negro surgeon in relation to the American College of Surgeons. In June 1945, Dr. Cave returned to the regents with the report of the committee, recommending that any surgeon that could meet the qualification requirements of the American College of Surgeons should be admitted to fellowship, and the motion carried. Four black senior surgeons were promptly admitted, without the formal application process, as fellows. The following year eleven more were admitted through the normal application and review process. Dr. Cave had operated with surgical swiftness. Applicants, however, were required to be members in good standing of the local AMA-affiliated society, and this effectively excluded applicants from the South and most border states. The medical society in Washington, D.C., for example, excluded black applicants, and thus the black surgeons from Howard were excluded from eligibility.

In 1951 the Harlem Surgical Society hosted a testimonial dinner for Dr. Cave that included many who had played or would soon play key roles in the civil rights struggle. The speakers included Dr. Wright, director of surgery at Harlem Hospital and chairman of the National Board of Directors of the NAACP; Walter White, executive director of the NAACP; and Dr. Montague Cobb of Howard University. Dr. Cobb would soon begin an inventive new campaign to end medical-staff barriers in voluntary hospitals. Two of those present, Aubrey Maynard and Farrow Allen, who had been inducted into the College in 1946, would save the life of the person who would come to embody that civil rights movement. In 1958, Drs. Maynard and Allen would be called upon at Harlem Hospital to remove a razor-sharp knife firmly embedded through the sternum whose point was lethally close to puncturing the aortic wall of Martin Luther King, Jr.

Dr. Wright, who would die a year and a half later, observed at the testimonial dinner, "Dr. Henry W. Cave represents America, American surgery and democracy at its best. He is, in the words of King Lear: 'One of God's spies who has taken upon himself the burden and mystery of things.'"[35] Many others would soon be called upon to play similar roles.

The Hill-Burton Wedge into the Voluntary Hospitals

For the NMA, just beginning their long and difficult struggle to get members in the front door of the white voluntary hospitals, a small crack in the door had opened. In 1946 the Truman administration pushed for national health insurance through the Wagner-Murray-Dingell bill. Part of the bill caught the eye of Senator Lister Hill of Alabama. With broad-based support, including that of the American Hospital Association (AHA), a separate bill was crafted providing matching funds to states and local communities for assessing the need for hospitals and financially assisting in their construction. The resulting Hospital Survey and Construction Act, or Hill-Burton Act, became law in 1946. Senator Hill, who would later sign the pledge of massive resistance to the implementation of the *Brown v. Board of Education* decision, crafted the bill carefully. Inserted in sec. 622(f) was a passage that would begin a national struggle that would last almost two decades.

> That the State plan shall provide for adequate hospital facilities for people residing in a State, without discrimination on account of race, creed or color, and shall provide for adequate hospital facilities for persons unable to pay therefor. Such regulation may require that

before approval of any application for a hospital or addition to a hospital is recommended by a State agency, assurance shall be received by the State from the applicant that (1) such hospital or addition to a hospital will be made available to all persons residing in the territorial area of the applicant without discrimination on account of race, creed or color, *but an exception shall be made in cases where separate hospital facilities are provided for separate population groups, if the plan makes equitable provision on the basis of need for facilities and services of like quality for each such group;* and (2) there will be made available to each such hospital or addition to a hospital a reasonable volume of hospital services to persons unable to pay therefor, but an exception shall be made if this requirement is not feasible from a financial standpoint.[36]

Such is the nature of compromise. Hill got the insertion of a phrase that permitted the construction of racially separated hospitals, while Robert Wagner, liberal senator from New York and key sponsor of the national health insurance bill, got the insertion of the phrase about providing a reasonable volume of care for those unable to pay.[37] Wagner was concerned about those lacking insurance, given the declining prospects for national health insurance legislation. He wanted hospitals receiving federal funds under the construction program to provide some assurances that care would be provided to those without the ability to pay for it. No one could figure out what the Wagner phrase meant, and no federal or state guidelines were developed. This provision was ignored until civil rights advocates rediscovered it in the early 1970s.[38]

No one had any trouble interpreting Hill's insertion. Most of the southern states proceeded with the construction of racially separate hospitals using the federal Hill-Burton funds. More significantly, however, the phrase inserted by Hill is the only one in federal legislation of this century that explicitly permitted the use of federal funds to provide racially exclusionary services. That fact would soon bring it much unwelcome attention.

The Wagner-Murray-Dingell national health insurance bill went on to be defeated in a bitter struggle perhaps matched only in its intensity by the Clinton health care reform effort in 1993. Dwight Eisenhower's landslide election in 1952 signaled an end to such efforts.

The Formation of a New Coalition

W. Montague Cobb, M.D., as a young professor of anatomy at Howard in 1947, got off to a rocky start in national professional association politics. In the bulletin of the District of Columbia, Medico-Chirugical Society, the only local medical society available to blacks, a bulletin he had served as editor, he had produced a scathing critique of the NMA's last annual meeting.

> The 52d annual convention of the National Medical Association, held in Los Angeles, August 18–23, 1947, was a painful exhibition of generalized inadequacy as tragic as it was convincing.
>
> If an organization exists because of the fact of racial exclusion and fails to compensate the effect of the exclusion or to fight the discrimination itself, what purpose does it serve? Over the years able chairmen and program sponsors have been repeatedly embarrassed, because after great effort to secure distinguished participants in most instructive programs, only a handful of physicians would attend, and tardily. In Los Angeles the oft-seen spectacle of criers going out from a near empty hall to drum up an audience for a speaker was more than once viewed again.
>
> Most deplorable of all was the consummately inefficient manner in which the meetings of the House of Delegates were conducted. . . . As a result of this colossal waste of time, major issues like financial provisions for medical care and measures against discriminatory practices in medicine received only the barest attention by the remnant of a very fatigued group.[39]

While much of this painfully accurate diatribe could well describe most professional meetings, it was not the kind of thing such organizations like to air in public. Unfortunately, the bulletin of the District of Columbia's black medical society was routinely shipped to Claude Barnett, director of the Associated Negro Press. Barnett's press service supplied copy for most of the black dailies and weekly newspapers across the country. Barnett, in turn, sent a copy of Cobb's review of the national meeting to the president of the NMA, J. A. C. Lattimore, for comment. An angry personal exchange of letters between Cobb and Lattimore followed. Cobb refused to back down and apologize.

It is to the credit of the NMA leaders that they managed to turn Cobb's cannon around and point it at the enemy. By the end of 1948, Cobb had assumed the editorship of the *Journal of the National Medical Association*. The former editor, Dr. John A. Kenney, had founded the journal and served as Booker T. Washington's personal physician. The change in editors signaled a significant shift in editorial policy. "The Integration Battle-Front" became a regular feature of the journal. For the next two decades Cobb, through his articles and editorials, served as the integration campaign's chief commander and master strategist. It was a role he often played, however, with less than enthusiastic support from the black physicians in the trenches.

For Cobb, all the bells and whistles went off with the *Brown v. Board of Education* decision on May 17, 1954. The date, as Cobb, editor of the *Journal of the National Medical Association,* observed, "now takes its place in the annals of freedom alongside the date of the Fourth of July on which the anniversary of the Declaration of Independence of the American colonies in 1776 is celebrated and the Fourteenth of July which commemorates the storming of the Bastille."[40] The NAACP Legal Defense Fund through Cobb now had a new partner in the NMA, both anticipating what the next logical step would be.

Cobb was well prepared to respond to the signal. He had become chairman of the National Health Committee of the NAACP as well as editor of the *Journal of the National Medical Association.* In a speech to the Forty-fifth Convention of the NAACP in June 1953, he announced the beginning of a new campaign, gleefully invoking Civil War imagery certain to enrage the southern opposition.

> As a logical step in its program to make the benefits and responsibilities of full citizenship available to all Americans, the National Association for the Advancement of Colored People today embarks on a campaign to eliminate hospital discrimination in the United States. This will be a long campaign, sure to be marked by many reverses as well as victories. But let us remember William Tecumseh Sherman, one of America's greatest generals. He never won a battle, but never lost a campaign. . . .
>
> The vast program of new hospital construction authorized by the Hospital Survey and Construction Act in 1946, presented the threat of foisting on generations unborn the entrenched ghetto hospital system, through the construction of new segregated hospitals. This possibility assumed realistic form in new hospital buildings erected in Tallahassee, Florida, in Atlanta, Georgia and in Memphis, Tennessee. It was necessary, therefore, for the N.A.A.C.P. to make its position unmistakably clear. This was done through action taken by the national Board of Directors of the Association in January 1952, when it directed that an N.A.A.C.P. Branch which had endorsed a new segregated hospital under construction would have either to withdraw this endorsement or have its charter revoked. The Branch rescinded its action. . . .[41]

The notorious basement ward for colored patients must be eradicated. But along with it must go the separate ward of all types, the relegation of Negro patients to the oldest and outmoded sections of buildings with new additions, etc., etc. The disruption of the sacred doctor-patient relationship effected when a Negro physician must leave his patient at a hospital door because he can not be a member of the staff, must be prevented. The subtle economic exploitation of the Negro by white physicians and institutions through racial bars in hospitals must be brought to an end.[42]

Both the NMA and National Dental Association (NDA) endorsed and announced their support of the NAACP campaign at their conventions in the same year.

The *Brown* decision was the culmination of a long-term legal strategy of the NAACP Legal Defense Fund to attack the "separate but equal" doctrine by forcing the letter of the law to be adhered to, requiring provisions for costly separate professional training, such as in law and medicine. In so doing, NAACP strategists hoped to compel the conclusion that integration was the only cost-effective option.

Robert Cunningham, editor of *Hospitals,* in an editorial in the June 1951 issue that included a series of articles on racial integration of hospitals, used the same approach, arguing that "in a time when our voluntary hospital economy is being challenged from within our country and our political idealism is being threatened from without, we cannot long afford the wastefulness of duplicated or inferior health facilities that become a burden to the economy, or the hypocrisy of social performance that falls short of our cherished ideals."[43] Public health care could be expected to be the next legal battleground, after publicly supported education, in the battle for parity.

In anticipation of such a challenge, a new public hospital was planned in Atlanta in the late 1940s. Finally opened on January 1, 1958, Grady Hospital consisted of two identical towers, one for whites and one for blacks, with essentially identical accommodations, including separate wards, cafeterias, emergency rooms, operating rooms, and even morgues. It had been assumed that the construction of separate but physically equal public-hospital accommodations would be a safe bet and would protect the city from legal challenges. Now all bets were off.

The Distinctive "Chicago Approach" to Integration

In northern urban centers, where health care providers were faced with accommodating a growing black population, the issues were different from those in the South. The potential implications of the *Brown* decision were far less straightforward. While most of the visible symbols of Jim Crow were lacking, the way in which hospitals and medical practices were organized in most northern cities assured a high degree of racial segregation. The efforts to end segregation followed a path outside the main-stream of national civil rights efforts in the 1950s and 1960s but perhaps more relevant to addressing the more subtle disparities of the present. Chicago was prototypical of these northern struggles for the integration of health care, but it had a distinctive "Chicago Style."

The Committee to End Discrimination in Chicago Medical Institu-tions, a loose collection of physicians and community activists, was organized in 1951 and initially focused on the admissions practices of Woodlawn Hospital, located in the racially mixed Woodlawn–Hyde Park–Kenwood section of the city. The hospital, in spite of its many empty beds, did not admit blacks, no matter how much money or insur-ance they had. While in some instances blacks might be admitted for emergency care, they would be placed in a private room and billed for the extra expense. A black patient with a skull fracture had been turned away at the hospital, only to die a few hours later.

Such practices were not unique to Woodlawn Hospital. The bulk of black hospitalizations in Chicago took place at the city's public hospital, Cook County, and the City's historically black institution, Provident, bypassing many other hospitals in closer proximity to black neighbor-hoods. Yet about half the black population had some form of private insurance. Members of the Brotherhood of Sleeping Car Porters and some of the meat-packing locals had better health benefits than most whites with employer-based coverage. Chicago's voluntary hospitals, however, insisted that they did not discriminate on the basis of race, and there was little evidence other than anecdotal stories to support the claims that they did. Dr. Herman Bundesen, president of the Board of Health in the City of Chicago, a strong and unusually independent curmudgeon in city and state politics, came to the aid of the Committee to End Discrimination, supplying them with birth and death certificate statistics on the area hos-pitals. The data showed that in 1953, 71 percent of all black hospital deaths and 42 percent of black hospital births in Chicago took place at Cook County. Only 2 percent of white hospital births in Chicago took place at Cook County. Eight other hospitals, including two public ones, accounted for almost all the other black hospital births and deaths. The remaining sixty-odd voluntary hospitals in the City of Chicago accounted for less than 8 percent of black hospital births and deaths.[44] As one of the participants on the Committee to End Discrimination observed, "We had this insiders joke that the only black births at some of these hospitals were those smuggled in the wombs of their white mothers and that the only deaths that occurred were black patients who had never been admitted but who ungratefully died in the emergency room awaiting transfer."[45] With the help of these statistics a city ordinance was passed in 1955 prohibiting racial discrimination in admission practices. Penalties for violations of the ordinance could include loss of tax-exempt status and even loss of license to operate.

Nevertheless, in spite of the ordinance and the continued prodding by the committee with updated statistics, little changed in the pattern of hospital births and deaths in Chicago, as one of the committee members observed.

> The data really ended the argument. Administrators would look at the numbers and say, "Oh, that's really bad, but we don't know anything about this, our doctors admit." That was totally disingenuous. In America doctors get their hospital staff appointments every year or two, at most, every three years. While there is something approaching tenure if you've been on a hospital's staff for say, twenty-nine years without a blemish, doctors are not always courageous and they sure knew that in some of those hospitals with the ghetto encroaching that it would be sacrilege to admit a black.[46]

Increasingly, however, the committee focused on the issue of staff privileges for black physicians as a way of breaking down the segregation in care and reversing the decline in the number of black physicians practicing in Chicago. In February 1961 ten black Chicago physicians filed a suit in U.S. district court against the state and local hospital and medical associations and fifty-six Chicago hospitals.[47] Unlike the suits brought in the South challenging the constitutionality of publicly financed segregation, this one challenged segregation's impact on the market. The plaintiffs argued that the refusal to provide staff positions to black physicians violated antitrust law. The majority of Chicago's black medical community, as one of the plaintiffs recalled, did not enthusiastically support the suit.

> When we instituted the suit, it was considered a very dangerous thing by many of our colleagues. We started with ten physicians but two dropped out. Some members of the staff of Provident stopped speaking to us. We were muddying the waters.[48]

If the plaintiffs had won, unlike the suits in the South based on constitutional violations, treble damages could have been awarded to members of the class represented by the plaintiffs. Three times the career loss of earnings of about three hundred black physicians in Chicago would have exacted a significant price on the city's voluntary hospitals (perhaps as much as $1 billion in current dollars). Instead, however, the judge appointed a hearing board (one representative from the plaintiffs, one from the defendants, and one appointed by the court) to hear the appeals of black physicians who felt they had been unfairly denied staff privileges. No one asked to come before the hearing board. As one participant explained,

> The result would have forced them onto the staff of a hospital where their survival depended on other doctors on the staff. They would be dependent on other staff physicians for referrals and the kind of extra duties they would be assigned. Nobody could expect a black doctor who had humiliated a hospital and its medical staff by forcing their appointment to thrive in that environment.[49]

In distinctive Chicago fashion, however, others were less reluctant. Perhaps mindful of the potential implications for Chicago black vote, Mayor Daley appointed a Special Committee on Staff Appointments for Negro Physicians. City power brokers on the committee included a representative of the Archdiocese of Chicago, the chief justice of the municipal court, two top executives from the larger voluntary hospitals, and some influential physicians. Two, a black surgeon and a physician who had been active in the Committee to End Discrimination, were appointed to add credibility to the process. The physician who had participated in the Committee to End Discrimination reflected on this experience.

> In a city of deals, we were put there to see how deals were made. If I ever write a book, the chapter on the committee will be called "The Meat Market." This is what the ruling class did to avoid the contradictions in the suit. These people, they'd sit down and tell what they had to offer that week. For example, "Mercy will take two light skinned pediatricians." I'm making this particular example up, but that's how it would work. Specialist surgeons were hard to place, because that was where the money was. To cut to the chase, at the end you could accurately say that any black physician that wanted an appointment at a predominantly white hospital had one. It would not necessarily be the one they wanted or be the one nearest where they practiced, but they would have one. They ended up placing about one hundred and twenty. About half the doctors did not accept the offer for placement. They tended to be the older doctors and in the most racially segregated and oppressed environments. They didn't want to go to the honkie hospitals.[50]

Its work completed, the Committee on Staff Appointments for Negro Physicians disbanded in July 1965.

The National Movement Is Organized

Meanwhile, armed with the *Brown* decision, encouraged by the new activism unleashed by the Montgomery bus boycott begun in December 1955, and under the joint auspices of the Council on Medical Education and Hospitals of the NMA, the National Health Committee of the NAACP, and the Medico-Chirugical Society of the District of Columbia, Cobb set about planning the first national conference on hospital integration in the fall of 1956. The conference had four stated purposes.

1. To bring together representatives of all the interests among hospitals, the public, the healing professions and government agencies, which are concerned with this problem.
2. To provide a complete, comprehensive picture of the situation throughout the country as it exists today through first-hand presentations from various regions.
3. To evolve in the atmosphere of common understanding and cooperation so created, recommendations and programs of remedial action which may be made known to the American people with the aim of securing widespread public support for their implementation.
4. To make available through publication of the Proceedings of the Conference in the Journal of the National Medical Association and in reprint form, a compact, authoritative reference on the subject of hospital integration which may have value both as information and as guidance for continuing efforts in this field in all parts of the United States.[51]

The "Imhotep Conference on Hospital Integration," named for the revered physician of ancient Egypt, Imhotep ("He who cometh in peace"), met March 8–9, 1957, at the First Presbyterian Church in Washington, D.C.[52]

Among the 175 registrants from twenty-one states were most of the black physicians and dentists who were or would soon become active in integration efforts. Dr. Paul Cornely, one of the organizers, was disappointed by the turnout. "It wasn't that great a turnout, even among our own people, and none of the leaders from the other professional associations you would have liked to have included in a coalition showed up."[53] Indeed, it resembled a meeting of pariahs. Neither Howard University nor the Department of Health, Education and Welfare (DHEW) was willing to provide meeting space, fearful of retaliation from powerful legislative appropriations committees. Even though the AHA, AMA, and ANA sent "observers," none of their leadership was represented. While the editor of *Modern Hospital,* Robert Cunningham, long an advocate of integration, did attend, neither the Catholic Hospital Association nor the Protestant Hospital Association sent representatives or showed any interest.[54]

Participants provided local reports on conditions related to the segregation of patients and medical staffs. Dr. Hubert A. Eaton of Wilmington, North Carolina, reported on his intention to fight in the courts for the right for staff privileges in the segregated, predominantly white hospital in Wilmington. Dr. Reginald Hawkins, a dentist in Charlotte, North Carolina, reported on his efforts to end separate and unequal conditions in the city's municipal hospitals. Most significantly, the conference unanimously approved the following action:

> Legislation [will] be sought which will amend the Hospital Survey and Construction Act of 1946 and its amendments so that the clauses which provide for separate provisions for separate population groups, be deleted since such clauses now appear unconstitutional in the light of recent Supreme Court decisions.[55]

A similar conference was held in Chicago in 1958; the following year the conference returned to the Presbyterian Church in Washington. By 1959, participation in these annual conferences had shrunk to several dozen hard-core followers. The conferences operated on a shoestring budget, fifteen hundred dollars, which was donated by the sponsoring organizations. Interest and attendance continued to flag at the conferences held in 1960 and 1961.[56] Although organizers of the conferences blamed the low attendance on the lack of promotion, there were three more troubling reasons for the decline in attendance: (1) the euphoria following the *Brown* decision had faded in the wake of massive southern resistance, (2) the black medical community was divided and ambivalent in its support of the effort, and (3) the student-led lunch counter sit-in protests of 1960 had yet to influence health professionals with their new passion and militancy.

Less resilient organizers would have probably abandoned the conferences after 1959. Nevertheless, a surprising breakthrough took place in 1961. The organizers had succeeded in attracting the interest of Senator Jacob Javits (R, New York). He introduced a bill that would eliminate the Hill-Burton "separate but equal" provisions. The introduction of the bill presented President Kennedy with a difficult dilemma. Kennedy had won the 1960 election by a narrow margin, and the black vote had made the difference between victory and defeat. Cobb took note of the problem, extracting a political commentary for his column in the *Journal of the National Medical Association. The Medical World News* on the delicacy of the situation the Javits bill now presented the Kennedy administration.

> If the liberal New York Republican makes a strong issue of this demand next year—when many fellow Senators will be fighting for re-election—it will present the Administration with a major dilemma: support amendment of the Hill-Burton Act and run a risk of wrecking the whole Government hospital construction program, or back away from the issue and invite political retaliation by Negro voters. . . .
>
> Sen. Lister Hill, powerful Democratic chairman of the Senate Labor and Public Welfare Committee and author of the hospital construction law, comes from Alabama where the medical school still allegedly practices segregation and former vice president of Emory, Boisfeuillet Jones is Secretary Ribicoff's top medical affairs advisor and a confident of Hill. All of these circumstances are making the Javits move extremely embarrassing to key Democratic leaders. While President Kennedy made civil rights one of the chief issues in his election campaign, many integration leaders have complained that he has been lagging on civil right legislation. . . .
>
> If Javits makes a strong issue of his proposed amendment, it will be difficult for Democratic liberals, especially in a congressional election year, to avoid taking a stand. The same will be true of the Administration. The one possibility may rest in Sen. Hill.
>
> The Javits proposal will be handled by Hill's committee. Regardless of the speeches made, many observers think this veteran of legislative skirmishes will find a way to avoid any action at all.
>
> Whatever happens, Senator Javits is putting a lot of people on the spot, the medical profession as well as the Democratic leadership.[57]

The Imhotep group, under Cobb's guidance, doggedly continued to push their three-pronged attack, which focused on finding a way to breach the defenses of the increasingly well-entrenched status quo. First, they could attack the problem by pushing through the Javits bill, which would revise the Hill-Burton legislation. This attack failed, because the bill never emerged from Hill's committee, as *Medical World News* had predicted.

Second, they could attack through the executive branch. DHEW had never dealt with a complaint of racial discrimination since the passage of the Hill-Burton Act, and it was unclear what actions could be taken. Complaints seemed to have little impact.

For example in November 1961, three representatives of the Old

North Medical Society of North Carolina, Drs. Armstrong, Watts, and Eaton, took a trip to Washington to present some of the facts about discrimination in hospitals to federal officials and to push for action. All three were resilient local leaders that had assisted in the birth of civil rights struggles in their local North Carolina communities. Arriving at National Airport, a crowded impersonal place for practitioners from rural North Carolina, they got an boost of support from an unexpected source. They managed to grab a cab. The black female cab driver immediately turned around and smiled.

> "How you, Dr. Armstrong!"
> "Hey sugar," Dr. Armstrong answered in surprise. "You know me?"
> "Yeah," the cabby answered, "I'm from Rocky Mount. You delivered me!"[58]

Their conferences with the under secretary of DHEW and with Justice Department and Senate staff were less reaffirming for these three physicians. They felt they had accomplished nothing. Nevertheless, the meeting must have left an impression with James Quigley, DHEW's assistant secretary. Dr. Watts was later contacted by him to assist in the training of civil rights inspectors for hospitals in the Atlanta regional office. The overall conclusion from the visits, however, was a discouraging one.

> The impression gained from conferences in the Department of Health Education and Welfare was that the anti-discrimination clause of the Hill-Burton Act had no teeth in it, that the "assurances" as to compliance on the part of the applicant had never been questioned and there was no procedure of checking on the validity of "assurances," nor was there any authorized course of action in case of violation to consider. It did not appear that the Department considered it its province to know what went on in hospitals after grants had been made nor was it anxious to become involved in this area.[59]

Finally, blocked on both congressional and executive-branch action, the only recourse was to push the attack through the courts, following in the tradition of the *Brown* litigation. That gambit was soon played. "On Lincoln's birthday, February 12, 1962," Cobb announced to the readers of the *Journal of the National Medical Association,* "eleven Negro citizens of whom six were physicians, three dentists and two patients, filed suit against two hospitals in Greensboro, NC, testing in this case the constitutionality of the anti-discrimination clause in the Hill-Burton Act."[60]

The Kennedy Administration's Dilemma

The Imhotep contingent and their new partners in the legislative branch were only vaguely aware of how deeply divided the new Kennedy administration was. They were struggling to develop a track record that would satisfy its commitments and debt to its black constituency, without incurring the political costs of a direct confrontation with powerful southern democratic legislators that would split the party. Surely there had to be something that could be done by executive fiat.

Harris Wofford, as special assistant to the president for civil rights, had the difficult task of finding some answers. During the 1960 presidential campaign, Kennedy had glibly promised that he would eliminate discrimination, "with the stroke of a pen." As president, he clearly did not want to risk a civil rights legislative battle that could destroy the fragile alliance with southern Democratic legislators and their constituencies. Yet, any politically safer executive action appeared elusive. An interagency subcabinet task force was set up by Wofford to develop a plan and implement it. James Quigley represented DHEW on this subcabinet interagency task force. In a report to Wofford on July 6, 1961, he acknowledged many of the agency's problems and the validity of criticisms by the NAACP.

> A survey of the Department's programs and activities indicates that there are instances where it could be said that "Federal money is being spent in ways which encourage discrimination." This spending occurs in a variety of circumstances and under a multiplicity of congressional authorizations.[61]

A DHEW staff study completed in January 1961 produced a long checklist of programs in the agency and classified them according to existing authority to take corrective action. Programs fell into three categories: (1) "Clear"—those for which authority to terminate funding in instances of racial discriminations appeared to exist in the authorizing statutes, (2) "Debatable"—those on which the authorizing statutes were silent, and (3) "Lacking"—those on which unchallenged provisions in the authorizing statutes explicitly sanctioned discrimination. Quigley observed in a memorandum that "in the effort to evaluate the authority to solve these problems by executive action, the staff study seems to have stirred up many more problems than it solved." The general counsel for DHEW, in a separate memorandum, attacked the exercise as hopelessly flawed and a

> fundamental misconception of the Department's legal responsibilities regarding the programs it administers and a misconception of the

relationship between these responsibilities and various possible situations that might be said to impair the constitutionally protected rights of individuals or discriminate against them in other respects. It is regrettable that the legal portions (Part II and III) were included in the Staff Paper without clearance by this Office.[62]

The general counsel's opinion was that, without explicit authorization in the legislation to withhold funds on the basis of discrimination, or without explicit rejection of the constitutionality of parts of legislation that permitted "separate but equal" use of federal funds, DHEW and the president had no authority whatsoever. Quigley concluded,

> The existence and extent of the present authority of the Department of Health, Education and Welfare to take corrective action to eliminate racial discrimination in the operation of its programs is, for the most part, anything but settled. Where it is settled, it would appear to be settled against the Department's ability to take executive action in this area. The two clearest instances involved the Land Grant Colleges and the Hill-Burton hospital construction program. The language in both statutes makes it clear that Congress intended to allow Federal monies to be spent in ways which would condone discrimination on the basis of race.[63]

Like the Hill-Burton Act, the second Morrill Act in 1890 included a similar phrase permitting the provision of funds to racially segregated colleges.

> That no money shall be paid out under this act to any State or Territory for the support and maintenance of a college where a distinction of race or color is made in the admission of students, *but the establishment and maintenance of such colleges separately for white and colored students shall be held in compliance with the provisions of this act if funds received in such State or Territory be equitably divided as hereinafter set forth.*[64]

The 1890 Morrill Act and the 1946 Hill-Burton Act blocked any executive action to prevent the use of federal funds in state or locally administered programs that discriminated on the basis of race. As long as their constitutionality was not rejected by the courts, there was no authority to prevent the use of federal money in ways which encouraged discrimination, unless specific provisions existed in the authorizing legislation.

In the meantime, the Civil Rights Leadership Conference, an um-

brella organization including most of the civil rights groups, had completed its own analysis, submitting a report to the White House at the end
of August 1961. It was an incisive and bruising critique. While the report
noted some positive efforts by the Kennedy administration, it observed,
"Nonetheless, we cannot fail to observe that the sum total of these actions
is dwarfed, and in fact nullified, by the massive involvement of the federal
government in programs and activities that make it a silent but nonetheless
full partner in the perpetuation of discriminatory practices."[65] The most
telling part of the argument, particularly for a president planning to run
for reelection, was a table showing by state the ratio of federal taxes paid
to federal dollars received in aid, allowing a comparison between eleven
southern and eleven northern states. The average for the southern states
was less than .50, for the northern states more than 1.5. In other words, the
federal government was the means by which northern taxpayers were massively subsidizing discriminatory practices in the South at the expense of
programs in their own states. For Public Health Services and other health
care programs, HEW had distributed approximately 120 million dollars to
the states in 1960. During the life of the Hill-Burton program the federal
government had supplied more than $1.3 billion to hospital construction
programs in states. The Civil Rights Leadership Conference report concluded, "In the light of Brown v. Board of Education and subsequent decisions, there seems little doubt that segregation by publicly assisted hospitals, particularly if governmentally operated, is unconstitutional."[66]

For the federal officials, of course, it wasn't quite that easy. As
Quigley pointed out in a November 1961 memorandum to Wofford,

> There can be no question about the constitutional and moral sound-
> ness of the position taken in the Leadership Conference Report that
> the Federal government ought not to contribute to the perpetuation
> of segregation and discrimination. As in many cases, however, the
> trouble lies in the implementation of this principle. Federal aid is not
> a monolith. In DHEW we have a variety of grant-in-aid programs
> that run from the mandatory formula grant to States for the support
> of such programs as Land Grant Colleges, public assistance, public
> health services, to the highly discretionary research grant which the
> head of our operating agencies can use if he wishes as an alternative to
> a research contract; that run from grants encrusted in tradition in
> their administration and the popular expectations based on them to
> those in new programs that are barely known. It is clear that the
> impact of an Executive Order that spoke to grants-in-aid and Federal
> assistance generally would vary greatly from program to program.
>
> Naturally, those persons in the Department responsible for the

administration of programs are concerned about the effect of such a sweeping Executive Order. They are concerned particularly about its effect upon programs supported by mandatory grants to States. There are many people dependent on the benefits and services provided through a host of complex relationships among State, local and private agencies. Without doubt, segregation and discrimination are practiced, in some form, by many of these agencies. Yet, apart from the field of education, no racial group as a class appears to have been seriously deprived of the benefits and services intended by Federal mandatory grant programs. Nonetheless, the heads of this Department's operating agencies are fearful that, in some States vital services would be disrupted by an Executive Order that would withhold Federal funds because of the inequities of segregation not wholly connected with the Federal Program.[67]

Quigley noted in the same memo that the "separate but equal" provisions in both the Morrill and Hill-Burton acts involved important legal questions that needed to be addressed by the attorney general.

Thus, in regard to the executive branch of the federal government taking any initiative to deny funds to states and local organizations because they discriminated on the basis of race, the entire federal bureaucracy had ground to a halt. Was the Hill-Burton "separate but equal" provision constitutional? If so, there was little room for executive action.

By the spring, Harris Wofford had grown restless. He had become the custodian of thousands of pens sent as a protest to Kennedy's failure to honor the promise of ending discrimination with the stroke of one. Other White House staffers didn't take kindly to the effort to humorously prod the president to action and would stop by Wofford's office whenever they needed some pens. In the spring, Wofford asked to be reassigned to the Peace Corps, and the pens were eventually donated to a home for the disabled. Wofford's position was abolished and his duties assigned to Lee White, an oil and gas lawyer on Special Counsel Ted Sorensen's staff.[68]

Burke Marshall, the assistant attorney general for civil rights, had a background as free of commitment to civil rights as Lee White's. Nevertheless, after months of waiting and indecision, the Justice Department finally saw an opportunity to take action. In a memorandum to Attorney General Robert Kennedy on April 9, 1962, Marshall wrote,

On April 3, we received formal notification from the N.A.A.C.P. of a lawsuit filed in Greensboro, North Carolina, seeking desegregation of the two hospitals there. The suit attacks the constitutionality of the provision of the Hill-Burton Act, and the regulations issued under it, which permit HEW to consider separate but equal hospital facilities as meeting the non-discrimination requirements of the statute. Under 28 U.S.C. 243, the Attorney General has a right to intervene in the suit. At present a motion to dismiss is set for May 18. I have consulted with the general counsel of HEW about the suit and with Nick Katzenbach. [Deputy Attorney General]. We all feel that you should intervene in the suit which is of importance to the hospital program, and are considering what position should be taken.[69]

On May 25, 1962, as the Sixth Imhotep National Conference convened at the Fifteenth Street Presbyterian Church in Washington, D.C., Dr. Montague Cobb, its chairperson, received an unusually explicit telegram describing a powerful but unlikely new coalition.

MAY 25, 1962
11:52 AM EDT
DR. W. MONTAGUE COBB
15TH ST. PRESBYTERIAN CHURCH
15TH AND R STS., NORTHWEST
WASHINGTON, D.C.
PLEASE EXTEND MY GREETINGS TO ALL THE PARTICIPANTS IN THE SIXTH IMHOTEP NATIONAL CONFERENCE ON HOSPITAL INTEGRATION.

AS YOU KNOW, THIS ADMINISTRATION IS TAKING STEPS TO ASSURE THAT NEEDED MEDICAL CARE AND HEALTH SERVICES WILL BE WITHIN REACH OF ALL AMERICANS. RACIAL DISCRIMINATION IN HOSPITAL PRACTICES IS OBVIOUSLY A BARRIER TO THE ACHIEVEMENT OF THIS GOAL.
DECISIONS OF THE SUPREME COURT HAVE MADE IT CLEAR THAT THE DOCTRINE OF "SEPARATE BUT EQUAL" IS DEAD—IN LAW AS WELL AS IN FACT. I AM SURE YOU ARE AWARE THAT THE ATTORNEY GENERAL HAS INTERVENED IN A FEDERAL COURT CASE, ARGUING THAT THE CLAUSE SANCTIONING SEGREGATION IN THE HILL-BURTON ACT IS UNCONSTITUTIONAL.

I AM HOPEFUL, AS I KNOW YOU ARE, THAT THIS ACTION WILL SPEED THE DAY WHEN ALL WILL RECOGNIZE THAT WE CANNOT AFFORD TO SQUANDER OUR RESOURCES ON THE PRACTICE OF RACIAL DISCRIMINATION AND THAT THE AVAILABILITY OF HOSPITAL SERVICES WILL NOT DEPEND ON THE RACE, COLOR OR CREED OF THE PATIENT.

I WISH YOU A SUCCESSFUL CONFERENCE.
JOHN F. KENNEDY[70]

The disparate strands of the story now converged on North Carolina and the City of Greensboro. One hundred years after the Battle of Gettysburg, a similar watershed in the civil rights struggle was unfolding.

CHAPTER 3

The North Carolina Campaign

> We have more small marginal farms than any other state and a lot of small town merchants. These are people angered about the economy, and that anger can be translated against blacks. Fortunately we have three very good papers: the *Raleigh News and Observer,* the *Charlotte Observer,* and the *Greensboro News and Record.* They and the University of North Carolina have done a good job of keeping the rats down in the holes.[1]

North Carolina, as this veteran state politician observed, has done a good job of keeping the "rats down in the holes." Long regarded as part of the more progressive "New South," North Carolina was seen by those on both sides of the regional divide in the civil rights struggle as the linchpin.[2] It was both the South's best defense of the status quo and the place where that mold was most likely to be broken. In regard to the racial integration of health care, the campaign in North Carolina was key. The battles often were quiet, personal ones. Similar local battles played out with minor variations in thousands of communities and hospitals across the country. The ones in North Carolina, however, stimulated and shaped the character of change and set many key legal precedents. This chapter describes health care's civil rights campaign in North Carolina and its key battle in Greensboro.

Three phases of the civil rights campaign in North Carolina are described in this chapter. The first phase was the struggle to integrate state and local medical societies; the second the early struggle to integrate hospitals in North Carolina; and the third the final, pivotal struggle in Greensboro. Each is described in some detail in order to capture the complexity and ambiguity that accompanied such struggles in professional and local communities across the nation.

The Stage Is Set

North Carolina did not become the focal point of the health care civil rights campaigns by accident. Media coverage and academic responses to racial issues in the state in the decades leading up to the civil rights era supported its progressive self-image. The three leading newspapers attacked the lynchings that took place in the 1920s and 1930s, demanding punishment of their perpetrators.[3] Frank Graham, a professor of history, assumed the presidency of the University of North Carolina in 1930, a state school with about twenty-five hundred students. He was able to build a loyal following and to transform the university into a strong moderating influence, insulated from the more reactionary forces in the state. Sociologist Howard Odum (noted for his efforts to develop a regional research and planning group), the University of North Carolina Press, and politically active faculty and students all flourished in that environment in the pre–civil rights era.[4] In the 1950s the University of North Carolina Medical School became a four-year program. Its rapid growth and prominence in the 1960s would exert a subtle civilizing influence on hospitals and medical practice in the state well beyond the technical and scientific.

North Carolina also had a key ingredient that was lacking in most other southern states, namely, black lawyers. There could be no local civil rights litigation without black lawyers. All of a black lawyer's clients in the South were black, and the local white establishment could not threaten them with the withholding business, because it provided none. Black lawyers could, however, be disbarred or face physical retaliation. Between 1930 and 1950 there were about a dozen black lawyers practicing in North Carolina, three regularly involved in civil rights law.[5] Limited as this capacity for litigation may seem, it was better than the situation in other southern states, which in some cases had but one or two black attorneys, who were often practicing only on a part-time basis.

Julius Chambers joined the ranks of this small band of pioneers, setting up practice in Charlotte in 1964. The University of North Carolina's first black law school graduate and the first of many NAACP Legal Defense Fund interns, his practice would handle most of the civil rights cases in North Carolina for the next two decades. North Carolina's reputation for civility and moderation notwithstanding, he saw his law office burned to the ground and his home and automobile bombed.[6] He would later serve as director counsel of the Legal Defense Fund before returning to his undergraduate alma mater, North Carolina Central University in Durham, as its chancellor.

In spite of the progressive image of North Carolina as a part of the New South, health care was as starkly divided along racial lines as anywhere in the nation. In 1961, 53 percent of all hospital beds in the state, some 15,438, were located in either all-black or all-white facilities.[7] The state psychiatric hospital system of 11,649 beds had, as specified by state law, two racially separate systems. Of North Carolina's general hospitals,

116 accepted both white and black patients, 27 accepted only white patients, and 11 served only black patients. One-quarter, or 3,688, of the short-term general hospital beds in North Carolina were located in racially separate facilities. The separate black facilities existed predominantly in those North Carolina cities large enough to accommodate such a division (i.e., Charlotte, Raleigh-Durham, Winston-Salem, Greensboro, and Wilmington). The acute hospitals that served both white and black populations did so on a segregated basis. These hospitals had white medical staffs and often restrictive admission practices for black patients. These restrictive admission practices made it impossible to determine how unequal accommodations were simply by counting beds. Both public funds, including Hill-Burton money, and private philanthropy supported the development of racially separate hospitals in North Carolina.

Reporting on these conditions, the North Carolina Advisory Committee of the U.S. Commission on Civil Rights in 1961 struggled for the elusive middle ground.[8] The committee had attempted to limit its focus to health departments, but there had been some complaints presented to the committee that hospitals obtaining Hill-Burton funds in the state had not maintained adequate space and beds for the needs of Negro patients. There were no state supreme court decisions related to the racial exclusion of patients. Persons requiring hospitalization, however, as the committee noted, are rarely in a position to litigate. While the committee's report noted several legal challenges that were currently in the lower courts, there was nothing to suggest that the state's hospitals, other than those in the state-run mental health system, were under much pressure to change.

Nevertheless, behind the scenes much *was* changing. In testimony to the Advisory Committee's Subcommittee on Medical Care, a representative of the Old North State Medical Society (ONSMS) made clear its intention to sue the University of North Carolina over the discharge of three black psychiatric patients. As a state-supported institution, the university hospital made an easier legal target than the private and voluntary hospitals and a less intransigent one. The hospital had maintained separate admission lists and thus quotas for the admission of black and white patients, ostensibly because of a concern about being overwhelmed by black admissions given the shortage of adequate inpatient care for this group across the state. This practice would quietly and unceremoniously change over the next several years.

> We filed a suit against the University of North Carolina when I was president of the Old North State Medical Society. We had gotten three young people admitted to the psychiatric unit. One weekend a

state senator got drunk, got the DTs, and was admitted. When he woke up, he was enraged to see the black patients on his unit that he had assumed was still segregated. He demanded that they get them out in a week. So the university told them they would have to leave in seven days.

So the Civil Rights Commission (North Carolina Advisory Committee of the U.S. Commission on Civil Rights) was having a hearing. I represented the Old North State at the hearing, and I described this situation. The head psychiatrists at the University of North Carolina said it has nothing to do with race; they found that they couldn't treat black and white patients in the same setting. I said, "Well, we're going to let the courts decide." Consternation went through the place. The gentleman who was conducting the hearing, he was a legislator. He called me Monday after that meeting to ask me if I thought it would be satisfactory for the Old North State, if we would withdraw our complaint, if they just quietly went on and integrated—that it would hurt the university and hurt them in getting grants if we made a big public to-do about it or published the fact that they had changed the university policy. I said, "We're not out to hurt the university, and it will cost us more legal fees, so if you will send me a letter to that effect that I can present to my committee . . ." And that's what they did. They sent a letter saying that racial discrimination no longer would be allowed in the university hospital system. They didn't relate it to our suit at all. We made a file of it. Floyd McKissick was our lawyer. He advised us to accept it and keep it under observation, so that if somebody came up with a complaint, we could trot it out. I think it cost us two hundred dollars to integrate the whole university hospital system. They decided that we had an issue. It was not our purpose to stir up controversy but to get change.

I will never forget this, though. There was a person at the commission hearing from Duke, and, of course, Duke was completely segregated. Nothing had been said about Duke. I got up and went to the bathroom. As soon as I relieved myself in the bathroom, there was this well-known physician at Duke. He said, "You're doing the right thing! Just keep on pushing." I knew what he was doing. He was trying to keep my attention on North Carolina![9]

The stark racial divisions that cut across health care clashed with North Carolina's progressive mystique and created an unusual chemistry. Compared to those in most other southern states, black businesses, universities, and cultural institutions had long thrived in the relatively supportive, albeit paternalistic, atmosphere of North Carolina. Particularly in the industrial centers of the central Piedmont region, these conditions had produced a growing, economically independent black middle class.

North Carolina Mutual Life Insurance Company, which had evolved out of several black mutual-aid societies of the nineteenth century to become the largest black-managed financial institution in the United States, was headquartered in Durham. Throughout the region blacks had access to steady, relatively well paying jobs in the growing tobacco-processing and textile mills of the urban centers. The faculty and staff of the racially separate colleges and schools expanded an educated middle class to a critical mass. Black physicians and dentists, seeking a congenial lifestyle and paying patients, began setting up practices in these towns after World War II. Patients flocked to them. In North Carolina, more progressive leadership had stimulated a growing independent black professional class that in some communities reached the critical mass necessary to push for the elimination of racial barriers.

Medical-Society Pressures for Integration

The pressure for change from black physicians and dentists began to build in the 1950s. It was clear that the deck had been stacked against them. The medical-staff bylaws of most hospitals in North Carolina, as in the United States as a whole, required that a physician applying for privileges be a member in good standing of the local county medical society. In North Carolina the bylaws of the state medical society explicitly restricted membership to white physicians. Since county medical societies were constituent bodies of the state society, the same restriction applied at the county level. Ensnared in a slow-moving shell game, white and black physicians who tried to end discrimination were constantly thwarted.[10] As one white Greensboro surgeon observed:

> It was catch-22. They were capable people. These were people who were as good or not better than we were. You had to belong to the county medical society, and it distinctly said white physicians only. They had them absolutely boxed out. It was unbelievable. They didn't have a chance![11]

Physicians in North Carolina as elsewhere lived in a relatively self-contained world where social and professional activities intertwined. It was a more professionally isolated world then than now, composed largely of rural, solo, fee-for-service practitioners. Events sponsored by the local and state medical society offered an all-too-rare opportunity for social interaction and relaxation among one's peers and took on an emotional and symbolic importance alien to most practitioners today.

> When I first joined the [state medical] Society in 1951 the annual meeting at Pinehurst was considered the highlight of the Society's year. Not only did the House of Delegates conduct business, but the general membership joined enthusiastically in attending all sessions, and members with their auxiliary wives took a very active part in the social side of the meeting. All members as well as invited guests from the AMA and neighboring states gathered in hospitality suites, and the formal banquet, filling the main dinning room at the Carolina, was the climax of the meeting. But by then a shadow was falling over these festive occasions.[12]

It was the shadow of a world that was changing. In the original 1903 bylaws of the Medical Society of North Carolina (MSNC) there was no mention of race in eligibility for membership, but *White* mysteriously appeared in the publication of the bylaws in 1925 and took forty years to remove that restriction. The Old North State Medical Society, established in 1887, the black counterpart to the MSNC and the oldest one of its kind in the United States, pressed for relief from the effects that exclusion from the white society imposed on its members. Meeting at Bennet College in Greensboro in 1951, the group drafted a letter to their white counterparts requesting that (1) MSNC enter into negotiations with the American Medical Association with the objectives of recognizing ONSMS as one of the AMA's constituent societies, and (2) should the first proposal be unacceptable, that individual members of ONSMS be admitted to membership in the MSNC. The ONSMS leaders preferred a group solution rather than individual integration into the existing county societies. The president of the MSNC urged the AMA to accept the first approach, but the AMA refused.

The AMA had been facing pressure for a decade from the National Medical Association and some local northern medical societies to bar from AMA membership state and local societies that discriminated on the basis of race. In 1950 the AMA House of Delegates passed a resolution urging that "constituent and component societies that have restrictive membership provisions based on race study this question *in the light of prevailing conditions,* with the view to taking steps as they may elect to eliminate such restrictive provisions."[13] This resolution, falling far short of the NMA demands, seemed partly motivated by the need to close ranks in the battle to block the Truman administration's proposal for national health insurance. The 1949 NMA convention had come close to endorsing the

Truman proposal, and its president had taken exception to the AMA's viewpoint, insisting that the NMA should do its own thinking and be concerned "with the masses of the poor and needy people who do not have adequate medical care."[14] In the delicate political balancing act in which the AMA was now engaged, it clearly could not afford to go on record officially sanctioning racially separate medical societies.

The ONSMS and the MSNC, excluded from the option that would leave both bodies essentially unchanged, now engaged in their own delicate political balancing act that would take another fifteen years to achieve some stability. At first the ONSMS president tried to reassure the white medical society. Stating that "the major aspiration of Negro physicians seeking membership in the State Medical Society is scientific advancement as medical men," he pledged to "prevent any attempt to acutely disturb present social customs and to aid in working toward a gradual and evolutionary situation."[15] It was, indeed, a gradual evolutionary situation. A president of a county medical society who pressed for the elimination of the term *White* from the bylaws at the annual meetings of the House of Delegates was continually frustrated.

> The eastern North Carolina doctors resisted. I was a delegate with one vote. We had some pretty tough old boys, but you expect that. The debate would drag out, and they would wait till I left the room to urinate and then they'd get the motion tabled to be brought up the following year.[16]

In the meantime, some of the larger county societies began to push on their own. A proposal forwarded by the Guilford County Medical Society to strike the word *White* from the bylaws was first debated at the 1954 state convention. The Mecklenburg Medical Society, the largest county society and one that represented the state's largest city, Charlotte, admitted a black to membership in September 1954. A unanimous resolution by the MSNC House of Delegates in 1955 then censured the Mecklenburg Society for "premature action" and instructed other county societies to "desist from taking any similar action until the State Society can accomplish a satisfactory program and policy to meet this situation."[17] A "satisfactory program and policy" seemed to hinge on inclusion in the "scientific" benefits of members and exclusion from the "social" functions. At the MSNC House of Delegates meeting in May 1955 such a resolution was proposed by the committee studying the issue. It was passed, but only after heated discussion. One member took the floor afterward, observing emotionally,

I believe that the State Medical Society as we have known it has had the first dagger put through its heart, and that it is now in the quivering process of its demise. But I believe the organization will have to live on under difficulties, if you please, and I certainly want it to live on.[18]

It was not just some of the older physicians who were disturbed by the proposal. The Carolina Hotel at the Pinehurst resort subsequently notified the MSNC that if a single Negro were made eligible to come to the hotel, the reservations for the next meeting would be canceled. In 1956 the society's president announced that the annual meeting would move from Pinehurst to accommodate the Negro physicians who wished to become scientific members. Blacks were permitted as "scientific" members to attend the meetings dealing with medical topics, but not the social functions. The meeting was relocated to hotels in Asheville.

Such accommodations, however, were not greeted with enthusiasm by the members of the ONSMS. The ONSMS executive committee passed a resolution recommending that members refuse to accept such "second class membership" and censured two of its members who had done so.[19] This event in 1957 made national news. In the wake of bus boycotts and other protests, the positions of the black physicians on the issue had shifted. One physician, writing in response to an offer of "scientific" membership in the Guilford County Society in 1960, observed in exasperation,

I am a native American citizen, trained in approved American institutions, and possess an unrestricted license to practice my profession within this state. I have no criminal record, and I have honorably and faithfully discharged my military obligations. I belong to a recognized Protestant faith, and I believe in the existence of a Supreme Deity. I grumble about taxes, but pay them just the same. I like baseball, good bourbon, and the Pirates. I love my four sons and seldom beat my wife . . . now why can't I belong?[20]

Something else was pushing at these physicians now in the wake of the lunch counter sit-ins in 1960. It was their children. One of the white physicians involved in the negotiations with the ONSMS representatives observed that "it was perfectly obvious that these doctors were having a terrific amount of pressure put on them." The black physicians explained that if they, while their children were participating in such things as sit-down strikes in eating places, accepted anything less than what was offered to others, they could not keep the respect of their children.[21]

Some of the white members of the NCMS were upset by the black physicians' growing intransigence. One physician and member of the executive council of the medical society noted emotionally in one of its subsequent debates,

> They are willing to come into the Society and dissolve our social functions. This matter has already partially dissolved our Society. The last year we were at Pinehurst we had around 1,200 doctors present. For the past two or three years we are running around 700. . . . Pinehurst is the ideal place in North Carolina to accommodate the Medical Society of the State of North Carolina.
> We have sacrificed for them our meeting place, our home. . . . They are unwilling to make any sacrifice for us . . . a sacrifice to participate in the Medical Society of the State of North Carolina. We are asked to bear the brunt of the whole thing, give them all the cake. . . . The majority of the Committee . . . has voted that we have gone as far as this Medical Society can go with honor and dignity until they . . . take some advantage of the opportunities that have been offered them.[22]

Some of the black medical leaders took a more humorous view of the predicament now faced by the MSNC.

> The interesting thing was that they had always met at Pinehurst. It had very nice facilities for playing tennis and golf. I don't think they were very substantive meetings. They had good attendance to come to the golf courses. When the board of governors passed a resolution saying that black physicians could come to the annual meeting (for the scientific sessions), Pinehurst threw them out. They said, "We don't want any black folks down here, no Jews and no dogs," or something to that effect! They started losing their constituency. Attendance at the annual meetings dropped to its lowest level in 1960. Here they were with no blacks attending, being forced to have their meetings elsewhere and losing attendance.[23]

The hard negotiations between the two groups began in earnest in 1961. The ONSMS asked for a meeting with an enlarged Integration Committee. A tough but respectful negotiating session followed, helping to clarify positions.

> We met with a Dr. Whitaker and his group somewhere down in eastern North Carolina. There were about eight of us in our group that went. I remember we tried to prepare ourselves for it. We didn't want

it to become a knock-down-drag-out bitter meeting. We had a very successful conference, and we left with mutual respect. Dr. Whitaker, who chaired the meeting, really became a friend.[24]

The ONSMS group asked for a meeting with the executive council of the NCMS. The meeting took place on December 9, 1962. According to the leader of the ONSMS delegation, Dr. Watts, "It looked like a lynching party. There were about fifty of them, and I was not happy about being there." Dr. Watts and his colleagues were, however, well prepared. The black physicians had watched television coverage of the Cuban missile crisis and discussed how John F. Kennedy had kept those discussions on track and were determined to match his approach to their own equally tense negotiations. Dr. Watts spoke briefly to the executive committee, careful to provide a dignified, face-saving "out," as Kennedy had provided the Russians.

> We are all sympathetic with the problems that you face in the prospect of the change in our community life. As educated and intelligent men, it seems that this adjustment, however, due to the winds of change, could reasonably be made with a minimum of fanfare. It may mean a change in the character of the social aspects of the meetings, or changes in meeting places. To recognize these problems as sensitive individuals we are willing to work in this area to the end that a minimum of embarrassment and no hurt would be experienced by anyone.
>   We feel that these problems can be overcome if our goals are correct and regard for one another is what it should be.[25]

A small but intransigent minority tried to use the two most inflammatory issues to sway the debate. One person had argued that "this action will do only one thing: it will allow Negroes to come to our dinners and to dance on the floor with our women," and another accused the ONSMS of having "taken a stand on the Medicare legislation that was diametrically opposed to the stand of the American Medical Association and this society."[26] Neither argument had any impact on the outcome. Finally, in May 1965, in an emotional session of the House of Delegates, a resolution striking the words *white* and *scientific members* from the bylaws and constitution of the society passed by well over the required two-thirds margin. The ONSMS had delayed litigating the issue pending the outcome of the vote, a move that was now unnecessary.[27]

In 1966 the AMA House of Delegates again defeated a resolution that would have expelled from the AMA constituent societies that engaged in discriminatory practices, but it did amend its bylaws so that those who felt they had been denied membership in a state or local society on racial grounds could now appeal that decision to the AMA.[28] By then the Carolina Hotel was begging the North Carolina society to return to Pinehurst, which it did in 1967. Yet, as one participant observed, "The popularity and social grandeur of the meetings in the early 1950s never returned. They have gone with the wind."[29] Pinehurst itself, however, seems to have survived. According to the current Fodor's travel guide, "Civilized decorum rules in the spacious public rooms, on the rocker-lined wide verandas, and amid the lush gardens of the surrounding grounds. Guests can play lawn croquet, shoot skeet or tee off on one of seven premier golf courses."[30]

The president of the ONSMS, who had participated actively in the negotiations, recalled a special greeting on his first visit as a participant at the Pinehurst annual conference.

> When I walked in the room, there were fifteen to twenty older gentleman who were past officials on the platform, and one was waving his hand off. It was Dr. Whitaker. His attitude was, I see you made it and I'm glad.[31]

In 1989, in a gesture intended to heal some of the old wounds from the struggle for integration, members of the ONSMS presented to Dr. Paschal, president of MSNC, a plaque for his courageous help, in the face of "strident criticisms by his peers," in breaking the tradition of medical segregation.[32]

Other events, however, had relegated the medical-society integration story to a minor footnote, a small brushfire beside an inferno.

Dr. Eaton Gets the Call

Perhaps the real health care integration story began with a telephone call to Dr. Hubert A. Eaton in Wilmington, North Carolina. Wilmington is located in the "down east" coastal plain of the state. This region was viewed, at least by those in the central Piedmont, as an underdeveloped backwater with racial attitudes and economic conditions akin to rural Mississippi. It lacked the progressive, albeit paternalistic, spirit of the Piedmont region. Yet, it was here that the campaign for racial integration of health care began. In the words of Dr. Eaton,

> Before the call that summer day in 1947, I lived quietly and uneventfully. I had a thriving medical practice, a family that gave me pride and comfort, a home with my own private tennis court. I was

working hard and playing hard and believed, at 31, I was set on a satisfying, predicable course for my life.

Then the lawyer called. I don't remember his name now, but he
explained that he represented a patient of mine who had been hurt in
an accident. A dispute over liability and expenses had arisen; a settlement could not be reached, so litigation was necessary, and the lawyer
needed my testimony.

. . . . I climbed the steps of the New Hanover County Courthouse in
downtown Wilmington, entered the back of a small courtroom and
made my way along the wall toward the front, where I could catch the
lawyer's eye. . . . He nodded and turned to the judge. "Your honor,"
he said, "Dr. Eaton has arrived. Can we take his testimony now?"
Neither the judge nor the bailiff realized that Dr. Eaton was colored,
so there was a moment of confusion while they looked for me. I
stepped from the wall, and the judge told me to come forward and be
sworn.

I pushed through the little gate in the balustrade that separated the
spectators from the rest of the courtroom. The bailiff beckoned me
toward the judge's bench, a high desk-like structure with a bottled-
water dispenser on the right and the witness stand on the left, near the
jury box. The American and North Carolina flags stood behind the
bench on either side of the judge. "Put your left hand on the Bible,
raise your right hand and say after me . . ." the Bailiff began. I reached
toward the shelf that stretched across the front of the judge's bench
for the Bible and saw two Bibles. Each was wrapped shut with a strip
of dirty adhesive tape. One was labeled "COLORED," the other
"WHITE." Segregated Bibles! I was stunned. . . .

That my children should grow up in a community that required
them to swear in court on a segregated Bible was unconscionable.
"I'm going to have to do something to change some of the things I
have seen in this town if I'm going to live in it," I said to myself. How
I would accomplish this was not yet clear to me but I knew I must
try.[33]

That resolution by Dr. Eaton to try would eventually lead to the first test
of the racial exclusion of physicians from staff privileges at a voluntary
hospital in the United States. Dr. Hubert Eaton had moved to Wilmington
after finishing his medical degree at the University of Michigan and completing a residency at Reynolds' Hospital in Winston-Salem. When he
began his practice there in 1943, there were two hospitals in Wilmington.[34]
James A. Walker Memorial Hospital provided about twenty-five beds for

black patients in a ward that had two toilets. The ward was in a building separated from the main hospital so that to reach the operating room, delivery room, or x-ray facilities, patients were exposed to the elements as they were wheeled across ninety feet of an open yard to the main hospital. No black physicians had privileges at the hospital. Community Hospital, a woefully inadequate one-hundred-bed facility with a deteriorating physical plant, provided care only to black patients by a medical staff that included both white and black physicians.

Wilmington, through Dr. Hubert Eaton, became the first testing ground for the emerging Legal Defense Fund and National Medical Association strategy. The news of the *Brown* decision in 1954 focused Dr. Eaton's attention on James A. Walker Memorial Hospital. He had accidentally discovered that year that, while James A. Walker was a "private" hospital, it paid no city or county taxes. Here was a wrong, he felt, that went deeper than unequal schools for white and black children. Didn't such arrangements violate the equal protection clause of the Fourteenth Amendment of the Constitution? (No state shall "deny any person within its jurisdiction the equal protection of the laws.") Wilmington's hospitals were both separate and unequal. Did voluntary hospitals fall under such a prohibition? Was James A. Walker Memorial Hospital a public or a private entity? Did policies racially segregating patients and excluding black physicians from the medical staff constitute state action? If James A. Walker Memorial did indeed function as a quasi public entity or "arm of the state" such actions would seem to deny equal protection under the law prohibited by the U.S. Constitution.

Eaton and three colleagues applied for privileges but were denied. In 1956 they filed suit in federal district court. The district court judge ruled in 1958 that the act of discrimination did not constitute state action. That decision was upheld on appeal to the court of appeals, and the Supreme Court declined to hear the case in 1959:

> We may not interfere unless there is State action which offends the Federal Constitution. From this viewpoint we find no error in the decision of the District Court for the facts clearly show that when the present suit was brought, and for years before, the hospital was not an instrumentality of the State but a corporation managed and operated by an independent board free from State Control.[35]

To everyone but Dr. Eaton and his Legal Defense Fund lawyers, it looked like the end of the road for the Wilmington struggle. An appeal to other black doctors in North Carolina for contributions to mount a new case brought only seven contributions, and the National Medical Association declined to provide direct support.[36] The court of appeals decision would seem to stand. Yet the suit, the first of its kind nationally, had started the wheels turning. It would be a matter of the right time and place.

Reginald Hawkins and Charlotte Memorial Hospital

Charlotte is North Carolina's largest city, and it presented a more conducive environment for pushing the civil rights agenda. The Mecklenburg County Medical Society, which encompassed Charlotte, had voted a black physician into membership in 1954, incurring the wrath and censure of the state medical society. The Charlotte hospitals presented a more clear-cut legal case for those seeking integration. Charlotte Memorial was a municipally owned, all-white facility. The city also operated a smaller, overcrowded, black hospital, Good Samaritan. Charlotte Memorial began to admit patients on a limited and segregated basis in May 1960, in response to hospital expansion plans and pressures from members of their medical staff. The policy did not change overnight. Charlotte Memorial refused the admission of a critically injured black youth in June. He was then taken to another hospital, where he died. In an awkward but revealing admission of error on the part of the emergency room staff, a hospital official explained, "It has been the hospital policy since 1949 to care for all severe accident cases, including Negroes."[37]

A dentist and Presbyterian minister in Charlotte, North Carolina, Reginald Hawkins, now pressed for integration. Hawkins showed up with NAACP pickets at Charlotte Memorial in 1962, demanding complete desegregation of treatment and training facilities at the hospital. It was remarkable in that it was one of the few times nationally that the behind-the-scenes legal, board, and professional society struggles over hospital integration actually spilled over into public demonstrations.

In the meantime, Hawkins filed a suit in U.S. district court against the North Carolina Dental Society in 1960. The suit picked up on the line of reasoning that Eaton's case in Wilmington had attempted to establish: that discriminatory nonpublic institutions could engage in "state action." While Hawkins had been denied membership in the all-white but nongovernmental North Carolina Dental Society, state law limited membership on the State Board of Dental Examiners to members of that society. Hawkins's suit also argued that the society participated in state action by serving to recommend dentists for employment at state institutions, and that "various clinics and hospitals operated by state, local or federal funds permit only dentists who are members of the NCDS to practice in their facilities." The initial response of the NCDS was to work toward rewriting state laws so as to change eligibility for the board of examiners to licensed dentists rather than NCDS members. Racial exclusion apparently mattered more than the society's control over such appointments.[38]

The Battle of Greensboro: The Turning Point

Greensboro, North Carolina, however, more by destiny than accident, became the right place and the right time. The battle in Greensboro represented a turning point in the campaign to integrate hospitals. Here and at this time the federal and the local community struggle converged. What happened quietly converted all of the courageous—but quixotic and largely ineffectual—protests of two decades into a battle that would leave the national health care landscape radically altered. Greensboro's battle captures all the richness and ambiguity of the American story of race relations. Perhaps more than any other community in the Piedmont region, Greensboro had long been a double-edged sword, attracting more ambitious blacks to the community with rising expectations but also frustrating these expectations and sparking protest.[39] For this reason, it is important to carefully set the stage.

Greensboro and the Civil Rights Struggle

Greensboro is, for anyone familiar with the civil rights struggle in the United States, "holy ground."[40] Now North Carolina's third largest city, with a population of about two hundred thousand, it was in 1819 the birthplace of the Underground Railroad. The local Quaker group was the most active and single-minded constituent member of the Manumission Society of North Carolina, assisting slaves to freedom in the North.

The Reconstruction period was a real reconstruction period in Greensboro more than elsewhere. Former slaves created a thirty-four-acre planned community, now incorporated as part of the city. Similar efforts led to the founding of two black colleges, Bennett College, a private Methodist school established in 1873, and the Agricultural and Mechanical College for the Negro Race, established by local business leaders in 1893 and later renamed North Carolina A&T State University. (A&T had received federal funds through the "separate but equal" provisions of the Morrill Act of 1890.) A&T remains the largest historically African American college in North Carolina.

During the Reconstruction period Greensboro was also the home of Albion Winegar Tourgee, a former Union officer, and judge in Greensboro. His fight against Jim Crow laws links his life efforts to the legal battle that would be waged over Greensboro's hospitals in 1963. Tourgee wrote the brief and planned strategy for the case designed to block Jim

Crow legislation, *Plessy v. Ferguson.* The case was begun by a "one eighth African blood," Homer Adolph Plessy, who sat in a train coach in New Orleans that a new state law reserved for whites. This well-crafted test case was eventually appealed to the Supreme Court,[41] which with its decision ushered in a wave of state Jim Crow legislation. Tourgee, by the time of his death in 1905, saw in operation a caste system of segregation. Yet two months after Tourgee's death, W. E. B. Du Bois and a gathering at Niagara, New York, would renew the struggle.

Most remember Greensboro, however, for the four A&T freshmen who entered the downtown Woolworth's and sat down at the lunch counter at 4:30 P.M. on the afternoon of February 1, 1960. There had been many similar protests, but they had happened in isolation, unnoticed and without impact. The Greensboro protest spread quickly to hundreds of communities across the South and border states. A new phase of the civil rights movement, largely student directed, had begun. As if to ratify the wave of seemingly coordinated protests that had already happened, a conference of the new activists at Shaw University in Raleigh two months later created the Student Nonviolent Coordinating Committee (SNCC). Marion Barry became the first president of the new organization. Jessie Jackson, a football star at A&T whom the original student protest leaders had recruited to help attract other students to their demonstrations, soon was catapulted to national prominence.

Health Care in Greensboro

Health care for Greensboro's black residents, relative to most areas of the country, was good. At least eight black physicians were practicing in Greensboro in the 1950s. An implausible sequence of events had provided blacks the hospital, L. Richardson, with the best physical facilities in Greensboro.

> L. Richardson Hospital was named for my grandfather. The name was the black community's decision and predated the contribution of the Richardson children to help with the construction of the hospital. He was an unusual man. Searching for a way to support his growing family, he had moved to Greensboro and bought a drugstore about 1912. He would fiddle around in the back room and come up with a series of patent medicines, of which only one really caught on, Vick's Vapor Rub. He was one of the few white people in those days interested in hands-on work with the black people. He taught Sunday school in the black community. People used to say that there were only two white people who could safely walk in the most dangerous

sections of the black community. One was this very large and mean Greensboro chief of police and the other was Lunsford Richardson. He died, ironically, in the flu epidemic of 1918, in the same epidemic that propelled the success of his patent medicine remedy, Vick's Vapor Rub.

The Richardson Company and Vick's Vapor Rub, under the direction of the oldest son, had progressed in the 1920s to the point where they could set up a foundation. The Richardson Foundation made a substantial contribution for construction of the hospital. As soon as the hospital was open, a member of the Richardson family served on the board. I served on the board until about 1968, when I was elected to Congress. We kept an interest in the hospital, but we were concerned about it getting too tied to the Richardson name and that it wouldn't get money from anywhere else. We didn't want to be the perpetual bailer-out. The hospital was doing very well. It operated at a high occupancy up into the 1960s and was breaking even, if not profitable.[42]

In the meantime, hospital development for the white community was stalled by the settlement of the estate of Moses Cone. After his death in 1908, the bulk of Moses Cone's substantial estate was to be used to endow a hospital. However, the allocation of funds for this purpose was delayed until the death of his widow, Bertha in 1947.[43] Moses Cone Memorial Hospital was not completed until February 1953. The three hospitals that served the white community in Greensboro prior to its completion were reluctant to renovate or rebuild, uncertain whether they could compete with the generously endowed new institution and not sure when it would be built. As one retired Greensboro surgeon lamented, "it set medicine in Greensboro back forty years."[44] St. Leo's, a Catholic Hospital that had provided some accommodation to blacks in a ward in the basement, closed the year after Moses Cone opened. Piedmont Hospital, a marginal proprietary facility occupying two floors above a drugstore downtown and serving only white patients, struggled for another decade before closing.

Of all of Greensboro's early hospitals, only Wesley Long Hospital, established in 1917, clearly survived the coming of Moses Cone. Dr. John Wesley Long in that year he wrote an apologetic letter to a colleague in Brown Summit: "I'm sorry I could not take the colored patient you referred recently. When the War is over, if we live through it, I propose making arrangements to accommodate the colored people. I have a large following among the better class of colored patients in this region of North Carolina."[45] In 1923, the *Greensboro Daily News* reported an incident in which a black with acute appendicitis was turned away from Long Hospital, asking whether under those circumstances Greensboro could be "considered civilized."[46] Long Hospital, which later converted to voluntary sponsorship, remained a white-only facility and a determined adversary in the integration battle waged in 1963.

The intentions of the new Cone Hospital in serving blacks were more ambiguous. Bertha Cone's only stipulation for the hospital was that it serve people regardless of ability to pay, which some interpreted as meaning both blacks and whites. As the new hospital was being planned in 1950, a local physician wrote the chairman of the Cone Foundation Board, Bertha's son Herman, cautioning him not to take any federal Hill-Burton money.

> Thinking further about your question as to whether or not to accept federal aid for your hospital, I at present am of the opinion that it would be better not to do. I am thinking primarily of the problem of race integration; and the complications arising from such steps as the government requiring admission of colored surgeons to the staff and having white nurses work under their direction. In the years to come such problems will be worked out; but we know the tendency of the present administration to force these issues. Incidentally, I would like to see you take over L. Richardson Memorial and develop it into a real good hospital for all your colored patients. So many hospitals are accepting federal aid and seem to feel it is necessary, I would like to see at least one big North Carolina hospital not tied up with the federal government in this way . . . for the sake of comparison if nothing else.[47]

That advice was ignored. The hospital applied for and received more than $1.2 million in Hill-Burton funds for the construction and expansion of the hospital over the next decade. On October 12, 1950, however, an offer to give L. Richardson Hospital to Moses Cone had been withdrawn. Instead, the board voted to continue to study cooperation between the two hospitals.[48]

In the early days of planning for the new Cone Hospital, the board was clearly divided concerning the issue of racial integration. The March 13, 1952, board meeting appears to have been a key turning point. Board president Herman Cone presented the following resolution with respect to the Negro policy of the hospital, which had been developed by the executive committee in accordance with instructions given at the last meeting by the trustees:[49]

WHEREAS, the Board of Trustees believes that The Moses H. Cone Memorial Hospital should be operated for the best interests of all people in this community, without regard to race but with due regard for the traditional customs of the region which it is to serve;

THEREFORE, the Board of Trustees adopts the following statement of principles:

1. That upon the opening of the Hospital, a portion of its beds and facilities shall be made available for Negro patients;
2. That this policy shall be administered with full consideration for the available facilities of this Hospital as well as other hospitals which have been rendering such splendid service in the community; and
3. That invitations to apply for membership on the initial medical Staff of the Hospital be sent to qualified physicians of all races.

In order to carry out these principles, the Director is given the following instructions as a guide for admissions until further notice:

1. That on the opening of the Hospital approximately ten beds be made available for Negro patients. This figure is based on the assumption that the Hospital initially will open only 96 beds located on the north end of the second and third floors. Before other beds are opened, the matter will be reviewed and policies will be restated.
2. That, in the case of adults, patients of one race shall be assigned to a room; and that, in case of children and infants, this matter shall be determined according to the sentiments of the individuals involved and their families.

There was a general discussion of the content of the resolution, and the board adopted the suggestion of the president to divide and consider the resolutions in sections. The first sections so considered were amended, possibly from suggestions of the board's legal counsel, who were present at all meetings, and passed unanimously. The first three paragraphs were amended to read,

WHEREAS, the Board of Trustees believes that The Moses H. Cone Memorial Hospital should be operated for the best interests of all the people of this community;

THEREFORE, upon the opening of the Hospital, a portion of its beds shall be made available to Negro patients.

The second item concerning "full consideration of the available facilities" was deleted all together.

The third motion, however, "That invitations to apply for membership on the initial Medical Staff of the Hospital be sent to qualified physicians of all races," did not have smooth sailing. The members of the medical board, when asked to express themselves on the subject, recommended strongly that Negro physicians not be invited to join the staff, recommending instead that Negro doctors be invited only to participate in the scientific activities of the medical staff without being members. The original motion subsequently failed by a vote of seven to five. The five trustees supporting the original motion, including three Cone family members, requested that their names be recorded as having voted in favor of the original motion. Herman Cone also requested that his name be recorded as having been in favor of the original motion, if he had been permitted to vote.

Evidently there subsequently was some slipup in sending out invitations for membership, because in their meeting of December 3, 1953, the trustees were presented with the question of how to rule on the application of Dr. Girardeau Alexander.[50]

> The Medical Board believed that an application from one Negro doctor should not be considered by itself, but that, instead, the Hospital's policies with regard to all Negro doctors should be considered. . . Recognizing the newness of the Hospital and the many problems arising in the initial organization of its present Staff, the Board believed it would be unwise to complicate this situation by adding the problems attendant with the appointment of the Negro doctors. Instead, the Board favored that the introduction of the Negro doctors to this Hospital be approached gradually and that the first step be the issuing to them of an invitation to attend certain selected meetings of the full Medical Staff and its services at which clinical material is usually presented. The Medical Board had, therefore, recommended that the application of Dr. Alexander be rejected and that the Medical Staff be permitted to send an invitation to the Negro Doctors to attend the specified meetings.

After a brief discussion, the board voted unanimously to reject the application of Dr. Alexander for appointment to the medical staff. The "specified meetings," as subsequent discussion made clear, were those "at which the presence of Negro doctors would least likely produce embarrassment, particularly to patients being exhibited."

The American Friends Services Committee (AFSC) had set up their

Southeast regional headquarters in Greensboro in the early 1950s. Its staff set about exploring approaches to breaking down racial segregation and discrimination in the region. The first administrator of Cone Hospital, Dr. Joseph Lichty, had told AFSC that he wished to build a completely integrated hospital with black and white doctors and nurses working together to serve an integrated patient population. However, Lichty reported to the group that the board of directors had been besieged by "the elite" of Greensboro society in opposition to such an approach.[51]

According to some who participated in the discussions, Herman Cone and other board members were concerned that the opening of Cone not adversely impact the existing hospitals, particularly L. Richardson.[52] The board of trustees, they argue, sincerely believed that if Cone Hospital accepted black patients directly, the census of L. Richardson would drop, possibly leading to its closure. Furthermore, the white leadership was probably also getting mixed signals from the black community. One of the community's black leaders put it bluntly.

> The reason the Moses Cone didn't integrate was that a lot of the black doctors thought that the black patients would leave L. Richardson and go to Cone. It would bankrupt L. Richardson. Some of the older docs fought it. Another thing, you could go to L. Richardson and operate whether you were qualified or not. At Moses Cone you had to be a specialist with the right credentials. So it was going to hurt their income.[53]

Whatever the reasoning, several months before the opening of the hospital the board adopted a policy carefully restricting admissions.

> The Moses H. Cone Memorial Hospital will admit as patients Negroes whose medical conditions require facilities and services available at this Hospital and not also available in L. Richardson Memorial Hospital. To be considered for admission, a Negro must first have been admitted to and be a patient in L. Richardson Memorial Hospital from which transfer will be made to this Hospital. To insure continuity of medical management, the patient will be admitted only to the service of the doctor on whose service he is a patient in L. Richardson Memorial Hospital.
>
> Request for transfer from L. Richardson Memorial Hospital to this Hospital is to be made to the Admitting Office by the Negro patient's physician. Only a physician who is a member of the Staff of both hospitals may make such request. Approval to make such request must first be obtained from the Administrator of L. Richardson Memorial

Hospital. Except in extreme emergency, request may be made only after the history and physical examination of the patient has been completed and recorded and all the necessary diagnostic procedures for which for which facilities are available at L. Richardson Memorial Hospital have been carried out.[54]

The board of trustees amended this policy on February 25, 1960, eliminating some of the bottlenecks created by such an arrangement.

In cases where in the judgement of the attending physician hospital-ization is required primarily for studies or treatment, facilities for which are not available at L. Richardson Memorial Hospital, direct admission to Moses Cone Memorial Hospital may be arranged with the prior approval of the Administrator of L. Richardson Hospital, provided final authority to approve such admissions rests with the Admitting office of the Moses H. Cone Memorial Hospital.[55]

Only white physicians had privileges at *both* L. Richardson and Cone, and relatively few black patients "required" such transfers. These sporadic transfers were accommodated in single rooms, rather than on a separate "colored" floor. The policy protected Richardson from direct competition with Cone and assured that Cone would care overwhelmingly for white patients. Generous, protective paternalism for a struggling black commu-nity institution, or simply a procedure to enforce the color lines? It is hard to assess the motives. The board members were, however, correct in pre-dicting the effect of direct black admissions to Moses Cone. After the bar-riers to direct admissions were lifted, L. Richardson struggled for several decades before finally closing as an acute-care facility, North Carolina's last historically black hospital.

Moses Cone, nevertheless, came to occupy the uncomfortable middle ground in a community rigidly divided along racial lines. The minutes of the board's executive committee during Moses Cone's first decade of oper-ations reflect the tensions surrounding that struggle which went well beyond the issue of staff privileges for black physicians and spanned the design of the facility, the hiring and accommodation of racially mixed staff, the accommodation of black patients and their visitors, its participa-tion in a nurse-training program, and the nature of its relationship to L. Richardson.

The Director reported on the progress of the construction of the Hos-pital, commenting particularly on the various proposals for changes which are under discussion with the Architect and Engineers. The majority of the details have been worked out. He recommended one change of a major importance, that the Canteen on the first floor be combined with the one in the basement, rearranged so it could serve both white and Negro patrons, and that a suitable dignified waiting room be provided for visitors of both races in the area vacated by the forgoing move. (December 14, 1950)

There was discussion about practices to be followed in connection with Negro personnel. The Committee requested more information about employment of Negro registered nurses in other hospitals. The Director was advised the he could try the plan of using only one serving line, but using separate dining rooms, for personnel of both races for those meals at which the number being served is small. (September 8, 1952)

The Director reported that the Hospital had engaged two Negro registered nurses who were to report the following week. These nurses had been assigned general duty care of all patients in the nursing divisions. He requested advice as to where these nurses should have their lockers and where they should take meals. It was decided that, for the present, the nurses would be assigned to locker rooms for Negro personnel and eat in the Negro dining room. (February 3, 1953)

It had developed that a small group of Negro personnel who are required to be on duty on Sunday have been conducting a short religious service. The group had selected a location for this service which was not appropriate. It was agreed that the Hospital should do nothing to discourage this activity but that it should be provided a suitable location on the ground floor. The volunteers room was recommended. (November 4, 1953)

A letter from the Medical Board, transmitting without recommendation a request from the Medical Staff that a separate area be designated for adult Negro patients, was introduced. The members were of the opinion that the Hospital's present policy of segregating Negroes only by room was affecting the Hospital's occupancy adversely. They believed an attempt should be made to comply with the recommendation of the Medical Staff. Therefore, on a motion with second it was voted that within the limits imposed by the physical arrangement of patient rooms and personal facilities, the Hospital will admit adult Negro patients to rooms on the extreme end of the north wing of

Division 2000 and that Negro patients and visitors will be directed to use certain specified toilets and lavatories. In complying with the foregoing policy, it was decided not to designate any area by sign reading "White" or "Colored." (December 30, 1953)

The Director reported on the conference which he and Mr. L. Richardson Preyer, Vice Chairman of the Board of Trustees of L. Richardson Memorial Hospital, had held with officials of the Agricultural and Technical College to learn the College's boarding and laundry arrangements for its students. [The two hospitals served as sites for training of nursing students from A&T and provided the students with meals.] (August 25, 1954)

[The Moses Cone Memorial Hospital print shop had supplied L. Richardson materials at 30 percent lower than market price.] The Chairman noted that doing this work was in conformity with the intent frequently expressed that this Hospital was to be a "big brother" to the Richardson Hospital. One member expressed concern lest the transaction offend commercial suppliers. (October 13, 1954)

These efforts to occupy a middle ground did not go unnoticed in the community and were a source of some sensitivity to the hospital. A survey conducted by one of the textile mills of their employees revealed minor complaints about racial integration, including "the use of colored nurses to a substantial extent; likewise, admission of Negro patients on the same footing as white patients, although this is more the exception than the rule."[56] This received a prompt and somewhat defensive response from the Moses Cone's board chairman.

> Actually there is no mixing of Negro and white patients in rooms, but there are no segregated wards at present, and we try to keep the few Negro patients we have in rooms at one end of one wing. Of course, they become mixed when being served in radiology, laboratory, operating room and obstetrics and delivery rooms. This can't be helped, and is exactly the same situation existing all over the South in general hospitals which do have segregated Negro wards.[57]

Even a hospital in as strong a market position as Cone walked carefully in the middle ground, fearing the flight of white patients and their physicians to their competition.

Greensboro's First Integrated Hospital

The concealed code guiding racial divisions in Greensboro was not etched in stone. Almost as a parable that perhaps should have been heeded, a miracle had taken place in 1948. Greensboro constructed and operated a hospital that year in which all race barriers disappeared. Many recalled that period as "Greensboro's finest hour."[58] For the tragedy that bound the community together was one that held the city's very future in a paralyzing grip. Greensboro's children were dying.

The worst polio outbreak in the nation gripped the city. "After consultation with the national Foundation for Infantile Paralysis it was decided that in order to receive the best care all patients with polio should be moved *from Greensboro's five hospitals to one central area.*"[59] In early spring 1948, fourteen patients were placed in what had been the gymnasium for the Overseas Replacement Depot during World War II. By late spring the census had grown to one hundred. Volunteer fire trucks with full crews stood guard around the clock to protect the immobilized children in the combustible wood frame structure. As this facility began to burst at the seams, convalescent patients were transferred on a temporary basis to the second floor of the former newspaper building in the city.

The community needed a more permanent convalescent hospital. In August, land was donated by Guilford County for a new hospital for convalescent patients. Locally $144,000 was raised from individual contributions in two weeks. In addition, local people donated construction materials and their labor. Union workers and nonunion workers contributed more than fifty-five hundred hours,[60] and a 132-bed hospital was built in ninety days. The real miracle was not the speed with which it was erected, but that both staff and patients were fully integrated racially. Even the school classes held for the children in the facility were integrated, six years before the *Brown* decision. While the National Foundation for Infantile Paralysis had insisted on a racially integrated facility, the National Foundation was in no position to impose their will on Greensboro. Greensboro's pediatricians and community leaders had followed their own instincts in the face of the crisis and created for a short period a single community out of a starkly divided one. Once the crisis passed, however, old patterns resurfaced. Some began to object to the white and black nurses eating together, and separate eating facilities were created. A white nurse who questioned the growing segregation in the facility was dismissed.[61] In 1955, the Salk vaccine began to be administered in a field trial to fifth-graders in Greensboro, and three years later the Polio Convalescent Hospital was closed. The real miracle, a social one rather than a vaccine, had ended long before.

Battle Cry on a Golf Course

A chain of events would begin that would profoundly alter the organization of health care across the United States.

On December 7, 1955, six days after Rosa Parks' arrest for refusing to give up her bus seat to a white passenger in Montgomery, Alabama, Dr. George Simkins, Jr. decided to play golf. Dr. Simkins, who had recently returned from Meharry Dental School to set up practice in his hometown, didn't have office hours that Wednesday afternoon. He corralled five old high school buddies and set out to play golf on the Gillespie Park Golf Course. A black golf course had been planned for Greensboro, but the area allocated next to the town's sewage treatment plant had remained an overgrown patch of weeds. The Gillespie golf course was owned by the City of Greensboro and leased to a private group for $1 a year. Without requesting permission, the six plunked down their greens fees on the counter and proceeded to tee off. Blacks did not play at Gillespie. Their game was interrupted. Dr. Simkins recalled the experience this way:

> We got to about the fifth or sixth hole and the pro came out. He wasn't there at the time we had stopped by the clubhouse. He called us everything under the sun and told us we better get off or something bad was going to happen to us. I had to keep a club in my hand for protection. He said, "Why are you out here?" I said, "I'm out here for a cause." "What kind of G damn cause?" he asked. *"The cause of Democracy!"* I answered. That statement made him all red and he was just mad. This fellow was cursing and cursing. Two deputy sheriffs finally came out. We told them we were not going to curse, we were not going to be violent, and all we want to do is play golf. This is a city-owned golf course, we're taxpayers and we have the right to play just like everybody else. It wasn't calculated, we just had said, lets go out and do it.
>
> That night the black police came and arrested us and took us to jail. My father came down and posted our bond. The city judge told us, now if you all will just drop this case he would just give us a light fine and that's it. I said, "No we intend to go all the way to the Supreme Court on this case, so you can do whatever you want to." So he fined us $15 and, of course, we appealed it.
>
> We had a judge from down East that was real anti. He said, "If you had come out on my place I would have probably got my shotgun. I'm going to give you all thirty days in jail. Take them away, Sheriff." He gave me hell for playing with guys who didn't have the same educational level as mine. One was a chauffeur, one was cab driver, one was a barber and so forth. He was trying to divide us.

In the meantime we had gone into federal court and gotten a declaratory judgement under Judge Johnson J. Hayes, who said that we had a right as taxpayers to do what we did. Anybody who fights for this country and pays taxes should have the right to use the city's recreational facilities. He gave them two or three weeks to integrate . . . Two days before integration was supposed to take effect, the club-house mysteriously burned down. The Fire Marshall went out and condemned the whole golf course. It stayed condemned for seven years. Of course that denied access to the white golfers, so nobody could play and that made them mad too. Finally after seven years it was opened on an integrated basis.

Simkins was not a member of the local NAACP at the time of the Golf Course Incident. The act, unlike that of Rosa Parks a few days earlier in Montgomery or the Lunch Counter sit-in in Greensboro's Woolworth in 1960, was not a carefully orchestrated effort to test Jim Crow practices. Simkins just wanted to play golf. Yet, it may well have had a much more jarring effect on the white middle class of Greensboro. They didn't ride public buses or eat at the Woolworth's lunch counter, but they did play golf. Now they couldn't play golf on the municipal course for seven years. When Simkins started something, he didn't stop. He soon joined the local NAACP, became its president and pushed hard. To most whites, during this period Simkins was just another "troublemaker." Increasingly, he won grudging admiration. "George and his group pushed all the time and you couldn't help admiring him . . . He just went ahead and did things that he thought he was entitled to."[62] This led him to Jack Greenberg and Thurgood Marshall at the NAACP Legal Defense Fund in New York. In retrospect, there would seem to be an almost inevitable logic to what would happen next.

In his autobiography, Jack Greenberg tried to explain why the Legal Defense Fund, whose image was that of a battler for the rights of the oppressed underclass, had devoted efforts to fighting for golf privileges for middle-class professionals.

Puzzling over why we had so many golf course cases in which plaintiffs were black dentists. Indeed the number of dentist-plaintiffs was disproportionately large. Black professionals wanted to play golf, like their white counterparts. They were different from later militant leaders whose goal was radical economic reconstruction. Some said dentists were socially active in order to gain status vis-à-vis doctors; others explained that their schedules were controllable and so they could set aside time for civil rights activities.

We debated whether to put resources into such cases, and decided we should. Dentists had rights too, every defeat of segregation contributed to its ultimate destruction, and last, but not least, these middle-class professionals were then the mainstay of the civil rights movement. Moreover, lots of people played golf, not just dentists and doctors.[63]

Some of this ambivalence is reflected in the correspondence between the Legal Defense Fund lawyers and Simkins. A letter from Thurgood Marshall to Simkins in August, 1958, admits to "searching our 'souls' as well as the law on this case and have reached the conclusion that we will be responsible for the costs of the record and brief on appeal providing that it is kept within reason. . . . One other point, you remember you assured me that you and the others involved were not financially able to carry these expenses."[64] A letter later in September, 1958, from Greenberg apologizes for the delay in getting back to him on the Golf Course case "because we have been quite tied up in some litigation involving Little Rock."[65]

The Gillispie Park Golf Course case, however, clearly paralleled the subsequent hospital desegregation case. The nine-hole golf course had originally been constructed in 1940 with federal WPA funds. Pressures from black citizens had eventually grudgingly committed City Council to half-heartedly build a Negro golf course, next to the sewage treatment plant. The legal and the personal issues, from Simkins' perspective, were the same.

The *Simkins* Hospital Case

A young student from A&T had come to Dr. George Simkins for dental care. His effort to treat that patient would lead from the examining room to Greensboro's hospitals, to the federal courts, and then to a chain reaction of events that would explode across the nation. Dr. Simkins reflected on his part of that story.

> A patient came into my office, a young A&T student. His jaw was swollen with an abscessed third molar. He had a temperature of 103. I said, "Young man, you need to be hospitalized." The hospital [L. Richardson] was one block from my office. I called up there to get him a room. They said, "I'm sorry, doc, we've got a waiting list of two or three weeks before you can get a bed." They actually had patients in the hallways. You had to walk a narrow path through the corridors because the patient beds were in the hallways. I called Moses Cone, and they had rooms over there, but they wouldn't take him. I called Wesley Long and the same thing. Then I called Jack Greenberg, who

had taken Thurgood Marshall's place. I said, "We got to really do something about these hospitals down here. It's a disgrace, a person could be dying." He said, "George, if you can get the black doctors organized and do some research and find out how much Hill-Burton funds have gone into building those hospitals, I'll take the case." I got busy and I got these young doctors I knew I could get signed on to be plaintiffs. When the older doctors saw the names, some of them signed and some of them didn't sign. I got each of them to put up fifty bucks for attorney fees. I worked the case up and found that both hospitals had been built with Hill-Burton funds. Then I gave it all to a local lawyer, but he would never file the case. I finally called Jack Greenberg. I said, "Jack, I think we've got a scared lawyer on our hands. This lawyer won't file the case." He said, "George, don't worry about it, I'll take care of it." He called a fellow named Conrad Pearson—he was a lawyer that worked with the NAACP in Durham—and said, "Conrad, you need to go over to Greensboro to file this case for us." The case was filed in the next two days.

We lost the case in Middle District Court. Judge Stanley ruled against us. In the meantime, Bobby Kennedy was then attorney general, and he intervened with a brief as a friend of the court. We appealed to the Fourth Circuit Court of Appeals in Asheville. Michael Meltsner from the NAACP handled the appeal and we won a three-to-two decision. The hospitals then appealed it to the Supreme Court, but the Supreme Court refused to hear the case.[66]

Some of the facts in the court case illustrate its legal significance. Moses Cone Memorial Hospital had received $1,269,950 in federal Hill-Burton funds for two projects (for its initial construction and then for an expansion and diagnostic and treatment center in 1960), or about 17.2 percent of the total cost of these projects; Long Hospital had received $1,948,800 in Hill-Burton funds for two projects (construction of their new hospital in 1959 and then for a laundry and hospital nurse training school in 1961), amounting to 49.6 percent of the total construction costs. As in case brought by Hubert Eaton over staff privileges, the case hinged on proving that the actions by the hospitals were state actions and thus bound by the Fifth and Fourteenth Amendments. In the Eaton case, James A. Walker Memorial Hospital had received no funding from the Hill-Burton program, while both Cone and Long had received substantial financial assistance. Moses Cone, in addition, had six publicly appointed board members and participated in a nurse-training program with two state-operated colleges.

Nevertheless, the intervention by Attorney General Robert F. Kennedy in U.S. District Court came as a surprise to both parties. The hospital attorneys were stunned. In objecting to the Justice Department's motion to intervene, they observed,

> The intervention sought by the United States in this case is apparently without precedent. The defendants have not been able to find any case in which the attorney general of the United States has ever sought to intervene in order to attack—rather than to defend—the constitutionality of an act of Congress; and the attorney general— through his representatives at the hearing before this court on May 14, 1962—conceded that he had also not found any such case. . . . That even if the action of the attorney general in this case does not directly flout congressional mandate, it is certainly calculated to disappoint congressional expectation; and that is clearly contrary to the purpose of and the tradition under Section 2403.[67]

The attorney general had his own interest in *Simkins.* He hoped to use it to break the pervasive gridlock of executive actions to prevent discrimination in the use of federal funds. His brief traced the court rulings from *Plessy* to *Brown* and to the current case. Attached to the brief was an affidavit from Alanson Wilcox, then serving as general counsel of the Department of Health, Education and Welfare. He had previously served as general counsel of the American Hospital Association, and before that as general counsel of the Federal Security Agency (predecessor to DHEW), where he assisted as technical draftsman for the Hill-Burton Act. His statement argued that voluntary hospitals functioned identically to public ones insofar as the Hill-Burton program was concerned.

Cone Memorial and Long Hospital proved worthy adversaries. They had their own network of support and substantial financial resources to protect what they defined as their interests. Cone Hospital, in particular, was well connected. Its administrator had received a copy of the Eaton decision in an envelope marked "personal and confidential" sent to him by the administrator at James A. Walker Memorial Hospital in April 1960.[68] Their lawyers had explored the possibility of the American Medical Association's filing an amicus curiae brief in their application for a writ of certiorari and with the American Hospital Association. The AMA had declined, apparently on technical grounds. Correspondence was also exchanged with the lawyers representing Grady Hospital in Atlanta in November 1963. As a public hospital Grady lacked the ability to argue the fine points of state action. Grady's lawyer reported to Moses Cone's:

We are attempting to argue that the hospital was unsegregated except insofar as sound medical practice dictates that the same should be segregated. In other words, we are trying to take the position that the primary concern of this institution is the treatment of the sick people and that segregation in a public facility such as our Hospital can be justified on the basis of sound medical practice. Frankly, we have serious doubt as to the validity of our position in view of more recent decisions of the Appellate Courts, but we, nevertheless, are trying to maintain this position.[69]

Falk, Carruthers and Roth, a respected Greensboro legal firm, present at all the meetings of Moses Cone's board since its inception, represented the defendants. "They gave it the works. We made a scrap out of it," reflected one of the hospital administrators at the time of the suit about their legal representation.[70] The overall legal fee for Moses Cone was more than thirteen thousand dollars, small by current standards, but large enough as an unbudgeted expense to create discomfort for the board chairman.

On March 2, 1964, however, the Supreme Court declined to review the U.S. Court of Appeals for the Fourth Circuit decision in the *Simkins* case. A disappointed Charles Roth, the lawyer handling the case for Cone Hospital, noted in a statement for the press, "The denial of certiorari represent the end of the line, and the hospital will naturally comply with the orders of the Court when issued." (The hospital had already "voluntarily" extended staff privileges to some of the plaintiffs.) The executive committee of Moses Cone Hospital, however, was not ready to submit meekly to federal interference. At a special executive committee meeting at Cone Hospital on March 11, 1964, the members unanimously passed the following resolution that the

President call a meeting of the Board of Trustees on Sunday, March 15, 1964 at 3 PM at the Hospital to consider a proposal that the Hospital return to the proper agency of the United States government or the State of North Carolina, all money received under the Hill-Burton Act, together with interest and thereby be relieved of any obligation under the orders of the Court entered as a result of the Hospital having received Hill-Burton funds.[71]

However, cooler heads and a more careful assessment of the hospital's options prevailed at the Sunday board meeting. The full board simply voted to continue existing policies until the official order was received from the federal court.

The Legal Defense Fund was predictably jubilant. "It will be an entering wedge for Negro physicians into mainstream medical practice in the South. We wait to see whether the medical profession will voluntarily follow the law or whether a long hard process of litigation such as we have had with schools will be necessary," Greenberg noted.[72] Asked for comment by the *Medical World News* on the earlier appeals court decision, Greenberg had said, "In principle it was as far-reaching in the medical field as the 1954 school desegregation was in its field." The *News* had added, "Most Washington observers share this view. But many of them feel that the effect on southern hospitals will be gradual not sudden. Hospital desegregation, like school desegregation, may have to be fought out case by case."[73]

In the meantime, something in the subsequent coverage in the *New York Times* had caught the eye of the attorney for Moses Cone Hospital.

[T]he high court's announcement was made while the whole issue that was partly involved in the lower court decision was pending in the Administration's equal rights bill on which the Senate had not even begun debate. Hence the effect of the Supreme Court's refusal to review that decision was to validate as mandatory under the constitution, a hotly disputed section of this legislation in advance of congressional action.

The usual procedure of the Supreme Court is to await the enactment of a legislative draft into law before passing on its constitutionality. In this instance it was known to all concerned—including the Court, which also reads the newspapers—that Senate opponents of this particular section (Title VI of the equal rights bill) were preparing a last ditch effort to legislate the exemptions which were outlawed in the lower court decision it allowed to stand. This being so and in view of the additional fact that the Supreme Court can indefinitely postpone announcing when it will review a lower court decision, it must be concluded that the Court was fully aware that its timing in the case would cut the ground away from the effort in the Senate to maintain in Title VI the exemptions authorized in the Hill Burton Act. . . . In sum, the Court departed from the usual by ruling, not that a statute passed by Congress was unconstitutional, but that a proposal about to be taken up would be if legislated."[74]

To a copy of the article sent to Cone's administrator, the hospital's lawyer, Charles Roth, had penned, "Harold, this helps explain why we got such prompt 'service' from the Supreme Court."[75] The Greensboro battle was coming to an end, but a new one on a national scale was just beginning.

CHAPTER 4

The Federal Offensive

> Simple justice requires that public funds, to which all taxpayers of all races contribute, not be spent in any fashion which encourages, entrenches, subsidizes or results in racial discrimination. Direct discrimination by Federal, State or local governments is prohibited by the Constitution. But indirect discrimination through the use of Federal funds, is just as invidious; and it should not be necessary to resort to the courts to prevent each individual violation.[1]

Title VI of his proposed civil rights legislation, President Kennedy argued, was not a heavy club. It simply clarified the authority of those who administered federal funds. This cautiously worded section of his message to Congress on June 19, 1963, arrived almost thirteen months after his telegram to Montague Cobb reporting the Justice Department's intervention in the *Simkins* case. The government's argument in *Simkins* was now embedded in Title VI of the proposed legislation. The subsequent journey of the *Simkins* case through the federal courts would shadow the journey of Kennedy's civil rights bill through Congress.

However cautiously worded the message, Kennedy's proposed legislation now swept him into a current that all his political instincts had resisted. He had barely squeaked out a victory in 1960, winning just 49.7 percent of the popular vote to Nixon's 49.5 percent.[2] Blacks had supported Kennedy with 78 percent of their vote. Without the black vote, Kennedy's fortunes would have been reversed: Nixon would have won 52 percent of the popular vote, carried Illinois and Michigan, and been elected president. The fragility of the Democratic coalition that had provided the slim margin of victory in the presidential election would almost guarantee a stinging defeat to Kennedy's proposed civil rights bill in Congress.

The legislative process has been crafted almost deliberately to guarantee the defeat of such legislation. Franklin D. Roosevelt, despite his landslide victories, had been unwilling to push even an antilynching bill for fear that retaliation by southern legislators would block all other legislative initiatives. The House committees operated as private fiefdoms, dominated by elderly chairmen protective of the seniority system. The powerful House Rules Committee could, in the event a bill cleared the other committees, prevent legislation from being considered on the House floor. Any civil rights legislation escaping the House would then face the Senate, where thirty-four of its one hundred members could talk it to death. Compromises to escape a filibuster would simply water down the bill to the point that it was meaningless, as such legislative efforts in 1957 and 1960 had shown. Southern Democrats in both houses earned their long tenure and powerful committee posts by the intransigence and skill they could display to their constituents in thwarting such legislation.

On the other side of the aisle, the Republicans lay in ambush. The last thing the Republican legislators wanted was for Kennedy to get credit for civil rights legislation. An election year was coming up. Both parties had strong civil rights planks in 1960, competing for the high moral ground on the race issue. Kennedy had failed to take the legislative action promised by his party's platform. The Republicans in Congress let the liberals in their party take the lead on the assumption that a strong bill would split the Democratic party. The conventional wisdom said that the southern and northern Democrats would devour each other, the Republicans would emerge as the majority party from this process, and Kennedy would go down to defeat in 1964.

The conventional wisdom, however, proved worthless. The House, the Senate, and the executive branch had little control over the real agenda. They were swept by more powerful currents into uncharted waters. The bus boycotts, the freedom rides, the sit-ins, all brought a rising tide that would not wait and could not be turned back. The rats, the violent segregationist elements that the ruling elite (according to the implicit accommodationist compromise) were supposed to rein in, had been flushed out of their holes. All thrashed and swirled together in the currents of the flood tide.

By 1963 the currents had become rapids, and then, over a precipice, the free fall began. In May 1963 Birmingham's Bull Connor turned high-pressure fire hoses and police dogs on children who were demonstrating against segregated facilities in downtown Birmingham. The children filled the jails and flooded the national news with images that stunned the nation. The marchers would not turn back. On June 11, Governor George Wallace stood in the doorway of the enrollment office of the University of Alabama, physically barring two black students. In a carefully choreographed performance, the National Guard was federalized and the two students enrolled. In a nationally televised address that same evening, Kennedy proposed his long delayed civil rights bill. Later that same evening, as if in response to the address, an assassin waited in the honey-suckle bushes across the street from the home of Medgar Evers, NAACP field secretary in Jackson, Mississippi. Medgar Evers was shot in the back with a deer rifle and died several hours later. On August 28, a nervous Kennedy administration played host to more than two hundred thousand assembled in front of the Lincoln Memorial in support of the civil rights legislation. Martin Luther King's "I Have a Dream" speech appeared close to cementing a new national consensus. Two weeks later, on September 15, a bomb at Birmingham's Sixteenth Street Baptist Church, where the protest marches had been organized, killed four young girls during Sunday school services. On November 22, John Kennedy, on a trip to mend badly damaged political fences in preparation for a difficult reelection campaign in 1964, was assassinated in Dallas, Texas. The free fall continued.

The Civil Rights Legislation

Kennedy's bill began its long, painful legislative journey in the chandeliered, high-ceilinged hearing room of the House Judiciary Committee on June 22, 1963. Seated at the horseshoe-shaped mahogany hearing table on its raised marble dais, the eleven congressmen of Subcommittee No. 5 began to shape the legislation. The pace and atmosphere of their deliberations belied the turmoil that swirled outside the room. In more than one hundred communities across the South and in bordering states demonstrations, riots, and white extremist reprisals, along with tense negotiations and some initial steps at the integration of public accommodations, were taking place.[3] Even the American Medical Association, meeting in Atlantic City that June, was picketed by physicians from the Medical Committee for Human Rights and felt it necessary to respond defensively to the challenge.[4] The hearings themselves lasted twenty-three days. The subcommittee called 101 witnesses, and their testimony filled 2,649 pages. The American Public Health Association and the American Nurse's Association, supporters since the mid-1950s of such legislation, were represented at the hearings. Other health trade and professional associations were absent.

In his own testimony to the subcommittee, Anthony Celebrezze, secretary of the Department of Health, Education and Welfare, struggled to explain the predicament faced by his department in withholding funds and the need for Title VI.

This title is of particular importance to the DHEW as administrator of over 100 separate programs—actually 128 programs—most of which involve allocations or grants to States and payments to individuals and institutions. By far the largest part of our operating budget goes to these payments. In 1963 such payments amounted to 3.7 billion. . . . In many of the formula grant programs, the Department is required to operate under conditions rigidly prescribed by statute; in other programs, the Department has great flexibility in determining who shall receive funds, in what amounts and under what conditions.[5]

According to the secretary, DHEW's authority to withhold funds for racial discrimination usually remained unclear. Celebrezze specifically mentioned the *Simkins* case. "The United States has intervened in a Federal court action, contending that the separate but equal provision of the Hill-Burton Hospital Construction Act is unconstitutional. This case is now pending in the Fourth Circuit Court of Appeals."[6]

After the Labor Day recess Subcommittee No. 5 began the final drafting or markup of the bill. A far stronger bill than the Kennedy administration had envisioned emerged from the subcommittee. Judiciary chairman Emanuel Celler apparently had planned to use its provisions as bargaining chips with the southern opposition. Although the Leadership Conference on Civil Rights was elated, the Kennedy administration was disgusted with the result and with Celler's failure to rein in the liberals on the subcommittee. The Republicans on the full committee happily stood by to let the administration do the dirty work and get the blame for watering down the bill. On October 15 and 16, Robert Kennedy, flanked by Burke Marshall and Nicholas Katzenbach from the Justice Department, testified before the full House Judiciary Committee, informing the press outside, "I want a bill and not an issue."[7] The liberals, however, seemed satisfied just to stake out an issue. On the other side, the southern Democrats were delighted to see a strong bill emerge from committee, as it was certain to be defeated by full vote in the House or Senate. A compromise bill, still much stronger than the initial one, was eventually thrashed out between the Republican leadership and the administration. Now, however, it would potentially die in the House Rules Committee.

Yet, the momentum was growing. Deputy Attorney General Katzenbach could report in materials requested and submitted after the last hearing, "The U.S. Court of Appeals of the Fourth Circuit has recently held the 'separate but equal' provisions of the Hill-Burton Act unconstitutional. *Simkins v. Moses Cone Memorial Hospital* was decided November 1, 1963. Title VI would override all such 'separate but equal' provisions without the need for further litigation and would give, to the Federal agencies administering laws which contain such provisions, a clear directive to take action to effectuate the provisions of Title VI."[8] On November 18 the bill was sent to the Rules Committee, whose archconservative chair was Howard Smith. The fate of the fragile bipartisan alliance hung by a thread. On November 22 an assassin's bullet in Dallas ended the life of the president.

At a joint session of Congress on November 27, in the stunned atmosphere five days after the assassination of President Kennedy, President Johnson pledged, ... "no memorial oration or eulogy could more eloquently honor President Kennedy's memory than the earliest possible passage of the civil rights bill for which he fought so long. We have talked long enough in this country about equal rights. We have talked for one hundred years or more. It is time now to write the next chapter, and to write it in the books of law."[9] Johnson added his own hands-on, flesh-pressing style of persuasion to the newly defined cause of a martyred president. The bill would serve both as a memorial to the slain president and as redemption for the southern politician who now occupied his office. The alliance with the House Republicans held together; the bill was forced out of the Rules Committee and onto the floor.

The brief floor debate in the House is most noteworthy for what was perhaps one of the most unintended consequences in legislative history. Howard Smith offered an amendment on the floor of the House inserting *sex* on various pages, thus adding gender to the list of discriminations prohibited (race, creed, color, and national origin) in the equal employment (Title VII) section of the bill. Rather than undermining the passage of the bill by making it too controversial, as was his intent, he thus effectively and significantly widened its political base of support.[10] A bipartisan group of five congresswomen embraced the amendment. Nothing would ever be quite the same again. The bill, essentially unchanged except for Smith's addition of the word *sex,* passed the House on a vote of 290 to 130 on February 10, 1964.

An epic confrontation now awaited the civil rights bill in the Senate. Compromise with the southern Democrats in the Senate had essentially been ruled out by the understanding with House Republican supporters that the bill would not be watered down and by Johnson's own awkward position. He could not, as the new president and as a southerner, appear to be gutting the slain president's civil rights bill. The only alternative was to force the two-thirds vote necessary for cloture to end debate and pass the House bill untouched.

Johnson used his own unique knowledge of the Senate and its members to needle people into action. The Johnson "treatment" combined that knowledge with threat and flattery. On the eve of the bill's introduction on the floor, the new president told Majority Whip Hubert Humphrey, "You have got this opportunity now, Hubert, but you liberals will never deliver.

You don't know the rules of the Senate, and you liberals will be off making speeches when you ought to be present in the Senate. I know you've
got a great opportunity here, but I'm afraid it's going by the boards."[11]
That may have done the trick.

On February 26, by a majority vote, the bill was placed directly on the
agenda of the Senate, bypassing referral to the southern-dominated Senate
Judiciary Committee. On Monday, March 9, consideration of the bill and
the Senate filibuster began.

A significant intervening event, the March 2 decision by the Supreme
Court refusing to review the *Simkins v. Cone* case and allowing the Fourth
Circuit Court of Appeals decision to stand, did not go unnoticed in the
Senate. On March 3, Senator Jacob Javits noted on the floor of the Senate,
"Mr. President, yesterday's decision by the U.S. Supreme Court refusing
to review the Hill-Burton anti-segregation ruling of the Fourth Circuit
Court of Appeals was a most welcome development for me. For many
years I have sought to eliminate from the Hill-Burton Hospital Construction Act this lingering vestige in Federal law of the long-discredited separate-but-equal doctrine."[12] Senator Javits then went on to insert into the
Congressional Record his correspondence with Secretary Celebrezze on
April 23, 1963, and his delayed response on February 11, 1964. Celebrezze
noted in that response, "If pending litigation results in a final court decision that the separate-but-equal provision of the Hill-Burton legislation is
unconstitutional, regulations will be changed to preclude grants for the
construction of separate-but-equal facilities. On the basis of the decision
of the court of appeals in *Simkins v. Cone* which is now on appeal, no
applications for the construction of separate-but-equal facilities are being
processed."[13] Senator Kenneth Keating from New York went on to add
his comments about the decision and to request the insertion of the *New
York Times* coverage of the decision into the *Congressional Record.*

Thus the initiation of Senate debate on the Civil Rights Act was recast
in the light of the *Simkins* decision. The provisions of Title VI could no
longer be dismissed as mere radical posturing, as they had been when they
were first introduced by Harlem congressman Adam Clayton Powell in
1946 and regularly reintroduced by him as amendments to subsequent
appropriations bills. The bill could no longer be dismissed as the calculated baiting of the fragile Democratic coalition by northern Republican
liberal legislators. It now had on it the official seal of the Supreme Court
and the Constitution.

During the filibuster southern senators tried to portray Title VI as a
sinister federal executive power grab. Now, in the wake of the court's decision in the *Simkins* case, that rhetoric had a hollow ring to it. Now Title VI
could in reality be portrayed as little more than dotting the *i*s and crossing

the *t*s in what the court had determined was the law of the land. While the rhetoric now seemed out of context, the southern filibuster still sought to ignite the broader fires of opposition.

Senator Gore of Tennessee, for example, argued,

> In my view, the power conferred in this bill could be used oppressively. If an administration is inclined to so use it, Title VI could be a sledge hammer provision. Federal aid permeates our whole system. We have already had an example in the State of Louisiana when aid was ordered cut off to the entire State. This is a hard-hearted, cold policy. It punishes innocent people for the commission of alleged wrongs over which they have no control. This is a power that the legislative branch should not vest in the executive branch without knowing just how and under what conditions it would be applied.[14]

Senator Sparkman of Alabama added his voice to the effort to ignite fears of an oppressive federal government:

> Mr. President, my opposition to Title VI grows from two firm convictions that I have, one about people, the other about government.
>
> I have always felt that in our Nation people are the most important element in our way of life. By the same token, I feel that government should be the servant, not the master of the people.
>
> Title VI tends towards placing people in the position of pawns in a massive life-size chess game with the government in control of the chess moves, sacrificing the pawns for the sake of political expediency.
>
> States attempting to protect their rights would have their people sacrificed by depriving them of the benefits of Federal programs.
>
> This terrifying possibility causes me to attack title VI with considerable relish."[15]

During the debate, proponents of the Civil Rights Act repeatedly referred to the *Simkins* decision in justifying the need for Title VI. Senator Humphrey, the majority whip, observed on one of the first days of the debate,

> If anyone can be against that, [Title VI] he can be against Mother's Day. How can one justify discrimination in the use of Federal funds and Federal programs? President after president has announced that national policy is to end discrimination in Federal programs and Federal assistance. But regretably, there has been open violation of these policies.

. . . Under the Hill-Burton Act, Federal grants are made to hospitals which admit whites only or Negroes only. The Civil Rights Commission, in its 1963 report reported that between 1946 and December 31, 1962, Federal grants totaling $36,755,994 were made to 89 racially segregated medical facilities. Of this a very small proportion— $4,080,308 and 13 projects—was for projects which admitted Negroes only; the rest had a "white only" label. One consequence of these Federal policies—which in this instance are required by Act of Congress—was stated by the U.S. Court of Appeals for the Fourth Circuit in a recent opinion:

Racial discrimination in medical facilities is at least partly responsible for the fact that in North Carolina the rate of infant mortality (for Negroes) is twice the rate for whites and maternal deaths are five times greater (*Simkins v. Moses H. Cone Memorial Hospital,* 323 F 2d. 959, 970 n. 23 [1963]). . . . Some federal statutes appear to contemplate grants to racially segregated institutions. . . . In each of these laws Congress expressed its basic intention to prohibit racial discrimination in obtaining the benefits of Federal funds. But in line with constitutional doctrines current when these laws were passed, it authorized the provision of "separate but equal facilities." It may be that all of these statutory provisions are unconstitutional and separable, as the Court of Appeals for the Fourth Circuit has recently held in a case under the Hill-Burton Act. (*Simkins v. Moses H. Cone Memorial Hospital,* 323 F. 2d 957 [C.A. 4, 1963] Certiorari denied, March 2, 1964). But it is clearly desirable for Congress to wipe them off the books without waiting for further judicial action.

. . . In all cases, such discrimination is contrary to national policy, and to the moral sense of the nation. Thus Title VI is simply designed to insure that Federal funds are spent in accordance with the Constitution and the moral sense of the nation.[16]

Senator Pastore of Rhode Island was also quick to site *Simkins* as a justification for Title VI.

Mr. President, why is Title VI necessary to the civil rights bill H.R. 7152? Let me explain. In the community of Greensboro, North Carolina, there are two excellent hospitals. They are numbered among the most modern in the area. This is due, in part, to Federal financial assistance. Under the Hill-Burton Act, one of these hospitals received $1,300,000 in Federal aid. That took care of over 17% of its construction costs. The other hospital accepted nearly $2 million from the Federal Government. This satisfied half the cost of its construction. They are two very good hospitals. But there is one thing wrong with both of them: The doors of these two hospitals would not open to a large segment of the Greensboro community. Their modern medical care was denied to those whose skin was colored—denied strictly and solely on the basis of the color of the patient's skin. The Federal funds that helped build these hospitals were raised, of course, by taxation— taxes paid by both white and Negro citizens. But the Negro in need of care could not get it at these hospitals simply because he was a Negro.

It was natural that such a flagrant case should be litigated in our courts. A month ago, on March 2, 1964, the Supreme Court, across the street, terminated this specific case of discrimination. The lower court, The Court of Appeals for the Fourth Circuit, had decided that the two hospitals involved could no longer decline to treat patients or refuse to admit doctors to their staffs strictly for racial reasons. . . .

The Supreme Court declined to review that decision; so it is the law of our land. Yet despite the effort of the Court of Appeals to strike down discrimination in the *Simkins* case, the same court was forced last week to rule again in a Wilmington, N.C., suit that a private hospital operated with public funds must desist from barring Negro physicians from staff membership.

That is why we need title VI of the Civil Rights Act, H.R. 7152—to prevent such discrimination where Federal funds are involved.

Title VI intends to insure once and for all that the financial resources of the Federal Government—the commonwealth of Negro and white alike—will no longer subsidize racial discrimination.[17]

Senator Pastore went on to summarize the intent of Title VI, making what was perhaps the most passionate argument in support of Title VI on the Senate floor.

Title VI is sound; it is morally right; it is legally right; it is constitutionally right. What will it accomplish? It will guarantee that the money collected by color-blind tax collectors will be distributed by Federal and State administrators who are equally color-blind. . . .

We all realize that segregation is a caste system imposing an inferior status on the Negro citizen from cradle to grave; but are we are also aware that Uncle Sam is a partner in the erection, maintenance and perpetuation of that system: The toll of "separate and most unequal" begins with birth of the Negro in a segregated hospital constructed with Federal funds.[18]

Titlc VI closes the gap between our purposes as a democracy and our prejudices as individuals. The cuts of prejudice need healing. The costs of prejudice need understanding. We cannot have hostility between two great parts of our people without tragic loss in our human values—without deep damage to our national decency and dignity—without threat to our manifest destiny in a world we have to accept for what it is—a world which has to accept us for what we are or aim to be.

Title VI offers a place for the meeting of our minds as to Federal money. It can recognize no prejudice. It affords a place for the meeting of our hearts, as prejudice must yield to our common purposes, our common progress and the common perfection of these United States.[19]

Finally, the longest debate in the Senate's history, more than 534 hours, was officially over. Senator Everett Dirksen, Republican minority leader, stood up and, paraphrasing the words of Victor Hugo, affirmed, "Stronger than all the armies is an idea whose time has come. The time has come for equality of opportunity in sharing in government, in education and in employment. It must not be stayed or denied." At 11:00 A.M. on June 10, the roll call vote for cloture began. California senator Claire Englc, terminally ill and in the advanced stages of cancer, was wheeled in on a stretcher for the critical vote. Unable to speak, he feebly lifted his finger to his eye. "I guess that means aye," murmured the clerk. Many of those on the Senate floor were in tears as the vote was recorded. The final vote was seventy-one to twenty-nine, far more than the required two-thirds.[20]

The Republican leadership in Congress—McCulloch and Halleck in the House, Everett Dirksen in the Senate, and a substantial majority of Republicans in both houses—supported the bill and assured its final victory. This should have bolstered a pro–civil rights image of the Republicans. That effect was mitigated, however, by Arizona Senator Barry Goldwater's opposition. Goldwater had been assured the Republican presidential nomination after primary victories that spring and argued that the bill "will require the creation of a federal police force of mammoth proportions. . . . These, the Federal police force and an 'informer' psychology, are the hallmarks of the police state and the landmarks in the destruction of a free society."[21] The debate was not over.

The Civil Rights Act of 1964 was signed in the East Room of the White House on July 2, 1964. Seven months before, John Kennedy had lain in state in the same room. Most of the leaders of the civil rights movement and the Republican and Democratic leadership in Congress were present. In front of the TV cameras at the desk, Johnson spoke slowly and briefly about the bill before signing it.

> Its purpose is not to punish. Its purpose is not to divide, but to end divisions—divisions which have lasted too long. Its purpose is national, not regional. Its purpose is to promote a more abiding commitment to freedom, a more constant pursuit of justice, and a deeper respect for human dignity. We will achieve these goals because most Americans are law-abiding citizens and want to do what is right.[22]

The Death of "Separate but Equal" in Hill-Burton

Even before the passage of the civil rights legislation of 1964, the Hill-Burton program changes stimulated by the *Simkins* decision had been put into operation. This involved a minor shock to the nation's hospital system and to the Public Health Service program. No new requests for racially separate facilities would be considered for funding by the Hill-Burton program. On March 9, 1964, appearing before the House Committee on Interstate and Foreign Commerce (which was considering a bill to amend the Hill-Burton Hospital Construction Act), Anthony Celebrezze, secretary of DHEW, referred to the Supreme Court's refusal to review the *Simkins* decision on March 2.

> Following last week's action by the Supreme Court, I have directed that the following additional steps be taken:
>
> 1. That we make permanent the earlier decision to approve no new applications under the "separate but equal provision" of the law;
> 2. That we require a nondiscrimination assurance in admittance from those pending projects approved on a "separate but equal" basis;
> 3. That we seek from all pending projects an assurance that there will be no discrimination on the basis of race, creed, or color in granting staff privileges; and
> 4. That the application forms to be used hereafter be amended to require of all applicants whose application has not been finally approved, a nondiscrimination assurance covering staff privileges and admissions, and that all portions and services of the facilities be made available without discrimination on account of race, creed or color.

> Finally, Mr. Chairman, consideration is being given to calling a meeting of the leaders in organized medicine in the hospital and other

appropriate fields, with the view toward implementing a program for voluntary compliance with these policies. I would hope that such a voluntary program would encompass not only Hill-Burton facilities but all hospitals in the United States.

Our urgent responsibility is to assure adequate health care to all Americans. I would think that none would deny that consideration of race or color has no place with regard to the ailing body or the healing hand. I believe that we have an opportunity to demonstrate a constructive and positive approach to assuring equal opportunity in this important area of health care that has wide significance in these changing times.[23]

The revised Hill-Burton regulations, citing the *Simkins v. Moses Cone Hospital* decision, appeared in the *Federal Register* on May 19, 1964. On August 18, 1964, President Johnson signed into law H.R 10041, an act extending Hill-Burton for five more years with the "separate-but-equal" clause eliminated and authorizing 1.36 billion dollars in additional expenditures over this period. Montague Cobb, serving as president of the National Medical Association, attended the signing ceremony.

More satisfying vindication for Dr. Cobb, however, had come earlier on July 27, 1964, at the final Imhotep conference. This time the hosts were DHEW and the White House. This time *all* of the top executives of the six key national organizations were present—the American Hospital Association, the American Medical Association, the National Medical Association, the American Dental Association, the National Dental Association, and the American Nursing Association. Although hosted by DHEW, everyone knew that this was a White House conference. All were expecting the president himself to appear to greet the assembled health care dignitaries. In walked Mr. Hobart Taylor, associate special counsel to the president. With a disarming smile, he stated that he was there at the request of the president to extend on his behalf greetings to the assembled group and the president's hope that all would cooperate in what would be explained to them. A black man was the president's representative: though his words were innocuous, his presence sent a message to the group.[24] Celebrezze in his own message graciously thanked the group for coming to discuss ways to eliminate racial discrimination in hospitals.

This is a job that must be done, a job that we in the Government cannot do alone, and a job for which I hope you will let us have your help. I hope that, before this day is out, you who represent the major health professions of the Nation, in cooperation with persons who represent this Department and its Public Health Service, will have had a fruitful exploration of ways for moving affirmatively toward that end. You are engaged in an important task and I wish you well.[25]

Embedding Title VI in DHEW

James Quigley, assistant secretary of Health, Education and Welfare, now faced the complex task of implementing Title VI of the Civil Rights Act. DHEW had grown rapidly since its inception in 1953, largely as a conduit of funds for constituencies. These constituencies included of course the individuals or groups represented by the senators and representatives, but also, increasingly, the organizations affected by or related to DHEW and its programs. The health-related constituencies included hospitals, medical schools, state and local health departments, allied health-training programs, research institutes, and their corresponding professional and trade associations. The *Simkins* case and Title VI of the Civil Rights Act had altered the chemistry in the relationship between DHEW and its constituencies. A federal purpose unrelated to the immediate needs and interests of these old constituencies had now intruded. A broad-based, well-organized, local, vocal new civil rights constituency had been activated and empowered. They demanded that a new federal purpose be served. The department was now caught in the crossfire of the debate that had raged on the Senate floor.

The final rules governing DHEW regarding implementation of Title VI of the Civil Rights Act of 1964 were published in the *Federal Register* on December 4, 1964.[26] A hastily pulled together interagency task force had worked on the regulations. Since DHEW would assume the bulk of enforcement responsibilities, the DHEW model, by default, served as the standard for all twenty agencies of the federal government having Title VI responsibilities. These regulations were modeled after other federal administrative enforcement procedures and have remained essentially unchanged to the present.

For the American health care system, Title VI regulations banned discrimination in any activities that used federal funds for training, employment, or construction. Discrimination was also banned among parties who had contractual relationships with entities receiving federal funds. Every recipient of funds would be required to provide written assurance of such nondiscrimination, and the assurances had to apply to the entire institution. Specifically, "In the case of hospital construction grants the assurances will apply to patients, to interns, residents, student nurses and other professionally qualified persons to practice in the hospital in which the grant is made, and to facilities operated in connection therewith."[27] The responsible department was to seek the cooperation of recipients in obtaining compliance, as well as to provide assistance and guidance to recipients in gaining voluntary compliance. Recipients were required to complete timely and accurate compliance reports, to provide access to records to the responsible department, and to provide information to beneficiaries to make them aware of the protections provided to them against discrimination as assured by the act. *What was not resolved, as it had not been resolved in the legislation itself, was what "discrimination" was.* Beyond a general recognition that de jure racial divisions in programs and services were banned, the details were left to the program agencies. The devil, as all parties soon learned, was in the details.

The Public Health Service was authorized by these regulations to conduct investigations to determine actual compliance in the funding programs it sponsored. Such investigations could be initiated by complaints by individuals or classes of individuals who felt that they were subjected to discrimination, or the department itself could initiate an investigation based on compliance reports or any other information that came to the attention of the responsible officials. Matters could be resolved informally, but the identity of those making the complaints would be kept as confidential as possible and intimidatory or retaliatory acts against those bringing complaints was prohibited. Noncompliance that couldn't be corrected by informal means would be subjected to a formal review process. An elaborate process of administrative review was spelled out, including the opportunity for hearings before final decision by the secretary. In addition, any such action by the secretary was subject to judicial review.

At a January 28, 1965, conference held under the auspices of the United States Commission on Civil Rights and attended by four hundred leaders of organizations receiving federal funds from across the country, Vice President Hubert Humphrey noted in his keynote address that the law was on the books and "enforce it we will," but that he was willing to "walk the last mile" to secure voluntary compliance. Secretary Celebrezze noted,

> The basic philosophy of our Department, set forth in these regulations, is not something new. As many of you know, we have been engaged in very intense efforts to bring about the elimination of discrimination in the programs we administer. . . . And, taking full advantage of the Court's decision in the Simkins case, we required that hospitals and nursing homes built with the aid of Hill-Burton funds be operated on a nonsegregated basis and that staffing privileges be extended solely on the basis of professional competence. . . .

The initial response to our letters of request for these assurances has been most gratifying and most encouraging. We appreciate the prompt returns and we appreciated, particularly, the good faith of all those who have demonstrated their earnest desire to reason with us and to work with us in righting these old wrongs. As President Johnson has said, "it is a challenge to men of good will to transform the commands of our land into the customs of our land." . . . We extend to you now our good will, our good faith, and our willingness to reason and, in addition, whatever financial and technical help that is in our power to provide.

Let no one see, however, in our exercise of reason an absence of resolve to obtain the absolute justice that the law—and our own principles require.[28]

The rhetoric, however, was speeding toward a head-on collision with reality. The overwhelming priority in DHEW was to use its funding leverage to bring about racial integration in the public schools. The bulk of the public schools in the South and in the border states remained segregated. Yet, as of January 1966, a year after the implementation of the Title VI regulations, not one case had been carried forward to the point of withholding funds from a local school district. The entire effort faced a growing credibility gap. Those opposing desegregation seemed determined to check any progress. The civil rights advocates saw DHEW as doing nothing in the schools. They expected more of the same in hospitals in 1966.

Meanwhile, outside the Beltway

Nevertheless, independent of this painful effort of the federal bureaucracy to reinvent itself through the promulgation of regulations, agency procedures, and reorganization, civil rights efforts in health care had developed a momentum of their own. Legal suits continued to be brought and won, forcing the issue against hospitals.

In Greensboro, the implementation of the court-ordered hospital integration proceeded smoothly. The first black patient to receive care at Long Hospital, Ms. Maggie Shaw, was admitted on May 6, 1964, shortly after the court order. She had a myelogram the following day and was discharged on May 9.[29] The event went unnoticed by the public and the hospital staff as a whole. Patients also began to be admitted to Moses Cone Hospital without incident. The national press had picked up the story, and Moses Cone Hospital now began receiving mail from outside Greensboro similar in tone to that which Simkins had received earlier.

You are all bound to know that Negroes always take a million miles when given one inch. It is in the nature of the race—God segregated every single thing. He made and man dare not change it. Read Genesis carefully. . . . The women patients and workers are in for danger not yet realized. Do you see in this clipping who is rejoicing? NAACP, King, etc. N.C. is too lovely to cater to them. They are already laughing at our stupidity. It was in the paper. Fight!

. . . When I visited your beautiful City a year ago, I fell in love with Greensboro and its lovely people. On the strength of this I planned to live there when my husband retires. But I changed my mind when I read the enclosed newspaper item. I can't understand your voluntary manner in this decision. You must realize as I do that integration will lead to intermarriage.[30]

As spelled out under Title VI regulations, Moses Cone Hospital received its first visit from the Department of Health, Education and Welfare Regional Office in Charlottesville, Virginia, on July 9, 1965. A complaint had apparently been passed on from the local NAACP chapter to the New York NAACP clearing house and then to DHEW. Moses Cone Hospital had received a call on July 6 informing them that two persons from DHEW would be visiting the hospital. The two visitors sat down with several administrators and the hospital's attorney and proceeded to go over a questionnaire concerning employment practices, placement of patients in hospital rooms, the number of black physicians on the staff, and the number of whites and blacks currently employed in various departments of the hospital. They were then given a tour of the facility. The specific admission policies that should be followed to assure compliance with Title VI were vague. During the exit interview the two DHEW staff persons indicated that if the hospital could show that at least some white and nonwhite patients shared semiprivate room accommodations, then that should be sufficient, along with some public notification (preferably in the local press) concerning nondiscrimination in the hospital, to satisfy compliance regulations. The hospital itself was struggling with the mechanics of even such token compliance. A draft of an admission questionnaire, asking the patient's willingness to share accommodations with a black, appears in the hospital's files next to the description of the DHEW Title VI visit and a suggestion that the racial indicator from the admitting form be removed altogether. The draft questionnaire stated:

We are trying to comply with the provisions of the Civil Rights Act of 1964. In helping us comply, will you please answer the following questions:

1. Are you willing to occupy a room with a person of the same sex but of another race or color?

Yes __
No __
Don't Care __

2. Would you object to being placed in a room with a person of another race or color?

Yes __
No __ [31]

In Wilmington, North Carolina, Dr. Hubert Eaton finally got a measure of satisfaction in his second suit against James Walker Memorial Hospital. The decision of the lower court was reversed by the U.S. Court of Appeals for the Fourth Circuit on April 1, 1964. The suit argued that the hospital was "performing the state's function and was the chosen instrument of the state and therefore bound by the provisions of the Fourteenth Amendment to refrain from the discrimination alleged in the complaint."[32] The key facts about the hospital considered that were absent in the earlier suit were (1) a reverter clause in the deed to the hospital by the city that permitted it to control the use of a facility that was originally established as public, (2) the hospital's exemption from city taxes, alleged to be more than fifty thousand dollars per year, (3) the hospital's use of eminent domain in an expansion project, and (4) the hospital's receipt of a variety of state and local capital-construction subsidies.

The painful ten-year legal battle for privileges, ignored by white colleagues at James Walker Memorial Hospital, was not, however, over. When the three physicians in the suit, Drs. Eaton, Gray, and Roane, applied for privileges, Drs. Gray and Roane were admitted to the courtesy staff, but Dr. Eaton's application was denied. Dr. Gray, now in poor health, died before admitting a single patient. Dr. Roane succeeded in admitting a few patients before the hospital closed and was replaced by a new county facility, New Hanover Memorial. Dr. Eaton went back to federal court asking that the board of managers of James Walker Memorial Hospital be found in contempt. Twenty-six members of the medical staff were then required to testify in court as to how they voted and why. The court could find no legitimate grounds for excluding Dr. Eaton from privileges. Eaton, however, never succeeded in admitting patients to James Walker Memorial Hospital. The legal delays and the hospital's subsequent closure made the issue moot. He was, however, granted privileges at the new county facility, New Hanover Memorial. Reflecting later on this period in his life, Eaton observed that

> the victory in this lawsuit established a firm legal precedent against the arbitrary denial of hospital privileges to black physicians and the segregation of black patients in hospitals receiving tax funds. Of all the barriers that I have helped to bring down, and all the civil rights victories I have won, the victory in *Eaton et al. v. James Walker Memorial Hospital* was the most significant and meaningful one and the one from which I received the greatest personal satisfaction.[33]

Southern medical schools and their hospitals, dependent on federal funds for research and teaching, also began to respond to increasing federal pressures on funding. A black southern medical school faculty member reflected on his own experiences at that time.

> When I came to do my fellowship in endocrinology in 1964, I was told by the division chief that he didn't want me going on the private side because some of the physicians were concerned about the reaction of their patients. I felt I had been signed on under false pretenses. I would have never signed on if I had known that I would be excluded from this experience.
>
> However, it turned out the [medical school] division was trying to get funds for a biometrics lab from the National Institute of Health. Dr. Fein, the leader of the site visit team from the University of Michigan, questioned the endocrine fellows first. We were all sitting at the table, all nine of us. At the end of the session Dr. Fein asked, "Are any of you unhappy about the training you have received?" I said, "Yes, I am. I have been told that I can't rotate on the private side because of my color." He said, "What did you say?" I said, "'I have been told I can't rotate on the private side of this hospital because of my color. He said, "Well, I'll see to that!'"
>
> The other fellows came to my support. I hadn't known how they felt before. A session with the senior faculty and chief of the division followed. The first question asked the chief of the division was, "Why can't Dr. Johnson rotate on the private side of the hospital?" No answer. I never heard the inner workings of what did and didn't get said after that, but I'm certain a lot of money got tied up in that discussion. One of the senior faculty for whom I was doing research called me and said, "I think you better stay away from the laboratory until the dust settles."
>
> Finally the chief calls me in. He says, "Dr. Johnson, do you really

want to rotate on the private service?" I said, "Look, I chose clinical medicine rather than research. I had wanted to be a nuclear physicist, but they weren't taking blacks at Livermore or anywhere else then. There are not enough black doctors. When there are an excess number, then let them worry about research. I don't want to be a rat doctor. I want to rotate on the clinical service of endrocrinalogy so I can take care of people."

I rotated. Clearly they accepted the money and me too. Otherwise, they would have lost a large sum of government money. It wasn't that they wanted me so bad, they wanted the money more. They needed a big stick waved over their head in order to do what was right in the first place.[34]

In Atlanta on July 1, 1965, Grady Memorial Hospital, which had become a national symbol of separate-but-equal health care, fell to the pressures of desegregation. Planned in the late 1940s, construction had begun in 1954, the same year as the *Brown* decision. In 1962, a local dentist, a physician, and other Atlanta residents initiated an omnibus lawsuit to open membership in the local dental and medical society and to desegregate care at Grady Memorial Hospital.[35] In compliance with a court settlement, on the evening of June 30, 1965, Grady Memorial's patients, who had been separated in the wards of the twin towers, were transferred to achieve integrated wards. Bill Pinkston, who had first come to Grady as a part of the accounting department in 1948, was promoted to associate superintendent in 1955 and to superintendent in 1964. By then the management of the hospital had recognized the inevitability of integration and had begun the process. The two racially segregated emergency departments had first been recast to serve male and female patients separately, but since many of the emergency medical needs of both males and females were the same, this had proved as inefficient as the racially segregated system. The two emergency departments were later converted to Medical and Surgical services. The clinics were gradually integrated. Grady started accepting black interns in 1964. The integration of the two nursing schools, involving separate dormitories, separate affiliations with colleges, and separate uniforms, was the last part of the transition tackled. The integration of the patient floors, however, was the largest and most publicly visible symbolic change.

On the night of June 30, 1965, we moved the patients all around. We just came in to rooms and wards and said, "You're being transferred to room so and so." We just pushed the beds around. I was scared to death. I couldn't talk about it. I didn't know what would happen. We didn't make any public announcement about it. Of course, the director of nursing and the chiefs of services were told. I thought we were going to have a terrible time. There were going to be pickets, maybe even a white uprising against the hospital. Not one damn thing happened. The next day, the papers simply announced that integration had taken place, "in perfect order."[36]

Across the country between 1963 and 1965 a subtle change had taken place in the racial dynamics of most hospitals, even in the Deep South. The focus became how to adapt to the changed conditions, rather than how to resist change. The balance of power had shifted on local boards and within administrations. *Simkins* and Title VI were now the law of the land. There would be no massive resistance. Most hospitals were willing to accept the gradual, at least token, change that would avoid the Jim Crow label that would could cut off the flow of public funding. Ironically, the same insulation that had earlier enabled them to withstand the pressures of black physicians and community groups to change policies now gave them the flexibility to act in their own self-interest in breaking down racial barriers. Public-school officials, with elected school boards, faced a more volatile environment that imposed political constraints on such effort.

The Passage of Medicare

Another matter in which self-interest clearly came into play was the pending Medicare legislation. Compliance with Title VI of the Civil Rights Act could serve as a key condition for receiving Medicare funds, which would mean the difference for most hospitals between comfortable financial surpluses and insolvency. Johnson had won a landslide victory in the presidential election of November 1964, a fateful watershed election that would realign both parties.[37] It also assured legislative action on hospital insurance for the elderly.

Most accounts of the passage of Medicare and Medicaid legislation in 1965 trace the history of our national health insurance debate from the early efforts to initiate public health insurance in World War I, through its consideration and elimination from the original Social Security legislation of 1935, to the death of the Truman effort with the Wagner-Murray-Dingle bill in 1949. They trace the subsequent incremental strategy of covering hospital costs for the elderly through Social Security to legislation first proposed by Oscar Ewing in 1951 as head of the Federal Security Agency (soon to become DHEW).[38] Other than the general ebb and flow of electoral politics, the struggle for national health insurance has been described essentially as a self-contained process of vested interests and advocates. In reality, the boundaries between the civil rights struggle during this period and the battle that led to the passage of Medicare were far more blurred in the minds of both the protagonists and the public at large. Medicare did not by accident follow by less than eleven months the passage of the Civil Rights Act. Nor was it an accident that less than a month after the passage of Medicare the Voting Rights Act became law.

The civil rights legislation and the Medicare and Medicaid legislation shared much more than just a point in time and a combined set of political events that provided an opportunity for action. The cast of characters in both efforts overlapped. The American Nurse's Association and the American Public Health Association were strong advocates of both pieces of legislation. The American Hospital Association played a more muted but supportive role in both. The National Medical Association, which had hesitated to openly endorse the Truman national health insurance proposal, now, as a spillover of their new activist civil rights role, became advocates for the passage of Medicare.

Yet, even for a civil rights activist physician in 1963, a year of widespread public protests, engaging in such activities was a foreign and awkward experience. Drs. John Holloman and Walter Lear, officers of the newly formed Medical Committee for Civil Rights (later the Medical Committee for Human Rights) struggled to recruit a core of physicians willing to picket the AMA convention in Atlantic City in June and with their own self-image as physicians. The thirty physicians that walked the picket line wanted the AMA's House of Delegates to speak out against segregation and discrimination in state and local medical societies and health care facilities in the South. Dr. Lear reflected on some of the ironies of the experience.

> We were very tentative and wary of using rhetoric that was too flamboyant. When I spoke to the press I told them, "You may call it a picket, but we call it a public witness." There was also a problem with the style of the "witness" for physicians. John [John Holloman] and I went to Atlantic City several days in advance to work it all out with police department. I had learned that if you work it out in advance and don't give them any surprises you are likely to get good cooperation. The biggest issue we had to discuss with the chief of police of Atlantic City had to deal with signs. Atlantic City has a law that says that there may not be anything permanent placed on the boardwalk. We explained to the chief of police, "We have these signs, and physicians can't carry signs." We wanted permission to have our signs on sandwich boards stationary on the boardwalk. The police

commissioner looked Mike in the eye and he looked me in the eye and then he said, "Yeah, you're right. Physicians can't carry signs.". . . The picture in the *New York Times* article that day shows us all conservatively dressed in dark suits and ties marching by the sandwich boards. That was the culture, even of radical physicians. It was just unprofessional.[39]

A meeting between the leadership of the American Medical Association and the National Medical Association on December 19, 1963, illustrates the dynamics of the political chess game being played out on the beyond public view. It was the third meeting of the two groups, which had been precipitated by picketing by the NAACP and representatives of the NMA at both the AMA's annual meeting in Atlantic City and its Chicago headquarters. The meeting, held in the boardroom of the AMA's headquarters, was civil but tense. The AMA president repeated the organization's 1950 position, which encouraged nondiscrimination in local medical societies but did not require it as a condition of membership in the AMA. The NMA president, Dr. Clement, then cited examples of racial exclusion in local medical societies and the AMA's own acknowledgment of such practices. Dr. Annis, the AMA president, countered by citing the loan guarantee program for medical students at Meharry and Howard, a program that had provided 158 loans, totaling $204,000, for which the AMA served as guarantor.

The AMA's leaders were troubled by the breach in the medical ranks caused by the NMA support of the Medicare legislation. In an effort then to shift the discussion and regain the offensive, Dr. Annis raised the issue of the NMA's support of medical care for the elderly financed through Social Security.

Dr. Annis inquired as to why the NMA opposed the AMA on this subject when all the other doctors in the country, with the exception of 51, [physicians] supported the AMA's position. The NMA, he stressed, was alone among national organizations of physicians in this respect.

Dr. Clement replied that the NMA supported the principle of Medicare because it considered it good legislation and was not in opposition to the AMA. The NMA's approach was positive and evaluated the proposal on its merits.

Dr. Annis freely acknowledged that there was no connection between the moral values inherent in the AMA's working to eliminate discrimination and the NMA's position on Medicare.

Dr. Cobb [NMA president-elect] pointed out that there was no relationship between majority opinion and truth. Columbus was a unique minority in 1492 in his concept that the world was round.[40]

At the annual convention of the NAACP in Washington, D.C., in June 1964, the nation's oldest and largest civil rights organization added its own weight to the passage of the Medicare legislation, which it described as "an essential weapon in our war against poverty."[41]

Dr. Hubert Eaton, president of the Old North State Medical Society, in 1965 explicitly attacked the AMA's alternative proposal as well as the efforts of a North Carolina doctor through the Medical Society of North Carolina to undermine popular support of the Johnson administration's bill.

We disagree strongly with our colleague, Dr Raiford, who has intimated that the Kerr-Mills program plus the available voluntary health insurance plans can provide adequate hospital and health insurance for our senior citizens. The deficiencies in the Kerr-Mills Medical Assistance for the Aged program as stated here and the limitations which most insurance companies include in policies offered to older people make these two approaches to the health care problem of senior citizens undesirable as well as inadequate.

We also take issue with Dr. Raiford concerning his statement that "We believe the people of North Carolina when they know the facts will agree that they don't want federal bureaucrats meddling in our hospitals and interfering with medical decisions that should be left to those who are qualified to make those decisions—your doctors."

To our Society, this statement seems to be an appeal to emotions. The scare of Federal control is the old and obsolete battle-cry of those opposed to legislation of this type but [who] can come up with insufficient logical reasons for opposing such programs. Hospital insurance under social security would give the government no control over hospitals and there is no basis for making such assertions.

The American Medical Association through its constituent Society, the Wake County Medical Society, said among other things in its advertisement in the Raleigh News and Observer on October 15, 1964, that "this program [Kerr-Mills] enables individual states, with federal assistance, to guarantee to every elderly person who needs it the health care he or she requires . . ."

The Negro physicians of North Carolina are forced to agree with the *News and Observer's* Editorial comment that the American Medical Association and its constituent societies are indeed "guilty of a cruel and unthinkable hoax by misleading thousands of old people about 'free health care' supposedly available to them."

The Old State Medical Society has cast its lot and thrown its support to the Administration's program of Medicare. We believe that the majority of Americans will do likewise.[42]

Montague Cobb testified as president and spokesperson for the NMA before the Senate Finance Committee in May of 1965, using his full medical authority as a leader of a national physician organization. He spoke of the great strides made in medicine and his organization's support of the passage of the administration's bill.

Our greatest problem now lies in finding ways to pay the costs of the medical care that modern knowledge has made possible. The principle that in our society every citizen, rich or poor, should be able to obtain the medical care he needs is not debated. The problem of financing has been accentuated by the fact that costs of medical care have risen astronomically in recent times and may continue to do so. Hospital stays, diagnostic procedures and many drugs have zoomed upward in expense, and the application of future discoveries and advances is likely to raise costs even further. Moreover, because we have in large measure been able to conquer and control the diseases and conditions which produced mortality in early life, a major portion of our armamentarium for restoring and maintaining health must today be directed at the latter years of the life span and for the benefit of the elderly members of our population, a segment which steadily increases in numbers and in population percentage.

For the past two decades legislation considered by the Congress has reflected a recognition of a deep concern for this problem of the costs of medical care. The many volumes which record the testimony of experts and interested persons on the subject [are evidence] that every possible aspect has been at some time examined. There has also accumulated a certain experience with some types of plans and legislation. Most of all, unflagging public interest in the problem is at a peak.

The National Medical Association firmly believes that more than twenty years of study, observation and experience are enough, and that the time has come for broad definitive action.[43]

Since so many of the opponents and advocates of both the Civil Rights Act and the Medicare legislation were the same, the rhetoric and the imagery in the civil rights debate and the debate over the passage of Medicare blurred together.

The connection between Medicare and Title VI was clearly understood by all sides. On April 13, 1965, Senator Harry Byrd, chairman of the Senate Finance Committee considering the Medicare legislation, received from Secretary Celebrezze the following reply to his request for clarification of this point: "The matter has been explored by the Department's legal staff. Title VI of the Civil Rights Act establishes a fundamental policy applicable to all programs receiving Federal financial assistance. The system of hospital insurance under the social security system will substantially strengthen the financial position of the hospitals of the nation. I am advised, therefore, that the new hospital insurance program will be subject to the requirements of Title VI."[44]

Both the Civil Rights Act of 1964 and Medicare legislation in 1965 were initially introduced by Kennedy and were advocated as memorials to a martyred president. Unlike many legislative initiatives that get watered down by the inevitable compromises necessary to assure passage, civil rights and Medicare legislation picked up energy and emerged as stronger and far more ambitious pieces of legislation than was originally envisioned. The benefits were expanded from hospital coverage to optional supplemental coverage of physician services, and Title XIX (Medicaid) was added along with Title XVIII (Medicare), greatly expanding coverage of medical expenses for the poor. Johnson greeted the final passage of the Medicare bill by the Senate on July 9, 1965, with a statement that, with the substitution of a few words, could have served to herald the passage of the Civil Rights Act a year earlier.

> The 22-Year fight to protect the health of older Americans is now certain—of swift and historic victory.
>
> For these long decades bill after bill has been introduced to help older citizens meet the often crushing and always rising costs of disease and crippling illness. Each time, until today, the battle has been lost. Each time the forces of compassion and justice have returned from defeat to begin the battle anew. And each time the force of increased public understanding has added to our strength. . . .
>
> I stood beside John Kennedy in the Senate in 1960 as he battled for the cause of justice, and watched in later years as his courage and his refusal to accept defeat gradually helped shape the forces which led us to this day.[45]

The bill was signed by the president on July 30, 1965, at the Truman Library in Independence, Missouri.

In retrospect, Somers and Somers, in their review of the passage of the Medicare legislation, appear to have come the closest to recognizing the symbiotic connection between the civil rights struggle from 1946 to 1965 and the struggle for the passage of national health insurance.

> Nineteen-forty-six may be considered a Rubicon in the legislative debate. By then, all major political and economic interests appeared to agree on the necessity for federal action to assure the availability of medical care. The controversy was now centered on two major differences: (1) whether the program should be administered by the states or the federal government; (2) whether medical care should be financed by social insurance as an earned "right" or provided only to the indigent based on a means test. For the next two decades dispute hinged on these issues, particularly the second, and Medicare has by no means fully resolved them.[46]

What the civil rights movement did for health care reform, if only for a brief fleeting moment in the middle of the 1960s, was to shift the balance toward the "federal" and the "rights" answers to these two questions. The images of Governor Wallace blocking the entrance to the University of Alabama and the police dogs and fire hose set loose on children in Birmingham were part of a new national consciousness. Few could advocate state and local autonomy in the face of such vivid defiance of the rights of blacks. In addition, the early years of the civil rights movement brought with it a yearning for reconciliation, less willingness to revert to the traditional means-tested formulas for the disadvantaged, and a reinvigorated advocacy for equal treatment. It was that shared chemistry, perhaps more than anything else, that permitted the passage and smooth implementation of the Medicare program. However briefly, the two currents flowed together.

Title VI Enforcement and the Beginning of Medicare

The Medical Committee for Human Rights (MCHR), the NMA, the Legal Defense Fund (LDF) and the other civil rights groups played a dual role with the federal Title VI compliance efforts beginning in 1965. They served as both its severest critics and closest allies. DHEW relied on them as an extended staff for the federal effort that had almost none. They brought complaints, provided volunteers and tested out field procedures that would later be adopted by the agency in conducting Title VI compliance investigations of hospitals for the Medicare program. MCHR responded to a variety of requests made by DHEW, as the following internal memorandums suggest:

I now understand that HEW has a need for complaints of racial discrimination and segregation from 10 or 20 Northern and Western hospitals. They need them quickly to enable them to get the effect of sudden impact, and voluntary compliance on a nation-wide basis, since they do not have enough personnel to visit and supervise 9,000 hospitals. The agency confidentially requests that MCHR release information about complaints to the press since this helps to get other institutions into line and the government is much more restricted than a private group in what they can say to the newspapers. (September 9, 1965)[47]

Please compile a list of northern physicians who went south and give to me immediately. The NAACP Legal Defense and Education Fund has been requested by HEW to seek out physicians who may be willing to go South and make hospital investigations at the expense of HEW. (September 29, 1965)[48]

The frustration of the activist volunteers, however, mounted over the fall. Nothing seemed to happen to the complaints that they developed, other than acknowledging their receipt. Almost three hundred complaints had been submitted. The LDF submitted a scathing memorandum to Secretary John Gardner, who had replaced Celebrezze in August, on December 16.[49] Except for four hospitals in Mississippi, which, in the ultimate gesture of defiance, refused to sign the form agreeing to not discriminate, no funds had been cut off from any facility. "In short," the memo observed, "the Department policy seems to be that if a hospital or state agency dispursing federal funds executes a piece of paper stating that it will not discriminate it is safe from a cut off of federal funds." Anticipating practices that would become widespread after the implementation of the Medicare program, the memo observed:

One of the hospitals complained about in the February 11, 1965 series of complaints, The Kings' Daughters Hospital in Canton, Mississippi, not only refused to comply with Title VI but has reduced the number of beds in the hospital so that no Negroes and whites will have to share rooms. Ironically, the hospital continues to receive funds from the Department to finance future expansion of its facilities and is presently constructing a new hospital building with Federal funds, which will contain only private rooms. Federal money had, therefore, been employed for the purpose of maintaining segregation and because all rooms will be private, will not add hospital beds to those available in the community.

In spite of the long list of complaints, the department, the LDF memo observed, "takes the view (privately) that it will be subjected to political pressure if it attempts to move against such hospitals." The lack of any staff or plan suggested that there was little commitment to aggressive enforcement. The memo noted that there was no specific appropriation for Title VI enforcement and the personnel involved had to be borrowed from other agencies. The LDF saw the need for a large staff in Washington and in the regional offices committed to civil rights enforcement. "These persons must be under the control of officials directly responsible for civil rights and not placed in operating agencies which do not have the confidence of Negro communities or sufficient experience."

> It is critical that the Department must make a firm policy decision that no funds under the Medicare program will be paid to hospitals, which are not in compliance with Title VI. . . . The Department should be given authority to employ (or borrow from other agencies) new staff. We recommend an increase of about 25 new staff members for the compliance office at DHEW in Washington and regional offices. In addition, we recommend that approximately 50 temporary staff members be borrowed from other federal agencies. The primary responsibilities of these new staff members would be to assure that only facilities in compliance would receive federal funds under the Medicare Program.

Representatives of the LDF, NMA, and MCHR had expected to meet in person with Secretary Gardner on December 16, 1965, to discuss the concerns expressed in the LDF memo. Failing to accomplish this, they held a brief press conference. The new president-elect of both the MCHR and the NMA, Dr. John Holloman, made the following statement:

> Hundreds of complaints have been filed. We took sad notice that 17 months after passage of the Civil Rights Act, after scores of complaints against medical facilities across the entire South, and glaring abuse after glaring abuse, it appears that only four hospitals in Mississippi, which refused to sign compliance forms with the Department have not received payments because of Title VI. The delays have persisted despite the obvious health disadvantages faced by Negro citizens. We expressed our disturbance over reports that HEW plans to bypass Title VI with respect to payment of individual doctors under Part B of the Health Insurance Law. Under this program, the Southern white physician who treats a Negro patent, who is a recipient of

Medicare funds, was last month offered the consoling advice of the American Medical Association—through its House of Delegates, that he does not have to desegregate his private treatment facilities—since Medicare money is going to the individual patient. Presently, under the Medicare Bill, there is no mention of the fact that hospitals in receipt of Medicare funds covering hospitalization of patients must provide service on a nondiscriminatory basis. We told Mr. Gardner that it will not be possible to implement the full scope of the health insurance and welfare medical assistance provisions, unless a bold and deliberate effort is made to bring all disadvantaged people and particularly southern Negroes into the mainstream of American medicine and health care. Therefore, we stressed that it is particularly important that the Federal funds to be spent on the Medicare Act should be spent in a non-discriminatory way; and, in no case should they be used to support segregated facilities.[50]

The coalition that had been involved in trying to push Title VI compliance for hospitals had the diagnosis right. As 1966 began, the law, the regulations, and the rhetoric surrounding Title VI enclosed a hollow organizational shell. The Title VI regulations had been in effect for less than a year, and the administrative response to these new regulations was still being organized. The assistant secretary, John Quigley, had the responsibility for supervising and coordinating the DHEW's Title VI activities. The Office of General Council would work with the assistant secretary in reviewing, approving, and providing final interpretations of Title VI policy. Both Quigley and the Office of General Council were located in the office of the secretary of DHEW. Title VI enforcement, however, was the responsibility of each of the five operating units or program agencies of DHEW.[51] The Social Security Administration was now gearing up for managing the Medicare program, which was scheduled to begin on July 1, 1966. Since Social Security was administered directly by the federal government and not through grants or contracts, it had not been involved in setting up any mechanisms for Title VI enforcement. Now, however, through its new responsibilities in establishing both conditions for participation and contracts with providers of medical services, the Social Security Administration acquired Title VI enforcement responsibilities that overshadowed those of any other federal agencies in both size and complexity.

The specter of attempting to enforce Title VI in the new Medicare program was mind-boggling. Many in the executive branch were convinced it would be foolhardy to enforce the nondiscrimination requirements of Title VI during the introduction of a massive new program for a vulnerable population of almost twenty million beneficiaries. Its success required the participation and active cooperation of most physicians, hospitals, and nursing homes in the country. Obtaining credible Title VI assurances from providers would require a program on a scale far greater than selectively responding to a few complaints. A well-organized, grassroots civil rights movement and a politicized black medical community would not tolerate the rubber-stamping of facility compliance; yet, the Senate and House Appropriations Committees, still controlled by southerners, were unlikely to respond either quickly or sympathetically to the expanded budgets and staffing needed to perform such a function.

The entire Title VI enforcement staff in January 1966 could at best be described as a token skeleton. Just as the Division of Education had established an Office of Equal Educational Opportunity, the Public Health Service had established its Office of Equal Health Opportunity to assure compliance in the programs it funded. A small skeleton staff also operated out of the assistant secretary's office, the Office for Civil Rights. Peter Libassi, as a special assistant to the secretary for civil rights, occupied this office. Robert Nash, a career civil servant involved in grants and contract administration, had assumed responsibility as director of the Office of Equal Health Opportunity. Most of the actual responsibilities as to administering programs were, however, the responsibility of the nine regional offices of DHEW. It was these regional staff from the Charlottesville, Virginia, office that had visited Moses Cone Hospital in July 1965.

DHEW's leadership was committed to the idea that the civil rights functions should be diffused throughout DHEW's operating divisions, embedded in its overarching mission. This was more than just noble rhetoric. For two critical years, the powerful members of the appropriations committees and the civil rights officials in DHEW would play a cat-and-mouse game. DHEW hid the staff and dollars going into civil rights compliance in the budgets of different divisions and agencies, while the chairmen pressed for centralization of these efforts into a single office, so that appropriations committees could control enforcement efforts more effectively.

Complicating things further was a budget process that made it almost impossible to quickly staff a new function.[52] In spite of the obvious indications of the need for increased staffing for civil rights, no substantial increase was requested in the budget submission for fiscal year 1966 (July 1965 to June 1966). The budget request had been processed well before the regulations, which were not officially approved until January 5, 1965. In January 1965 there were fewer than twenty persons involved with Title VI compliance efforts in DHEW.

One person, in fact, represented the entire infrastructure of DHEW devoted to Title VI enforcement for health-related programs. Robert Nash had previously served on the ad hoc interagency task force responsible for developing the Title VI regulations over the previous six months and his responsibilities would now be focused on the implementation of those regulations in his agency. He would now organize and direct the health-related Title VI activities in DHEW.

There were ominous similarities between this effort and another federal initiative, the Freedmen's Bureau, which had been implemented exactly a century earlier. This was an agency hastily patched together in 1865, with a staff that had only a vague idea of what needed to be done. It was exposed to repeated public attack, congressional investigations, white southern opposition, and inadequate funding. In 1869, responsibilities for addressing the problems of the freed slaves were shifted to the states and the Bureau was abandoned. A century later, in the fall of 1965, the backlash from an effort by DHEW to withhold funds from the Chicago school system raised questions about the administrative competence of the department and the will of the administration in enforcing Title VI. The Department had failed to follow its own regulations, miscalculated the political clout of Mayor Daley and had been forced to back down.

Secretary John Gardner tried to stem the damage. In a memorandum to the administrators of the operating agencies he clearly put the burden of responsibility on the shoulder of the agencies.

> This is too important to be treated as anything less than the highest of priorities in our total program. . . . The key is adequate staffing. We must assign as large a part of our staff resources to this activity as required to assure effective administration. . . . Title VI nondiscrimination requirements are an integral and essential part of all administrative responsibilities in every applicable program in the Department. The heads of each operating agency will be held responsible for meeting this requirement along with all other requirements.[53]

In short, DHEW as a whole was somehow to become a civil rights enforcement agency. Staff could be reassigned to do this function. By January 1966, the Public Health Service staff now assigned to Title VI had grown to about ten. In January it became clear that the regulations shaping the other conditions for participation in the Medicare program, scheduled to begin July 1, would include assurance of Title VI compliance. Nash's group drafted a plan for providing such assurance, which was approved by the end of February. DHEW still had no department-wide systematic compliance procedures and no systematic national compliance program. It had yet to conclude a single enforcement action or terminate assistance from a single noncomplying recipient. It had no staff for reviewing the Title VI compliance of hospitals applying for participation in the Medicare program.

Civil rights activities in the executive branch as a whole were still undergoing reorganization. The final parts of the reorganization did not take place until February 10, 1966, with the shifting of the Community Relations Service from the Commerce Department to the Justice Department. Johnson had dissolved the Council on Equal Opportunity, established in February 1965 and headed by Vice President Humphrey, to coordinate issues related to the implementation of the Civil Rights Act of 1964 . The Justice Department would assume overall responsibility for coordinating enforcement, but the agency directly involved in administrating specific program funds would assume primary responsibility and accountability. This basic principle had been pronounced by the president to his cabinet officials on March 25, 1965.

> I want to make one thing unmistakable and indelibly clear to every department, every agency, every office and every employee of the government of the United States.
> The Federal Service must never be either the active or passive ally of any who flout the Constitution of the United States.
> Regional custom, local tradition, personal prejudice or predilection are no excuse, no justification, no defense in this regard.
> Where there is an office or an officer of this Government, there must be equal treatment, equal respect, equal service—and equal support for all American citizens, regardless of race, or sex or region or religion. . . .
> I am asking the heads of each department to communicate this to every office and officer, whatever their rank or position in the Federal Service, and to take all appropriate measures to assure full compliance with the spirit of the law that governs and guards us all.[54]

The importance of driving Title VI enforcement down into the agencies was reinforced by the restructuring of civil rights functions that was approved by the president on September 24, 1965.

> A cardinal principle underlying these recommendations is that whenever possible operating functions should be performed by departments and agencies with clearly defined responsibilities, as distinguished from interagency committees or other interagency arrangements. Thus, the prime consideration running through my study and these recommendations is that each officer and employee of

the Federal Government who administers a Federal program recognizes that he is responsible for making certain that the program is administered without discrimination. Every person who contracts on behalf of the Government with private parties must recognize that he is responsible for nondiscrimination in Government contracts.[55]

As Johnson well understood, concentrating civil rights enforcement efforts within the operating agencies was also a way to hide the troops from a counterattack by their legislative oversight committees.

The Office of Equal Health Opportunity and Medicare Enforcement

The Office of Equal Health Opportunity (OEHO), set up in the Surgeon General's Office of the Public Health Service, had been established to fulfill the president's mandate. Its life would be a remarkably short one for a bureaucratic agency, less than two years, but long on accomplishments. For many of the civil servants who worked for the Office of Equal Health Opportunity during this period, it was the high point of their careers and a period that they looked back to with pride and more than a little nostalgia. During January and February 1966, the Johnson administration had finally come to closure about the most troubling and controversial question concerning the implementation of the Medicare program. Should Title VI be used to force full racial integration of hospitals, or should the issue be soft-pedaled? Health care was such a personal and private matter. Even the lunch counters had yet to be fully integrated. There were good reasons to defer dealing with the issue. Yet the opportunity to use the new Medicare dollars to break down racial barriers was also tempting.

The implementation of such a program was a massive undertaking by itself. Almost twenty million elderly citizens needed to be enrolled, and successful implementation relied on the cooperation of the nation's hospitals and physicians. There were efforts in some local medical societies to boycott the program; these could spread rapidly. School desegregation was bogged down by continuing massive resistance. A thirty-year battle to gain health care coverage through Social Security, so close to victory, could be lost in the resulting firestorm. No rational program manager would want to add the goal of desegregation to the responsibilities of implementing such a complex program in ten months.

For Lyndon Johnson, however, it was a test of will, a narrow window of opportunity to prove there was substance to his rhetoric. For Johnson and for many of those involved in executing that will, it was a decision driven more by passion than reason. At some point before March 1966, in a meeting in the White House between Secretary Gardner and President Johnson the commitment was made.[56] The implementation of the Medicare program ceased to be a technical task and became a crusade.

Robert Nash had, after January 1965, assumed responsibility for the implementation of those regulations within the Surgeon General's Office of the Public Health Service. It was his office that had shaped the questions asked by regional staff people at Cone Memorial Hospital in July 1965. During the first eight months of 1965 Nash's office had received and attempted to investigate about 225 similar complaints against hospitals and had begun work on a reporting form.[57] In January 1966 the Public Health Service had about ten full-time equivalents assigned to Title VI. The July 1 initiation date of the Medicare program loomed less than six months away. The responsibility for certifying facilities for Title VI compliance had been assigned to the Public Health Service and Nash's Office of Equal Health Opportunity. No one had an accurate list, but it was assumed that about eight thousand facilities would need to be brought into compliance with Title VI by July 1, 1966.

On March 4, 1966, as had been approved up the chain of command to the president, a letter went out under the signature of the surgeon general of the Public Health Service to every hospital in the country informing them that the Public Health Service had been given responsibility for assuring Title VI compliance for all hospitals receiving any federal funds and that participation in the Medicare program would be dependent on compliance with Title VI. A description of the guidelines for compliance, which had been published a year earlier in the American Hospital Association's *Journal*, was enclosed.

Hospitals in compliance with the Act are characterized by absence of separation, discrimination or any other distinction on the basis of race, color or national origin in any activity carried on in, by or for the institution affecting the care and treatment of patients.

Specifically the above would include (but not be limited to) the following characteristics:

1. The hospital provides inpatient and outpatient care on a non-discriminatory basis; all patients are admitted and receive care without regard to race, color or national origin. Declaration of an open admission policy may not be sufficient to effectuate compliance in some instances, particularly where the hospital has served only or primarily patients of one race. Where there is significant variation between the racial composition of patients and the population served, the hospital has a responsibility to determine the reasons

and to take corrective action if they are due to discriminatory practices.

2. All patients are being assigned to all rooms, wards, floors, sections and buildings without regard to race, color or national origin. In communities with non-white population, this results in biracial occupancy of multi-bed rooms and wards and use of single bed rooms on a nondiscriminatory basis.

   Patients are not asked if they are willing or desire to share a room with a person of another race. Transfer of patients is not used as a device to evade compliance with the Act.

3. Employees, medical staff and volunteers of the hospital are assigned to patient services without regard to race, color or national origin of either the patient or employee. Courtesy titles (Mr., Miss., Dr.) whenever used, are being used throughout the hospital including patient care areas and news releases announcing admissions, births, deaths, etc.

4. The granting of permanent or temporary staff privileges is carried out in a non-discriminatory manner. Staff privileges are not denied professionally qualified personnel on the basis of race, color or national origin. Removal of staff privileges or other disciplinary actions shall not be based on race, color or national origin.

5. Non-discriminatory practices of the institution include all aspects of training programs, and require recruiting and selection of trainees at both predominantly white and Negro schools. The same recruiting procedures are used at all such institutions. Third parties are not permitted to select trainees on a basis which, if done directly by the hospital, would be violative of the Civil Rights Act. These requirements apply to interns (medical, dental, OT, PT, dietician), residents and training programs such as graduate nurse, practical nurse, medical technology, x-ray technology, etc.

6. All services rendered by the institution, its employees or vendors to patients or to others are provided without regard to race, color, or national origin. This would include:

   A. Administrative services (admissions, medical records, fiscal, etc.).
   B. Medical and dental care for inpatients and outpatients (all specialties—clinical, diagnostic or other pathology services).
   C. Paramedical care and ancillary and supportive services (food, pharmacy, social services, laundry, toilet facilities, waiting rooms, entrances, exits, snack bars, gift shops, visiting hours, doctor's lounges). Patients and visitors are using all cafeteria

facilities without regard to race, color or national origin; no dining facilities are used only by "custom" or "preference."

7. Employees and medical staff have been notified in writing of the hospital's policy for compliance with Title VI of the Civil Rights Act.
8. Hospitals which have recently changed from discriminatory practices have taken steps to notify those who had previously been excluded from hospital services (e.g. letters to Negro physicians or physician organizations and Civil Rights leaders, notices to newspapers, posting of signs in hospitals, etc.).
9. Hospitals which have had dual facilities to affect racial separation have either converted one of them to a different purpose or have taken steps to change the traffic flow so that they are actually used biracially.[58]

Also enclosed with the letter was Assurance Form 441, to be signed by the administrator indicating compliance with the conditions described above, and a questionnaire to be completed. The administrator was asked to return the form and the questionnaire by March 15. "We will review the questionnaires as they arrive, and if any deficiencies are noted we will let you know so that you can take any necessary action to correct them. . . . Representatives from the Department of Health, Education and Welfare Regional office and State agencies will be visiting hospitals on a routine periodic basis to supplement this information and to be of further assistance in resolving any problems that may arise."[59]

Only those in the Office of Equal Health Opportunity could fully appreciate the magnificent audacity of this opening move. Many of the hospitals, as inspections of complaints in the previous year had shown, were far from complying with the standard. Noncompliance was not limited to any region. Some had engaged in deliberate ruses to frustrate inspections. As James Quigley had observed in a speech to the American Hospital Association meeting the previous August, many administrators welcomed the opportunity that Title VI gave them to work with their boards in ending discriminatory practices. Yet, according to Quigley, there were plenty of exceptions.

We have, for example, listened to explanations that no Negro babies were in the nursery because all Negro mothers preferred to nurse their babies—therefore all Negro babies "roomed-in" with their mothers.

We have met men who said they no longer segregate Negro patients; they now *reserve* a section of the hospital especially for Negroes (thus implying preferential treatment, incidentally). We have had hospital administrators state that Negroes were *not required* to use special entrances and exits of the hospital but *prefer* to use the entrance that used to have a sign marked "colored."

We have had a spokesman for the community tell us that no Negro was willing to serve on the Board of Directors of a community hospital because no Negro was public spirited enough to accept such an assignment. . . .

One institution removed "Colored" and "White" signs from their rest rooms and installed locks on the doors—and then issued keys only to white staff. And—as perhaps the ultimate step in our education to date—one hospital deliberately placed Negro and white patients in the same rooms, closed the Negro dining room and integrated the nursery for the benefit of the review team—and then promptly shifted everything back to business as usual as soon as the review team left the city.[60]

What if the hospitals didn't return the assurances and forms? What if a boycott was organized? Some of the local medical societies were developing plans to organize boycotts anyway. A few key southern politicians could have organized such an effort more easily than they had organized the massive resistance to school integration. What if the administrators just lied? There was no way the OEHO could audit approximately eight thousand facilities by the June 30 deadline. What staff they did have was unprepared and untrained for such investigative and adversarial assignments. Yet, Johnson appeared adamant about two things: (1) the Medicare program would begin on schedule—there could be no "bureaucratic" delays; and (2) all Medicare providers would be in full compliance with Title VI. What emerged was something equivalent to a children's crusade that actually seemed to work.

Secretary Gardner directed the temporary reassignment of 750 people to the Office of Equal Health Opportunity from all areas of the DHEW bureaucracy. Robert Ball, commissioner of Social Security, was instructed to provide some ten thousand square feet and support for the operation. In a sleight of hand that would avoid dangerous delays in seeking supplemental appropriations, salaries and travel costs would be paid out of each employee's home agency budget. Each division chief would recruit a quota of volunteers to assist in the Medicare Title VI certification process. If there were not enough volunteers, staff were to be drafted.

The "volunteers" trickled into OEHO in February and March, while

OEHO began the effort to recruit more permanent staff. It was a strange, ragtag army. There were bench scientists, veterinarians, local field managers from the Social Security Administration, Public Health Service nurses, pharmacists from the Food and Drug Administration, researchers from the National Institute of Health, and even "a medical officer from the Indian health service complete with an Eskimo secretary."[61] For some, it was just another assignment. For others, however, it was much more. Some DHEW "volunteers" had picketed discrimination in housing and public swimming pools in suburban Washington on weekends in the early 1960s. Now there was an opportunity to do something for a cause they believed in during work hours.

Some of the recruits from outside of government had a longer history in the civil rights movement. Frank Weil was an early recruit. He had served as national secretary for the American Veterans Committee and had worked since 1946 on integrating facilities surrounding military bases. Medgar Evers had written a letter of acceptance as a board member to the American Veteran's Committee the night before he was murdered, and Weil had used his influence as an officer in a veterans' organization to make sure Evers was buried in Arlington National Cemetery, and not in a segregated cemetery in Mississippi. Weil worked for civil rights in Mississippi in the summer of 1964. "I got shot at but they missed, although Hertz was somewhat miffed when I turned in a car with bullet holes," he reflected.[62]

Robert Nash was the right field commander for this remarkably fierce and passionate volunteer bureaucratic army. He reportedly told one of his recruits, "If I don't want to take on a hospital, I'll refer it to General Counsel for advice. Three months later they'll get back to me with a reason why I shouldn't do anything. If I want to take on a hospital, I'll just use my own lawyers and do it."[63]

The logistics of managing this army, however, were mind boggling. OEHO was located in the DHEW North building on the mall below the Capitol. The secretary's office in DHEW North housed Peter Libassi's Office for Civil Rights. This small office was responsible for coordination of all the Title VI activities in DHEW. The bulk of the physical facilities for the OEHO Medicare campaign, however, were housed in four different buildings in the Social Security Complex in Baltimore. Yet things got done.

By the middle of May an additional 120 staff persons had been trained in compliance work in the field. The president had begun receiving regular weekly updates from the OEHO, passed through Libassi to Special Assistants to the President Joseph Califano and Douglass Cater. The first update, pulled together on April 20 (a little over a month past the deadline imposed on the providers by the surgeon general's March 4 letter), was encouraging. Out of the 8,550 letters sent out to facilities, 4,932 had responded with completed assurances, reports that raised no red flags and had been forwarded to Medicare. Another 1,805 hospitals had not responded, and 1,813 were still being processed. A list of the nonresponding facilities was being prepared to be circulated to local Social Security Administration district managers for telephone follow-up, and to local public officials and to private organizations such as senior citizens groups.[64] A breakdown of Title VI compliance by state on April 30 revealed a not unexpected pattern of noncompliance in key southern states. In these states the majority of the hospitals had either not responded or had existing discriminatory practices.

A White House staff memorandum to the president from the director of emergency planning on May 23, 1966, reveals growing concern over whether the bluff of Title VI enforcement in Medicare was really going to work.

> You asked that I review the circumstances as of July 1 when Medicare becomes operative with relation to hospital availability under potential civil rights limitations.
>
> For practical purposes compliance with Title VI by hospitals will be complete in all States except Alabama, Louisiana, Mississippi and South Carolina. Alabama and Mississippi are probably not to be greatly improved; Louisiana and South Carolina may be.
>
> Options are limited:
>
> 1. Civil rights requirements be waived for an additional period of time on the proposition that the health of the people is the first consideration. Such a waiver would obviously encourage resistance.
> 2. Refuse financial contributions in some more recalcitrant areas as a demonstration that resistance will not be allowed and, for the moment, ignore other non-compliance.
> 3. Ban all financial assistance to all non-complying institutions.
>
> Secretary Gardner and his staff are doing all that can be expected and may gain additional success before June 30.
>
> Governor George Wallace is now trying to get the southern governors to a meeting and is encouraging hospitals in his own State to refuse compliance. Where there are gubernatorial elections, his conduct poses a real problem.

I recommend that a final course of action not be determined until we are closer to June 30, to give Secretary Gardner's force maximum opportunity to succeed. I do not believe that we need fear a "scandal" that might have resulted from nation-wide non-compliance.[65]

In the meantime, OEHO's ragtag volunteer invisible army continued to plug away. For many, it was a magical time when nothing was impossible. Each implausible success inspired even more audacious approaches toward accomplishing the next one.

I showed up in Baltimore at Social Security, where we were going to set up operations. That same morning an emissary from the commissioner of Social Security came and asked, "What do you need?" I said, "I need about six lawyers, and I've found that your switchboard doesn't know that we're here, and I've had some difficulty getting calls."

"Well, as to the lawyers," he said (he looked at his watch and it was now about 11:00 A.M.), "do you mind if they don't report until after lunch?" I said, "No, I don't mind at all, thank you." The next morning there was a phone on my desk that was so direct I didn't have to dial 9.

After about six weeks we needed to decentralize the files, which were all in Baltimore, and we needed to get them to the regional offices where they could be used. The day we needed to do this, there was a civilian pilot's strike, and we couldn't send them by airmail. We delivered the files to Charlottesville and New York by car. I got an idea. I didn't consult anyone, I just did it. I told six of the senior public-health officers on my staff to go home and put on their uniforms. We cut military orders for them and sent them up to Andrews Air Force Base in a truck with the files. We cribbed orders similar to those used by the Pentagon and had the surgeon general sign them with his alternate title of vice admiral. Nobody was going to question the orders of a vice admiral, particularly if you couldn't understand the initials after his name! The next day the other six regional offices had their files.[66]

The field investigations forged ahead in a tense and alien environment.

We would fall back on Social Security investigators in difficult cases. Robert Ball, the Social Security administrator, provided us everything we asked for. At first if we got into rough stuff we called in the FBI. But it never seemed to work. They always said everybody was in compliance. They didn't seem to find any problem with segregation.

You would go into a town and you would immediately be followed by state police or local cops. A lot of the lower-paid employees in hospitals were blacks, and you couldn't be seen talking to these people or they would be fired the next day. . . . You would make the arrangements secretly in advance. You'd go into something like the local dry goods store. The cops usually wouldn't follow you into the store, or, if they did, you'd go into the ladies' lingerie department. A cop in uniform was usually unwilling to go into ladies' lingerie, and you'd go down the stairs and out the back door, and your contact would take you to the meeting. There, the local NAACP or a church group would meet with you and with some of the black employees of the hospital. They'd go over the floor plans of the hospital with you and show you where the black lunchroom was, and you'd learn about the other things, like the doctor that would bring in his maid to occupy a bed and so forth. You'd then go on the visit and the hospital administrator would take you on a tour. You'd go down to the basement where you knew the black staff cafeteria was, and he'd say, "Well, why don't we go up this way?" and you'd say, "No, we'd like to go this way." You'd then walk into the shabby black staff lunchroom.

Nothing was organized, and we knew we had to be selective about where we went if it all was going to get done. We'd call on black physicians to help. Dr. John Holloman, who was president of the National Medical Association, was hired on a part-time basis and would spend a day a week with us making calls to local physicians in the South to find out the problem spots. We'd talk to a network of civil rights organizations. We relied to a large extent on contacts with community groups.

You'd get a little nervous in some communities that were tense. You'd kind of try to let slip that you were with the FBI because we figured they would be less willing to mess with us.

We'd go to work in the morning in Baltimore, and by 9:15 two or three mornings a week there would be a phone call, and one of our investigators had been stuck in jail. The usual charge was driving a stolen car. What they did was, whenever a rental car was late being returned, the rental-car company files a stolen car report. When the car is turned in, they file another report saying the car has been returned. The local police department keeps active the first reports but does not act on the second. They know you're coming, and they make sure you get one of the "stolen" ones. Sometimes he doesn't make it to the hotel. Sometimes he does, and they just arrest him if he's difficult on the visit to the hospital—if, for example, you ask to see the chart of the patient in the biracial room who is really one of the physician's maids. If the gracious lunch at the country club doesn't make you less persistent, then the next time you got in the car, you were jailed! Sometimes the detailed "volunteer investigators," the veterinarian or the dentist from the Public Health Service, would panic.[67]

By June the momentum had begun to shift. Enough facilities had complied with the requirements, however reluctantly, that it became clear that the Feds weren't going to back down. There was an increasing confidence and seat-of-the-pants aggressiveness on the part of the investigators. Investigative teams did not stop at the visible symbols. Confederate Memorial Hospital in Louisiana was told, for example, that they must not only take the "white" and "colored" signs off the doors but that they must also label them "Entrance" and "Exit" and fix the door handles accordingly. They were also told not just to take the "colored" and "white" signs out of the waiting rooms, but to label one "main waiting room" and to cordon off the other one, putting in a sign in saying "overflow waiting room—to be used only when the main waiting room is full." For six months I got monthly reports from a union steward whose union was in the Civil Rights Leadership Conference about how the signs were working."[68]

Two telegrams came from a town in North Carolina to OEHO, one from the black and one from the white hospital, wanting to know what they needed to do to comply and become eligible for Medicare. MERGE, said the one-word telegram sent to both in return. The hospitals dutifully set about doing just that, in less than six weeks.

Word was received through its informal network of civil rights workers that, even though some of the hospitals in Louisiana were making an effort to comply, the Red Cross blood bank still segregated the blood supplies. A telegram was apparently sent to the Louisiana Hospital Association, indicating that unless the blood bank was integrated, *all* the hospitals in Louisiana that used this blood supply would be out of compliance with Title VI and thus would be ineligible for a Medicare provider agreement. There was no attempt to check the legality of such a position with the General Counsel's office, no attempt to buck the decision up the chain of command. It was just sent. More significantly, there was no effort to file a protest. The blood banks were integrated overnight. "We were really doing something. We really felt useful."[69]

In the midst of all of this activity a key southern senator and opponent of the civil rights law wrote that he wanted to establish a policy that if the senior physician and the treating physician agreed that integrated room assignment would be detrimental to the health of the patient, OHEO would not insist on that requirement. The office wrote back indicating that they required only one physician's statement. The implication was that if a physician didn't certify this, it was perfectly all right to randomly assign rooms. "He did us a great favor," observed one of the staff who had been struggling at the time with the issue. "We didn't want to kill people, we just wanted to reform them." The policy, based on OEHO's response to a southern senator's inquiry, served as the first utilization review guidelines for hospitals established under the Medicare program. The policy established a new complicating diagnostic condition, one that required special patient management in the hospital—racism. Physicians almost never exercised this newly granted medical authority to diagnose and treat this condition (perhaps more out of their irritation with the extra paperwork than social convictions!). However, in so doing, they collectively produced the largest miracle cure in twentieth-century American hospitals.

As the deadline drew near, Hubert Humphrey asked whether there was anything he could do to help, even if it was just checking forms. He was put to work making phone calls. On the instructions of the president he called the mayors of cities where there remained concern about hospitals. According to a June 18 memo to the president by Douglas Cater, Humphrey had made calls to the mayors of Baton Rouge, New Orleans, Greensboro, Nashville, Knoxville, Houston, Jacksonville, and Dallas and expected to complete calls to the cities in Alabama over the weekend. A follow-up letter had been sent by the vice president to each of the mayors along with the DHEW status report on the hospitals in his city. "He reports that the Mayors have been uniformly appreciated of this effort and are ready to cooperate,"[70] reported Cater.

Lyndon Johnson did not spare the hospital industry from the "treatment" he had earlier subjected legislators to in securing passage of the Civil Rights Act. On June 3, Johnson received the Award of Merit from the National Council of Senior Citizens in the White House Rose Garden and used the occasion to turn up the heat on the more recalcitrant community hospitals who had yet to comply with Title VI requirements for Medicare. "It is fitting that we should come together once more on the eve of a great new era for older Americans. Next month the medical care program that you and I labored so long and so hard for will become a cherished reality. . . . I have asked you this morning—you and every one of your local organizations to get in there and help all that you can. Alert your hospitals to the requirements of the law, particularly the nondiscrimination requirements of Title VI. Encourage them to meet those requirements."[71] On June 15 at a meeting of hospital and medical leaders, the last of more than two thousand meetings that federal officials had participated in with local medical societies and hospital officials over the previous year, President Johnson was even more direct.

> Never before, except in mobilizing for war, I think, has any government made such extensive preparations for any undertaking as we have made in connection with medical care. . . . Now we all know there are going to be problems. One of them arises from compliance with the laws of the land, specifically the Civil Rights Act. In some communities older people may be deprived of medical care because their hospitals fail to give equal treatment to all citizens and they have discriminatory practices.
>
> Well, we believe the answer to that problem is a simple one and that Congress has given it in the law itself. We ask every citizen to obey the law.
>
> A majority of hospitals—we think now more than 80%—have already assured us that they will. And I am hopeful that most others—when it is understood and when it is explained—will make an attempt to come into compliance. But we cannot rest easy as long as any of our older citizens lose their rights because of hospital defiance or because of delay.
>
> Now we are going to hear about those cases. Mr. Rayburn, who served here 50 years, used to say that it is typical of the American people to give more recognition to a donkey that will kick a barn down than to a carpenter who will build one.
>
> That applies to all our people. And to those who still stand outside the gates I want to say this: Please comply. If you discriminate against some older citizens in your community, then you make it very difficult for the whole program.
>
> The Federal Government is not going to retreat from its clear responsibility and what the Members of Congress have written into the law. And I hope that you will not retreat either.
>
> So you are here today to help us make this reality clear to your communities. Because there is always a last minute hope that we can "fudge it" a little bit and we can prolong it and "it won't be necessary." Now that is one problem and it is a serious problem for the 20 percent group, as you can see.[72]

During June the workload and pressure on the OEHO staff grew. "Everyone worked eighteen to twenty hours a day. We used a hotel room near Social Security just to shower and change clothes." Another staff person just moved a cot into his office, putting his marriage on hold, which miraculously survived.

On June 23, the president was briefed on possible emergency plans for dealing with the states with noncomplying hospitals and the fear of a surge in demand. In Mississippi compliance remained at 20 percent. Compliance in Alabama and Georgia now stood at 51 percent and 53 percent respectively. If Medicare patients were unable to receive essential treatment from the recalcitrant hospitals, it could do serious damage to the new program and its aggressive stand on Title VI enforcement. It was clear now, however, that there would be no backing down. The emergency plans for noncomplying states were as follows:

1. In a serious emergency, the individual can receive treatment in a non-complying hospital and Medicare will pay for it.
2. In a life-endangering emergency, Federal hospital facilities can and will admit civilians under Medicare. Since such Federal facilities are clearly insufficient, however, Cohen [Wilbur Cohen, assistant secretary of DHEW] recommends no action at this time to create a public expectation that will cause patients to show up at Federal facilities.
3. In individual instances, the Secretary of the Armed Services can admit a person to a service hospital. This constitutes a stand-by authority which you can use for "compassion" cases, but clearly is not workable across the board.
4. By executive order, you can establish a new admission policy for Public Health Service and Armed Services hospitals, but *not* VA hospitals. This covers only a very few empty beds in the South. Nationwide, it covers a sizeable number. I have asked Cohen to develop a plan for using these as an emergency reserve.[73]

Peter Libassi was in charge of keeping communication open with Congress concerning the hospital compliance program as the final deadline approached. Libassi, as one of the OEHO staff persons observed later, was in the impossible position of trying to direct the civil rights efforts of the department while at the same "keeping peace on the Hill." In a memo to the White House on June 28 he outlined the DHEW's activities on the Hill related to the hospital compliance program.

The Secretary met with eleven Senators and staff representatives of 35 offices. . . . The Department has completed meetings with the following [congressional] delegations: Louisiana, Alabama, Virginia and North Carolina. The Mississippi, Georgia, and South Carolina delegations were contacted but meetings could not be arranged. Senator Stennis attended the Alabama meeting but was not willing to arrange a meeting with his delegation.

These four meetings followed the usual pattern with the Senators and Congressmen objecting to the Department's policies as they understood them. Where their assumptions as to [D]HEW's positions were erroneous, they were corrected (the Department does not require a quota of Negroes in a hospital nor a Negro and white patient in every room).[74]

On June 30, 1966, the eve of Medicare implementation, President Lyndon Johnson made the following statement inaugurating the program.

MEDICARE begins tomorrow.

Tomorrow, for the first time, nearly every older American will receive hospital care—not as an act of charity, but as the insured right of a senior citizen. Since I signed the historic Medicare act last summer, we have made more extensive preparation to launch this program than for any other peaceful undertaking in our Nation's history.

Now we need your help to make Medicare succeed. Medicare will succeed—if hospitals accept their responsibility under the law not to discriminate against any patient because of race. More than 92 percent of the beds in our Nation's general hospitals are already in compliance with the law. . . . This program is not just a blessing for older Americans. It is a test for all Americans—a test of our willingness to work together.

In the past, we have always passed that test. I have no doubt about the future. I believe that July 1, 1966, marks a new day of freedom for our people.[75]

It had been a remarkable demonstration of the nation's ability to work together. More than one thousand hospitals had been quietly, uneventfully, and successfully desegregated. The American Hospital Association, state hospital associations, DHEW officials, state health departments, local mayors and city officials, senior-citizens groups, civil rights groups, hospital board members, nursing staffs, administrators, medical staffs, and congressional delegations and their staffs had all worked to achieve a quiet revolution. A key part of our national life, one essential for the healing not only of bodies, but also of the body politic, one that had lagged behind on racial integration, was now showing the way. Its successes had helped close the growing credibility gap produced by the failures of substantial progress on the desegregation of public schools. Maybe, just maybe, we meant what we said. It was the high-water mark of converging national consensus. Just out of sight, far more difficult tests lay ahead.

CHAPTER 5

The Federal Retreat

Things Fall Apart

Just as the Medicare program started, other things began to unravel. Racial divisions that had been closing widened again. The unprecedented growth of the U.S. economy in the 1950s and 1960s slackened, and budget deficits widened. The rising economic tide that lifts all boats had begun to ebb. A sense of limitless possibilities that had propelled Johnson's vision of programs for the Great Society now met with increasing skepticism. The cost of the Vietnam War, itself a product of that optimism, cast a growing shadow.

Among the country's black leadership, tensions resurfaced between those who supported a path of separate development and those who supported integration. The visible symbols of Jim Crow that had helped to mobilize people both across racial lines and within the black community itself began to disappear. Rising expectations bumped up against a core of white intransigence and stark inequities that remained a part of American life. Increasingly, many blacks felt that in abandoning separate institutions such as schools and hospitals they were giving up too much to get too little. The balance of influence shifted back toward the Booker T. Washington wing of the country's black leadership, advocating separate development, or what was now called Black Power.

Urban riots rather than nonviolent protests now captured the media spotlight. The nation endured four summers of riots in urban ghettos, beginning with one in North Philadelphia in August 1964. Martin Luther King's assassination in Memphis on April 4, 1968, set off the last wave of riots of the decade.

The conflict spread to college campuses. At the A&T campus in Greensboro, students protested in the turmoil following King's death. National Guardsmen arrived in armored personnel carriers. Sniper fire came from the A&T campus; the National Guardsmen returned the fire, and three police officers were wounded. Black student protests spread in 1969 to Cornell, Swarthmore, UCLA, University of Pennsylvania, Rutgers, San Francisco State, Harvard, and many others. The protests spread to urban high schools. The police riot at the Democratic Convention in 1968 and subsequent Vietnam War protests all added to the sense that the glue that held things together was dissolving.

Civil rights organizations that had emerged in the early part of the 1960s fragmented under these new tensions. Quentin Young, who became president of the Medical Committee for Human Rights in 1966, reflected on this transformation.

> There was a strong nationalist trend among the [southern] blacks. They wanted us to go back north. To our credit, we did that. Our membership went way down, but we had a glorious second phase. We played an important role in occupational and women's health. We continued to work on racism in our own backyard. It's different, however, to take on your colleagues.
>
> The second phase, or postsouthern phase, involved work with a lot of Freedom Centers that provided health services. In Chicago we had about a dozen. We had Black Panther and Hispanic clinics. They enjoyed significant support among medical students. The Black Panther Clinic was a classy place to be. All the kids at the clinic were counterculture, antiwar, and dressed grungy. They used to give me a hard time because I dressed in a tie and a suit. I had enough problems and didn't want to make a statement with my clothes. One day the director of the Black Panther Clinic called everyone into the recreation room for a special meeting. "You are confusing the people," he announced to the group. "From now on, I want you all to put on a shirt and a tie and dress like physicians."[1]

The struggle to end divisions in health care after the implementation of Medicare reflected this chaotic and troubling middle passage. It can be seen as a microcosm, a parable of the larger failure to end many racial divisions. This story and its lessons is one that echoes without final resolution up until the present.

OEHO and the Last Campaign

The arrival of the July 1, 1966, Medicare deadline presented the Office of Equal Health Opportunity with three problems. First, roughly six hundred of the more intransigent hospitals remained as visible, embarrassing symbols of Jim Crow, challenging the credibility of the enforcement efforts. As of midnight on June 30, 1966, 6,593 hospitals had received Title VI clearance, and 327 other applicants were awaiting clearance from remaining Title VI concerns. About three hundred other hospitals had chosen simply not to apply for Medicare certification and remained, at least in theory, outside the sphere of influence of the federal government. Second, hospitals represented just the tip of an iceberg. Below the surface loomed a complex private medical world. That world involved physician admission practices to hospitals and their relationships with nursing homes and specialists as well as a complex, almost impenetrable system of financing and cross-subsidies. There could be no equal health opportunity without addressing the racially disparate impact of such subtleties. Finally, the two-front war continued. OEHO had to deal not only with the intransigent hard-core hospitals and the complexities that underlie the medical-care system, but also with the largely hostile congressional committees that provided oversight and approved their budgets.

Harvesting the Remaining "Low-Hanging Fruit"

OEHO began to implement the procedures worked out for dealing with noncomplying hospitals. They dealt with the easiest cases first, "the low-hanging fruit." The easiest of these were the facilities that had failed to execute the Title VI assurance form and complete the public health form describing their facilities' operations (HEW Form 441 and PHS Form 4867). It was as if they had said, "Go ahead, I dare you to try to enforce this." Monday, July 11, 1966, letters went out to three hospitals under the surgeon general's signature saying that their applications for the Medicare program had been deferred. The three hospitals, two in Mississippi and one in Tennessee, had not submitted the required forms, despite repeated requests. The letter further advised them that unless they responded within fifteen days they would be sent a notice of opportunity for a hearing to decide whether their eligibility for Medicare and other continuing programs should be ended. It also said that state agencies would be notified and welfare medical funding could be ended. In a process that would become routine, copies of this notification were also sent to the White House and the attorney general, along with the names of their senators and congressional representatives.

Hospitals that persisted in providing clearly identifiable separate accommodations for black and white patients were easy targets. Letters were sent to the Fifth Avenue General Hospital in Huntsville, Alabama, and the Hampton General Hospital in Varnville, South Carolina, by August 1. Fifth Avenue General had yet to adopt and announce a policy that it would admit blacks, and Hampton General, "despite extensive negotiations, is segregated throughout, including wings, patient rooms, waiting rooms, dining rooms, etc."[2] On August 24, thirteen additional hospitals in Alabama, Georgia, Louisiana, Mississippi, South Carolina, and Texas were sent similar notices. Most were small—only three had more than seventy-five beds, and one had only eight. Many were vestiges of an earlier era of medical care and would eventually close.

On November 23, eighteen hospitals, after all efforts to negotiate voluntary compliance had been exhausted, were sent notices of the opportunity for hearings. These eighteen were a motley assortment of renegades. Only six had more than seventy-five beds. One, a 75-bed tuberculosis sanatorium in Louisiana, continued to send black patients to the dilapidated older wings of the facility. Greenwood LeFlore Hospital in Greenwood, Mississippi, a 176-bed city- and county-owned facility, had maintained a separate wing on the first floor for blacks with a separate entrance. When rooms in this wing were filled, black patients were simply placed in the hallways, and the hospital had been unwilling to modify this policy sufficiently to assure assignment of beds on a nondiscriminatory basis. Clarendon Memorial Hospital, a 55-bed county facility in Manning, South Carolina, had been completely segregated at the time of the initial deferral letter. At a subsequent meeting in Washington between the OEHO chief and the hospital administrator, also attended by Senator Strom Thurmond, many issues were resolved. "However, the hospital adamantly refused to stop assigning patients on a segregated basis, insisting that Negroes and whites *preferred* to remain segregated."[3] Jefferson Davis Memorial Hospital, a 150-bed facility in Natchez, Mississippi, dug in its heels over the same issue.

Among the hospitals sent hearing notices in November, Newton Hospital in Newton, Mississippi, a 40-bed county hospital, attempted to circumvent integration with more subtlety. The hospital assigned its private paying patients to private rooms on a nondiscriminatory basis. However, the black welfare patients were assigned to a basement corridor, while the white welfare patients were distributed elsewhere. Many hospitals in all regions of the country would soon use Medicare funds that covered capital costs to rapidly expand private room accommodations.

All but these few exceptions among the hospitals that had applied for Medicare participation moved at least far enough to get initial clearance from OEHO. The lure of the Medicare and Medicaid dollars was strong enough to ensure at least this initial compliance.

However, some voluntary hospitals were determined to avoid such controls, even at the cost of Medicare participation. Some of these facilities were able for a short time to find loopholes that assured a continued supply of federal dollars in spite of nonparticipation in the Medicare program. Some tried to take advantage of the emergency care loophole provided in the final days before the implementation of Medicare.[4]

The Medicare program was directly under the control of the secretary of DHEW. Federal funds from other sources, such as CHAMPUS (Civilian Health and Medical Program of the Uniformed Services), flowed to hospitals not participating in Medicare. CHAMPUS provides payment to civilian medical providers for uniformed services personnel, their dependents, and retirees. The lack of direct control over the purse strings of such programs sometimes called for more devious tactics, as one of the more inventive staff members of OEHO recalled.

> I was really able to exercise my predilection for the unconventional approach. We got a call from a hospital in Meridian, Mississippi. It was a hospital that was run by nuns that had complied very early. They complained that they were losing their shirts to a nearby hospital that had decided not to comply with Title VI to receive Medicare funds so they wouldn't have to desegregate, but was getting a great deal of money through the CHAMPUS program. A person on my staff was a retired colonel. First, I got him an invitation to speak at an American Veterans Association meeting in Jackson, Mississippi. This gave him the authority to wear his uniform on the way there and back. The job he had was to inspect the hospital that had the CHAMPUS money. The hospital jumped immediately to the wrong conclusion we wanted them to jump [to]. They thought the Department of Defense was bearing down on them and began to integrate their facility.[5]

OEHO, however, was not alone in pressing the issue, even in situations where hospitals had attempted to insulate themselves carefully from Title VI enforcement by refusing to participate in the Medicare or Medicaid programs. The old Roper Hospital had originally opened in 1856 as Charleston's first community hospital and had eventually served as the primary facility used by Charleston's black population until its closing in 1957. The new Roper Hospital was opened in 1946 and served Charleston's white population. Following the passage of the 1964 Civil Rights Act, the chief of the medical staff had brought a motion to the governing board to sign a compliance agreement. Unlike most hospitals in the nation where such motions were presented, this one was defeated. The board did not want federal interference with hospital policy and voted to cease receiving federal funds of any kind. The Justice Department, however, eventually sued the facility. The suit not only forced Roper to integrate its facilities, but also to end discriminatory hiring practices. The suit argued that Roper's cafeteria and snack bar served visitors from other states and thus fell under the provisions of the interstate commerce clause of the legislation. Such places were subject to Titles II (interstate commerce) and VII (employment) of the 1964 Civil Rights Act.[6] In March 1969, the U.S. district court accepted the Justice Department's reasoning and ordered an end to discrimination in both employment and admissions at the facility.[7]

The Campaign for the Integration of State Hospitals

Largely overlooked in the initial wave of certifying acute general hospitals for Medicare were the state psychiatric and tuberculosis hospitals in southern states that had historically maintained racially segregated arrangements for patient care. These were also easy targets. They were state facilities and thus clearly fell under the federal constitutional prohibitions denying any citizen equal protection through state action. These segregated facilities were confined to the South and so presented a convenient political target for the Johnson administration. Only the states of Virginia, Alabama, and Mississippi resisted.[8] All the other southern states, however haltingly, had begun to integrate their facilities. A number of states had originally argued for "freedom of choice" plans, the notion that the individual patient should be given the right to choose whether they wished to receive care in the black facility or be cared for in the white one. Marilyn Rose, assigned to OEHO at the time as its legal counsel commented about such "choice,"

> The "freedom of choice" issue was to us quite bizarre, even as applied to patients in general hospitals. A black witness in one of the early hearings (concerning the use of "freedom of choice" in general hospitals) testified that he did not "choose" that his daughter be placed in the white wing of the hospital (or in a double room with a white patient) because of the risks taken by such a choice. "Who knows what would be done to her in the hospital after making such a choice." To us, it was even more ridiculous [in psychiatric hospitals]—people were being confined in these institutions because they lacked the capacity to make rational choices.[9]

In Virginia, Alabama, and Mississippi many state mental health officials engaged in largely mock battles with OEHO staff calculated to avoid political retaliation for decisions to integrate state facilities, which the health officials generally supported.

This appears to have particularly been the case in Virginia, the first state system tackled by OEHO. Investigation teams, which included a psychiatrist, had documented the referral system in Virginia. Blacks, no matter where they resided, were sent to the hospital in Petersburg, while whites were assigned to one of three other hospitals, usually in closer geographic proximity to where they lived.

In late October 1966, Bob Nash and Marilyn Rose met with Dr. Shep, chairman of the Department of Psychiatry, and other psychiatrists at the University of Virginia Medical School, who were clearly interested in solving the problem. Although the official DHEW position defined the consequences much more narrowly, Nash took the negotiating stance that *all* federal funds to the university would be jeopardized by the department's participation in the state system through their residency and internship and other programs. Nash knew better—and so did the psychiatrists, most likely. Dr. Shep indicated that he thought the governor would be very concerned about the loss of all federal support for the university. Shortly after the meeting, Nash learned that the governor's office had ordered the freedom-of-choice plan dropped and wanted the matter to be settled along the lines suggested by OEHO. Reflecting back, Rose interpreted the meeting as a ritual designed to limit the political damage for the governor.

> I suspect the whole meeting was a set-up. High officials in the Governor's office, if not the Governor himself, wanted the matter settled, and needed an excuse to drop the freedom of choice plan. Nash believed in, and wanted, the result, and used the opportunity to get it. At that time I felt that I could not advise him in front of the University of Virginia psychiatrists that he was misstating Department policy (although I must confess that I liked the result). However, not everyone in Virginia government agreed with the position of these psychiatrists and the Governor; at the meeting I attended with Nash in Richmond to sign the negotiated settlement, the Assistant General Counsel of Virginia who was handling the matter for the State bitterly characterized the agreement as "Appomattox."[10]

As state-operated facilities, they were accountable to state governors. Unfortunately, the governors of Alabama and Mississippi saw them as emotional symbols that could be manipulated for political gain. Alabama and Mississippi presented far more serious challenges to the OEHO than Virginia. During the first part of 1967 OEHO was involved in a difficult test of wills with Governors Johnson of Mississippi and Wallace of Alabama.

Alabama would not budge. An inspection team that included Dr. Hunt, a psychiatrist and retired associate commissioner of mental health in New York state, surveyed the state facilities. They first visited Bryce Mental Hospital and Partlow State School for the Retarded in Tuscaloosa. These facilities predominately provided facilities for white patients, with a smaller, inferior facility for blacks. The inspection team then proceeded to Searcy Hospital outside of Mobile, Alabama's black state hospital.

Services for patients at Searcy were custodial and the general wards were horrid. At Searcy there were only five doctors, four of whom were foreign doctors (whose primary language was not English). They were not licensed in the United States. The fifth psychiatrist was the Administrator, who was elderly, obviously not conversant with modern psychiatry and seemed to be running a southern plantation. A visit to the wards suggested to me what one might have found in the 19th century, at a time when mental patients were warehoused. The wards looked like prison cells. It was a scene out of . . . Kafka.[11]

Governor George Wallace was initiating a run for the presidency in 1968 as a third-party candidate, riding the growing backlash against integration. Alabama's state hospitals had begun to desegregate in 1966 but all were ordered to resegregate by Governor Wallace. Subsequent investigations revealed that the Montgomery facility segregated patients by room, sections, eating areas, and recreation programs. On January 13, 1967, OEHO sent notice of an opportunity for a hearing to the State of Alabama.

Alabama's mental health facilities are completely segregated. Searcy Mental Hospital is a grossly inferior and inadequate mental institution for Negroes and Bryce Hospital is the more up-to-date white only institution. Partlow School for mentally ill children is completely segregated internally, and shockingly inferior care is provided Negro children. Unlike even Virginia and other states which have made some effort to comply with Title VI, Alabama defiantly resists any and all change. The State mental health agency began to comply with Title VI by desegregating Partlow School and ordering transfers of patients from one hospital to another, but this policy was reversed by the Governor's office and the facilities remain as segregated today as they were in mid-1964. The Superintendent of State Hospitals has noted in official correspondence with PHS that the institutions are not in compliance with Title VI.
Alabama frankly admits its mental health complex is out of compliance but refuses to consider reasonable measures to change this status. It is expected that a notice of opportunity for hearing will not result in new negotiations, but we hope that this, together with parallel Title VI and judicial actions in the state, may result in some change.[12]

The hearing officer issued his decision, recommending that federal funds be cut off. The state appealed to the secretary of DHEW, who supported the decision of the hearing officer. The State of Alabama filed a lawsuit against the secretary in federal court. (The local chapter of the NAACP also filed suit on behalf of black patients under the Fourteenth Amendment in the same court, and the cases were consolidated.)

Several aides at the Bryce Hospital in Tuscaloosa had told the investigators about an elaborate tiered salary structure that gave white aides more than blacks, male aides more than females, and those who worked at the white facilities more than those who worked at the black one. The judge ordered the State of Alabama to release the information on the salary structures, and Rose returned to Bryce Hospital in Tuscaloosa to collect the information on the employment records. The visit was cut short because of snow, which spared her from becoming a victim of retaliation for her efforts.

> I got on the Interstate and drove much below the speed limit because of the snow. Nevertheless, after a short time, my car was wobbling and skidding. I drove slower and slower, but could not stop the skidding. I got down to 10–15 miles an hour, but could not stop the skidding. At one point my car turned around on the highway. Luckily there was virtually no one on the road, because of the snow. Realizing that I was barely controlling the car, I continued to drive as slow as I could until I reached the first exit and got off, blinking my emergency lights to warn other drivers. There was a gas station at the bottom of the ramp and I pulled into it. A young man came out of the station, and yelled at me something like "your right front wheel is almost off the car!" He checked the wheel and said that the lugs (or most of them) were gone. Had it not been snowing, I would have been going over 60 miles an hour, and could have been killed or badly injured.[13]

Mississippi, however, represented the most difficult test for OEHO. Inspections of the facilities by OEHO investigators began in May 1967. The state mental-health system consisted of three facilities. One, Ellisville, provided care to white mentally retarded patients. Another facility provided care for the white mentally ill, with a black patient population of less than 1 percent. A third facility, Whitfield State Hospital, provided care for black and white mentally ill patients in segregated units as well as black mentally retarded patients. In 1966, Governor Johnson had ordered a reversal of plans to desegregate the facilities.[14] State officials stood firm in negotiations with OEHO, arguing for their freedom-of-choice assignment policy that left all facilities racially segregated, except for token black admissions to the two white facilities. State officials in Governor Johnson's administration argued that the racial segregation in the Mississippi State Insane Hospital was of therapeutic value to the patients. In any event, the OEHO investigators described a far-from-therapeutic situation at the Mississippi State Insane Hospital's Whitefield facility.

> The investigation team, which included one psychiatrist, found considerable evidence to support racial discrimination in three major areas: (1) segregation of patients; (2) restrictive admission policies; and (3) differential services and benefits. An especially poor situation was found in the treatment of 802 Negro retardates. They were segregated in a special annex of the Whitfield facility, where they are provided no testing, education, training, or vocational rehabilitation, despite the fact that many could lead potentially useful lives on the outside. White retardates, in comparison, receive an advanced program of training and rehabilitation.[15]

In his subsequent negotiations with the executive secretary of the Mississippi Board of Trustees of Mental Institutions, Robert Nash shared the integration plan worked out with the State of Virginia. The notice of hearing was prepared in mid-June 1967 and was awaiting the surgeon general's signature when it hit a snag that cast a shadow over the federal civil rights offensive. Rose reflected on the events.

> That evening some issue related to welfare appropriations came up, and Wilbur Cohen (Assistant Secretary of DHEW at the time) apparently agreed to stop the Notice from going forward in response to some promise or threat to the welfare appropriation. The Notice of Hearing sat for seven months in my office; I finally got permission to mail it to Mississippi in December 1967 after the welfare appropriation issues had been resolved. Those of us in the civil rights programs were quite angry that the civil rights considerations would take a back seat. When I finally got the notice out, Hudspeth (the Mississippi official in charge of the state hospital system) called me and asked, "What took you so long?" I responded, "You know, and I know and Senator Stennis knows what took us so long." He laughed and said, "well I couldn't do anything until I got it, you knew that."[16]

In general, the federal government lacked the leverage of the Medicare dollars in dealing with the state mental hospitals that it had with the acute hospitals. While not directly connected to the Medicare program, the total federal dollars provided to Mississippi's state mental health system, including Veteran's Administration, the National Institutes of Mental Health, and the Department of Agriculture, totaled approximately a half million dollars. OEHO had even less leverage on the six segregated, state-owned tuberculosis sanitariums in Alabama. Only about fifteen thousand dollars in federal support, through the Department of Agriculture's Surplus Commodities Program, was going to these facilities. However, a half-million-dollar Hill-Burton grant application was pending to one facility that could have been rejected if an acceptable settlement was not reached. The "low hanging fruit" were now all picked. The easy victories had been achieved and momentum was shifting. Extracting victories out of the federal civil rights initiatives got harder.

The Stalemated Offensive

Even more difficult to address than the intransigence of some of the smaller renegade general hospitals or the state facilities in Mississippi and Alabama, however, was the more sophisticated resistance of some of the larger and more politically connected voluntary general hospitals in the South. OEHO now had to deal with the Title VI–certified facilities that were "poor performers," facilities willing to go just far enough to assure the continued flow of Medicare funds.

Druid City Hospital in Tuscaloosa, Alabama, became the first test case. Nineteen separate contacts and notifications had been made to the hospital in an effort to correct discriminatory practices. Druid City Hospital was a trendsetter and not a backward, marginal facility, as were many facilities involved in earlier enforcement actions. The rationale for confronting Druid City Hospital was set forth in a memo to the Justice Department.

> It is a large modern hospital to which a number of medical facilities in Central Alabama look for guidance. For example, two years ago Druid City undertook to convert its entire facility into private rooms to avoid any possibility of biracial room occupancy and a large number of other hospitals in the surrounding area followed suit. The private room plan proved unworkable under Medicare so Druid City and the others have resorted to "tokenism" in their room assignments. Druid City is thus an ideal case with which to litigate the "tokenism" issue because many other hospital administrators will be looking at this case. We expect that the issues and personalities involved in this case will result in considerable local interest and publicity.[17]

In other areas hospitals were more successful in avoiding room assignment issues through conversion to private rooms. For Druid City as well as many other facilities, the room assignment requirements represented a temporary inconvenience, to be corrected through new hospital construction now, ironically, generously subsidized by the same federal Medicare and Medicaid programs that were the basis of enforcing Title VI compliance.

Hospitals, however, could not only manipulate accommodations to minimize the mixing of the races within a facility through the construction of private rooms, they could also, indirectly, influence who presented themselves for admission to the hospital in the first place. The Committee to End Discrimination in Chicago Medical Institutions in the 1950s found that the admission practices of staff physicians could assure a remarkable degree of segregation of patients without the hospitals establishing official Jim Crow policies or engaging in any overtly discriminatory acts, such as refusing the admission of a black patient with private insurance. Physicians in larger cities have staff privileges on more than one hospital and can choose where to send each of their patients. They are reluctant to violate informal norms, for doing so could adversely affect their chances for reappointment. Physicians, or at least the payment for their services under Part B of Medicare, were exempted from Title VI. The general counsel of DHEW did, however, conclude that the hospital was legally responsible for the discriminatory referral practices of physicians on their staff. The theory was that hospitals granted privileges and thus were legally responsible for the admission practices of their physicians. That theory received a brutal defeat in the federal government's last offensive in Mobile, Alabama.

The Last Offensive

In the dark early morning hours of Sunday, January 27, 1967, in Mobile, Alabama, Dr. Jean Cowsert was apparently awakened by the sound of glass breaking in her kitchen window. She was found dead at 7:00 A.M. by her front steps, clad in pajamas and a bathrobe, fatally wounded in the chest by a single shot from a foreign made 38-caliber revolver.[18] The weapon, owned by Dr. Cowsert, was found underneath her body. Two days later, the death was ruled an accident. The coroner noted that there was "no evidence in the case of any intent nor any evidence of a second party involved."[19] Surrounding her death and unknown to those investigating it, however, swirled a bitter, protracted test of wills between the federal government, Mobile's largest hospital and its medical staff.

Up until 1965, medical and hospital care in Mobile had been divided strictly by race. The 540-bed Mobile Infirmary, the dominant institution in the region's social and medical hierarchy, served whites only. The 35-bed Saint Martin de Porres Hospital served private paying blacks of Mobile and was the only facility where black dentists and physicians could obtain privileges. Two additional hospitals with antebellum roots served both races: Mobile General Hospital, a 247-bed county facility for the indigent and Providence Hospital, a 262-bed facility operated by the Daughters of Charity of St. Vincent de Paul. Care in these two facilities was strictly segregated by race.[20] If, for example, there was an overflow of black patients in West Wing 7 at Providence Hospital, they were supplied with beds in the hall, even though beds lay empty in other white sections of the hospital.[21] The hospitals of Mobile served a population of about 500,000 of which one-third was black.[22] Following a pattern common to most Southern metropolitan areas, all four hospitals were located within a few blocks of each other, enabling white physicians, who crossed the boundaries of race, religion, and income in their practices, efficient access to the different accommodations custom prescribed for their patients. All four of these facilities had received substantial federal funds for their construction from the Hill-Burton program.

The four hospitals in Mobile, however, were among the 327 still awaiting Title VI clearance on June 30, 1966, as were slightly less than half the hospitals in Alabama. Among the four Mobile hospitals, Providence had made the most significant progress toward integration of its accommodations. In August 1965, the local civil rights group withdrew its complaint against Providence Hospital, informing federal officials that the facility had followed a determined policy to comply with Title VI.[23] Yet, these steps proved painful ones for Providence, whose census dropped significantly as white patients shifted their admissions to the Mobile Infirmary.[24] As the July 1, 1966, deadline drew near, a public meeting, arranged by Mobile's Mayor Joseph Langan with Dr. Leo Gehrig, the Assistant Surgeon General, and more than one hundred Mobile physicians, hospital board members, administrators, and civic leaders was held at the Mobile's Civic Auditorium on June 27. Perhaps reluctant to single out individual hospitals in a community for certification and, possibly, exacerbate the problem that Providence had already experienced, the OEHO had yet to certify any of the hospitals in Mobile. Providence, Mobile General, and Saint Martin de Porres finally received Title VI certification for Medicare funding on July 1. The Mobile Infirmary, the city's largest and best-equipped facility did not.

The decision not to certify the Infirmary plunged OEHO for the first time into the angrier and murkier waters of Title VI enforcement in medical practice. Yet, as one Mobile hospital administrator reflected, the advantage that the South had in integrating its health care was that there was nothing subtle about the way patients were segregated. This was certainly the case with the hospital admission practices of Mobile's physicians. During the last six months of 1965 only ten of the ten thousand patients admitted to the Mobile Infirmary had been black.[25] The Infirmary had admitted every patient referred by its medical staff, which included the majority of Mobile's physicians. Physicians were simply choosing to refer their black patients to facilities different from those of their white patients. From the perspective of the Mobile Infirmary, they were in full compliance with Title VI. From the perspective of the staff of the Office of Equal Health Opportunity, providing Title VI certification to the Infirmary would be tantamount to endorsing segregation. Similar hospital referral patterns existed in many communities. Chicago, as described in chapter 2, for example, had maintained a pattern of strict de facto segregation of its hospitals through the admitting practices of its physicians up until the 1960s.[26] OEHO hoped that the Mobile Infirmary case would serve as a test of the responsibilities of hospitals to assure that the admitting practices of their medical staffs was even handed. Enforcement of Title VI for hospitals would be an empty gesture if physicians, either through their own judgments, the implicit threat of loss of staff privileges or the fears of their patients, continued to selectively admit on the basis of race. OEHO, however, had touched a raw nerve. Beneath the surface lay more complex and subtle, racially disparate, patterns of practice that persist to the present in shaping specialty referrals and rates of therapeutic interventions.[27]

Dr. Jean Cowsert had been drawn into these angry and murky waters. An internist, she had graduated first in her 1954 class of the University of Alabama Medical School, one of two women in a class of sixty-two.[28] She had returned to her native Mobile in 1959 to practice and in 1966 had become president of the Providence Hospital medical staff, the first woman to hold that position. Described by various colleagues who recalled her as bright, aggressive, abrasive, and a bit of a loner, she had been instrumental in getting Providence Hospital to become the first in Alabama to participate in the Professional Activities and Medical Audit Program, an early precursor to current computerized medical auditing and profiling techniques. She was also a recent convert to Catholicism and a close friend of the administrator of Provident Hospital, Sister Andrea Hickey, who had initiated efforts to eliminate the racially segregated accommodations at Providence.

Dr. Cowsert's subsequent actions influenced OEHO's decision to block Title VI certification and to use the Mobile Infirmary as a test case. She had medical staff privileges at Mobile Infirmary and, as a participant in its staff meetings, served as a confidential informant to OEHO. In the vernacular of the cold war, equally appropriate to the cold war waged over racial integration, she was a mole. Dr. Cowsert was one of the persons that brought to the attention of OEHO the use of a loophole that had permitted the Infirmary to receive substantial Medicare payments beginning in July 1, 1966, for "emergency" admissions. The Social Security Administration quickly clamped down on this practice.[29] She was also probably one of the "confidential but reliable informants" referred to in an October 1966, letter from the local civil rights organization to DHEW. That letter accused the director of the hospital and leaders of its medical staff of working clandestinely to avoid complying with Title VI of the civil rights act. It accused them of "desperately but suavely defying the law relative to the acceptance of Negro patients and integration of its medical staff and personnel, other than on a token basis."[30] These were charges that Mobile Infirmary officials continued to vehemently deny. Some of the Mobile Infirmary's medical staff, however, had apparently vowed to never admit a black patient to the Infirmary. In an effort to focus pressure on this segment of the medical staff, OEHO repeatedly requested data on admission by race broken down by individual physician. The Infirmary refused all these requests. Dr. Cowsert, however, had apparently assisted in providing a confidential list of Infirmary Medical Staff members who were most emotional and active in opposing black admissions to the Mobile Infirmary. The list included twenty six physicians and was forwarded by the local Civil Rights group to the Director of OEHO on December 20, 1966.[31]

As the months without Medicare payments for the Mobile Infirmary dragged on, positions hardened, participants became more embittered and the pressure for some kind of settlement mounted. More than one hundred beds and an entire wing lay empty at the Mobile Infirmary.[32] The local paper published scathing editorials accusing DHEW of fashioning racial integration demands into "a blackjack for bureaucrats to wield in the Medicare program."[33] The Infirmary focused its significant political assets on DHEW. Delegations including Senator John Sparkman (D, AL), Mobile's Mayor Joseph Langan, and Representative Jack Edwards (R, AL) and pressure from Senator Lister Hill (D, AL), however, failed to break the impasse. Governor George Wallace weighed in describing the denial of a Medicare certification of the infirmary as not only "heartless but the most immoral act I can imagine" and demanded a congressional investigation.[34]

In December 1966, however, DHEW responded to these pressures by agreeing to conduct a top-level review of the Mobile Infirmary case and taking control away from the embattled OEHO. Deputy Surgeon General, Dr. Leo Gehrig, would return to Mobile in an effort to negotiate a settlement in early January 1967. In preparation for the visit, OEHO staff briefed Dr. Gehrig. In addition to the admission statistics, Gehrig was provided off the record information, including the identity of the Infirmary's medical staff informant, Dr. Cowsert. Meetings were held at the Infirmary with Dr. Gehrig during the first two weeks in January. Gehrig returned to OEHO in Washington towards the end of January and met with OEHO staff, believing that he had crafted the outlines of a workable settlement. In the course of that meeting, Gehrig reported that he had had the opportunity to talk with Dr. Cowsert on the phone from his hotel room. The OEHO staff was aghast, since those familiar with Federal civil rights investigations in the South at that time had to assume that such phone calls were monitored.[35] Less than two weeks later, early on Monday morning on January 28, Robert Nash, the Director of OEHO in Washington received a call from an administrator at the Mobile Infirmary, informing him of Dr. Cowsert's death. As OEHO's legal counsel at the time reflected later.

> The coroner's report was that she was accidentally shot, apparently having tripped, and shot herself. To this day I do not believe that finding. It seems too coincidental. What led the hospital administrator to call Nash about this incident, unless the word had gotten out that she was an informer? I am not implying that the administrator had anything to do with her death; there is nothing I ever learned which would indicate it. But if he knew she was an informer, others knew, and the knowledge may very well have come from the telephone call through the hotel switchboard ten days earlier.[36]

The Infirmary was soon notified of "interim" Title VI certification that would provide Medicare payments to the hospital retroactive to February 1, 1967. There had been no formal negotiated settlement, but the Mobile Infirmary numbers had improved somewhat. The number of blacks admitted to the Infirmary in January 1967 had increased to ninety and there was the possibility the Medicare payments could make the numbers improve significantly. OEHO staff had strongly opposed Gehrig's idea of interim certification. The Infirmary's medical staff had not budged and refused to agree as requested by the Deputy Surgeon General "to take the necessary steps to correct the pattern of segregation" and claimed that the request was "unethical."[37] They had unanimously rejected Gehrig's two preliminary proposals, (1) a temporary ninety-day certification plan and (2) that the Infirmary reiterate its nondiscriminatory policy relative to patient admissions and take disciplinary actions against members of its medical staff who violated that principle. The Board of the infirmary had again declined to be pushed into the position of monitoring and disciplining the admission practices of its medical staff. The *Mobile Register,* echoed local displeasure noting in an editorial that, Dr. Gehrig's proposal "actually makes it conclusive that any HEW claim of withholding certification for reasons other than bureaucratic displeasure, because the medical profession objects to performing as a parrot-like mouthpiece for rush-act mass integration of that hospital is entirely without foundation."[38]

While OEHO continued to insist publicly that it was a provisional arrangement, most knew otherwise. The lesson of the Medicare program, as with many federal funding programs, was that it is far easier to get institutions to do things in exchange for payments and far harder to take such payments away once the payments have been made. The Infirmary received full Title VI certification for Medicare beginning in July 1967. On June 28, 1967, the home of J. L. LeFlore, the leader of the local civil rights group that helped orchestrate the hospital integration efforts in Mobile was fire bombed. In the last six months of 1967, the census of the Mobile Infirmary hit a record of 93 percent and plans were completed for a six-story addition.[39] The death of Dr. Cowsert and the federal civil rights offensive that was somehow connected to it faded even from local memory.

The decision to certify the Mobile Infirmary for Medicare funds shocked many in DHEW and the broader civil rights community. In the wake of what seemed to be the virulent pressure mounted on behalf of the hospital and its physicians, it was tantamount to capitulation. The Mobile Infirmary case had offered an opportunity to review more systematically the issue of discriminatory physician-referral practices in the pending hearing. As Rose concluded later, "The referral practices issue was dead after the Mobile cave-in."[40] The tide had turned, and the Feds were now in retreat.

The Nursing-Home Title VI Program Flounders

The turn of the tide most dramatically affected Title VI enforcement in nursing homes, scheduled to begin participation in the Medicare program January 1, 1967, six months after the start of Medicare and just as the federal government had begun to cave in the Mobile Alabama confrontation. Title VI enforcement in nursing homes fell apart before it got started. Many saw enforcement in nursing homes as straying across a fuzzy boundary between the public and the intimate private lives of citizens. The private nursing-home industry—although it could hardly be called such in the early 1960s—was not dominated by massive standardized national and regional chains, as it is today. Many nursing homes were owner-operated converted houses that had evolved from facilities begun in the 1930s by nurses or poor widows who took in boarders. For many, these nursing homes fit the image of the fabled "Mrs. Murphy's boarding home." Mrs. Murphy was a powerful imaginary figure created by southern opponents to the Civil Rights Act during congressional debate. Her boarding home was an image created by opponents of Title II, the public-accommodation provisions.[41] She became a powerful symbol of white womanhood, whose honor was to be passionately defended. Surely the bill would not force such poor women, trying to eke out a meager existence, to have black men live in their homes? No one, including Kennedy and Johnson, was willing to go that far. Nursing-home patients in the early 1960s looked like boarding-home residents. There were few external controls on placement. None of the rules governing payment eligibility that were later to be created in the Medicare and Medicaid programs were yet in place. Most of the patients were really residents, frail elderly ones who needed a home. Furthermore, few private patients, and none supported by public funds, could afford single rooms. Was the federal government going to force race-blind room assignments? Johnson was apparently troubled by that question and saw a clear distinction between the standards that should be imposed on medical facilities and the homes in which people lived.

Such issues aside, the timing and operational constraints imposed on the Office of Equal Health Opportunity militated against enforcing the letter of the law for nursing homes. By January 1967 most of the momentum that had been part of the initial startup of Medicare was lacking. Most of the "volunteers" who had staffed most of the field investigation effort for hospitals had returned to their normal assignments. More than six thousand nursing-home facilities applying for Medicare certification filled out assurance and compliance forms, similar to those used for the hospitals. President Johnson apparently had decided not to enforce compliance in nursing homes, to rely on paper assurances alone. One of the persons on OCR's staff responsible for the program observed that it "was not a success . . . because we didn't change much."[42]

The nursing-home industry concluded that so long as discriminatory practices were not flaunted, there would be no intervention by federal officials. The following Louisiana newspaper account illustrates one strategy adopted: On January 1, 1967, facilities were magically transformed into nondiscriminating institutions.

> Intention to comply with the 1964 Civil Rights Act by eliminating all forms of segregation was announced today by 29 nursing homes in this area seeking to participate in Medicare.
>
> The nursing homes, all members of the Louisiana Nursing Home Association, made the following statement:

The governing boards of the listed extended care facilities have met and passed individual resolutions that effective Jan. 1, 1967, their institutions will be operated on a nondiscriminatory basis. This means that effective Jan. 1, 1967, and, thereafter, all facilities and services of the individual institutions will be available to all patients and employees on a nondiscriminatory basis.

Waiting rooms, public toilets, dining facilities, recreation rooms and room accommodations will be available without regard to race, color or national origin. This action will enable the institutions to continue receiving federal funds necessary for operation.

The listed institutions urge all public users and employees of said institutions to cooperate in this program so that the transition will be smooth and we can continue our mission of serving the aged of our community.[43]

Even if Title VI had been rigorously enforced in nursing homes, federal officials were in a far weaker position with nursing homes than with hospitals. Neither Medicare nor Medicaid offered the financial imperative for nursing homes that they had for hospitals. Medicare coverage for nursing-home care rarely accounted for more than 5 percent of a nursing home's income. Payments by state Medicaid programs were far less attractive than those to hospitals. More than half of the income of most nursing homes comes from out-of-pocket payments by residents and their families. There were no Title VI issues related to nursing homes that served private patients exclusively, and the states themselves, rather than the federal Medicare program, administered Medical Assistance programs. Many nursing homes simply chose not to participate in Medicare or Medicaid.

Strong advocacy by local black physicians and civil rights groups could have compensated for the lack of pressure from the federal government. Such advocacy, however, was absent. For physicians, nursing-home privileges were not worth fighting over. Nursing homes accounted for little income, did not serve as a source of professional development, and did not provide diagnostic and therapeutic support services essential to physicians' practices. For local civil rights groups, nursing homes were not a burning issue either. How could restricted access to a place no one wanted to go to be defined as a social injustice in desperate need of remedy?

Physician Practices Remain Outside Title VI

Even farther outside the reaches of the federal civil rights enforcement effort lay the practices of individual physicians. As participating providers, central to decisions about the use of services in the Medicare program, physicians themselves, one assumes, would have to comply with Title VI. But as a practical administrative matter, enforcing compliance would have been a daunting task. The sheer numbers—almost 150,000 office-based physicians participating in the Medicare program, the bulk in solo practices or small two- to five-person groups—made enforcement difficult to conceive. Defining what might constitute Title VI compliance was complex. What would constitute discriminatory practices? How would the racial composition of the practice be considered? the practice location? the pattern of treatment? Even if a defensible definition of compliance could be established, how would officials collect information? Furthermore, what would be the benefit of intervening in what was viewed (in the 1960s) as a personal and private relationship between a physician and his or her patient? Would patients benefit from pressure on physicians to treat those whom they did not want to treat?

As to the political realities at the time of the passage of Medicare, imposing any kind of Title VI requirements on medical practices was inconceivable. Local medical societies, state societies, and the AMA were powerful political forces and reluctant, if not openly hostile, participants in the Medicare program. Even if one could devise convincing and persuasive answers to all of the above questions, any attempt was certain to fail and was never a real prospect.

A contorted, but much desired, legal rationale for exempting physicians participating in the Medicare program from accountability to Title VI had been patched together by DHEW's general counsel in 1965. The most extensively debated part of Title VI had been the exclusion of federal insurance or guaranty from its reach. Senator Long of Louisiana had provided the final compromise, offering the following amendment.

> Nothing in this subchapter shall add or detract from any existing authority with respect to any program or activity under which Federal financial assistance is extended by way of a contract of insurance or guaranty.[44]

The original intent for the inclusion of the Long amendment in the 1964 bill was the fear that Title VI might be used to attack discrimination in housing through federal insurance programs for home mortgages and bank deposits. Ironically, federal laws now impose far stricter nondiscriminatory controls and reporting requirements on such lending institutions than they do on health care providers.

DHEW general counsel, however, chose to define Part B of Medicare as a private "contract of insurance" with its subscribers and not a direct grant of public funds. General counsel had argued that Part B represented an indemnity insurance policy in which cash payments were made directly to the beneficiary. Such "contracts of insurance," the argument went, were excluded from coverage. The exemption of Part B from Title VI coverage was vigorously challenged by the Civil Rights Commission in 1974 and again in 1980.[45] The Civil Rights Commission argued that Part B was not a federally subsidized, individually purchased health insurance. It was a program funded from federal general revenues and payroll taxes and thus subject to Title VI requirements.

Whatever basis existed for DHEW's position in 1965, it has become increasingly attenuated with time. Far from being an "indemnity insurance policy" in which the beneficiary receives direct cash payments, Medicare has required physicians to accept direct payment or assignment from Medicare. State Medical Assistance programs have stepped in to subsidize the premiums of medically indigent persons eligible for Medicare benefits. An increasing percentage of Medicare beneficiaries are enrolled in HMOs that receive pooled funds from both Part A and Part B as capitation payments. In addition, physician practices have been purchased by hospitals currently being transformed into "integrated delivery systems." In larger medical markets, less than a handful of such systems now dominate the provision of medical services. Computerization and consolidation have transformed what was at the start of the Medicare program an administratively impossible task into one that would be, at least as to mechanics, simple.

Yet, in what was perhaps the most ironic twist of all, some state medical societies in 1967 appear to have actually used the blanket exemption of private practice physicians from Title VI Medicare and Medicaid certification as a added membership benefit to encourage physicians to become dues-paying members. The following is excerpted from a November 1967 dues solicitation newsletter from the Indiana State Medical Association (ISMA).

FEDERAL GOVERNMENT AND STATE WELFARE departments agree that physicians who are members of the Indiana State Medical Association need not certify that they are in compliance with the Civil Rights Act of the Federal government. Arrangements have been made with the State Department of Public Welfare and approved by the Federal government that those physicians who are in good standing with the Indiana State Medical Association will not have to sign affidavits or other statements or certify that they are complying with the Civil Rights Act. It is deemed that if they are a member in good standing with this Association that they are automatically complying with the Civil Rights Act.

PHYSICIANS NOT MEMBERS of the Association have been listed with
the State Department of Welfare and will be required to sign an
affidavit certifying that they are in compliance with the Civil Rights
Act of the Federal government.[46]

The administrative and political compromises necessary at the time of the
implementation of the Medicare program had indeed borne some strange
fruit.

OEHO's Death Struggle

Title VI compliance for nursing homes and medical practices were set
aside, however, as OEHO faced a debilitating political struggle for survival. A test of wills had begun with the House and Senate Appropriations Committees in the spring of 1966. In April, the House Appropriations Committee had reduced DHEW's request for its Title VI budget
and ordered a reorganization of the operation. The committee was
annoyed. It did not like Title VI scattered all over the department at different agency levels, supported by funds from a variety of accounts in a
way that it could not be effectively controlled. The House Appropriations Committee directed DHEW to centralize the entire Title VI operation in the Office of the Secretary. Secretary Gardner argued for a decentralized approach, recognizing the import of the lethal cat and mouse
game being played out with the appropriations' committees of Congress.
In a March 15, 1966, memo, Assistant Secretary Wilbur Cohen acknowledged in writing what many staff in OEHO understood was the administration's strategy.

At the hearings yesterday before the HEW–Labor Appropriations
Subcommittee, Chairman John Fogarty indicated his strong intent to
pull out all of the money and positions for civil rights enforcement in
the separate places where they are now and lump them in one appropriation. He also indicated (with Congressman Denton's support)
that the total item might then be assigned to the Justice Department
and the appropriations subcommittee handling the Justice Department appropriation bill.
    Whatever merits this proposal might have it has one serious defect:
*It will highlight the substantial number of positions involved in civil
rights enforcement and serve as a basis for cutting the appropriation and
the number of positions.* If the appropriation is cut you can expect the
civil rights groups to demand that the Administration put on a big
campaign to get the money restored. If it is not restored, the Admin-

istration will be criticized for not vigorously enforcing the civil rights program.

I believe Secretary Wirtz might be able to influence Congressman Fogarty to postpone action on this proposal. Fogarty seems very convinced of the desirability of doing this. Denton seems convinced that all civil rights compliance activities should be handled by the Department of Justice. Fogarty is very critical of the HEW budget because of the decreases and "small" increases. He called it the worst HEW budget he has seen since he came to Congress. I feel reasonably certain he will want to cut some of the small items the Administration wants and increase some of the items for health research and education.[47]

The appropriations committees were largely controlled by the southern opponents of integration. Richard Russell, senator from Georgia, helped lead the opposition against the Civil Rights Act. He had long been a member of the Senate Appropriations Committee and assumed its chairmanship in January 1969. As Libassi noted in his own cover memo to the White House:

Such action would seriously cripple the civil rights program not only for this Department but also for the government as a whole. Regardless of the explanation, the budget cut would be interpreted as a step to curtail, if not eliminate efforts to secure compliance with Title VI of the Civil Rights Act and would have the government wide effect of slowing down all activities.[48]

In 1966, Secretary Gardner had stalled, agreeing that the centralization of civil rights enforcement in DHEW would be studied and gaining some time and flexibility in carrying out such a reorganization. In the spring of 1967, however, the noose tightened. Congressman Fogarty of Rhode Island, chairman of the House Appropriations Committee, renewed his demand for the reorganization. The not-well-veiled threat was that if DHEW wanted to receive its full twelve-billion-dollar appropriation from Congress, it would do what was requested. Libassi saw the consolidation as an opportunity to cement his relationships and make peace with the many members of Congress who were irritated with the Office of Equal Educational Opportunities efforts. The reorganization was announced in the *Federal Register* on October 19, though the transfer of functions had begun in late summer and would continue into the winter months. Robert Nash, director of OEHO, resigned, and his counterparts in the other operating departments of DHEW either resigned or refused reassignment to the centralized Office for Civil Rights. John Gardner resigned as secretary of DHEW on March 1,

1968, and was succeeded in office by Wilbur Cohen. Libassi resigned a month later, following Gardner to the Urban Coalition. The brief, turbulent life of one of the most productive organizational change agents in the history of federal bureaucracy had ended.

With the death of OEHO, civil rights ceased to be a part of the defining vision for the DHEW. For Cohen, a skillful and resilient congressional tactician, the civil rights program was an albatross. Cohen argued that minorities in the end would benefit more from improvement in basic programs such as Medicare and Medicaid than from aggressive enforcement of Title VI. Such aggressive enforcement would jeopardize getting important social legislation through Congress and getting substantial appropriations for important social programs.[49] This did not prevent southern opponents in Congress from pushing forward their own aggressive counteroffensive. At the end of September, Cohen was protesting the effort in joint conference committee concerning the Health, Education and Welfare Appropriation Bill (H.R. 18037). The effort would recommend adoption of the House-passed language originally proposed by Congressman Whitten of Mississippi to prohibit the department from using these funds to carry out aspects of their legal responsibility under Title VI.

At the end of October 1968, Cohen was strongly urging that the entire civil rights function be shifted to the Justice Department, as had been advocated two years earlier by Congressman Denton of the House Labor–HEW Appropriations Subcommittee. The Justice Department and White House staffers argued against this move, citing "the leverage which program administrators have to bring about compliance with the law."[50] The Justice Department argued that "the proposal would separate from the agency granting Federal assistance those persons who have to deny and terminate it. Much of the information obtained by the Federal government in passing upon applications would be lost if the compliance function were separated."[51] Yet through the centralization into a single office, that connection had already been severed. Title VI had become the pariah of the executive branch, isolated in an orphan office that nobody wanted.

Johnson's lame-duck administration was now a shattered shadow of its earlier self. The roller-coaster ride seemed to have hit bottom. Nixon would win a narrow victory in the November 1968 presidential election. It would be his turn, in the words of one of the slogans adopted by his campaign, "to bring us together."

A Rocky Beginning for the Office for Civil Rights

The newly formed Office for Civil Rights (OCR) got off to a rocky start in the Nixon administration. Nixon's own track record was one of politically driven ambivalence. Still smarting from his defeat in 1960, a defeat produced by the black vote for Kennedy, Nixon actively wooed blacks into his administration. He pushed through Congress legislation supporting the Philadelphia Plan, requiring black quota hiring in federal construction, a proposal earlier abandoned by the Johnson administration. Nixon increased the budget for the Office for Civil Rights and other civil rights agencies fourfold. (At least in regard to the Office for Civil Rights, some of these changes were a reflection of congressional pressure to force staff allocated to civil rights activities back "onto the books.") OCR made substantial progress in education, and by the time of Nixon's resignation in August 1974, the South was well along the way to having the most racially integrated public schools systems in the country.

In retrospect, however, Nixon's victory in 1968 led to a reversal of emphasis. For much of the southern congressional leadership, Nixon's election signaled payback time. Southerners wanted a go-slow policy for school desegregation, and the "Southern Strategy" preoccupied the administration during its first term.[52] Nixon spoke out against busing and made several controversial Supreme Court nominations, trying to build a growing southern Republican constituency. One of these nominations, Judge Clement Haynsworth, had written the dissenting opinion in the narrow (three-to-two) *Simkins v. Cone* decision in the court of appeals. Judge Haynsworth had argued that the majority decision was both unprecedented and unwarranted, that the majority was distorting the purpose and operations of the Hill-Burton Act, and that nothing like the operations of Moses Cone Memorial and Wesley Long Hospitals was "state action" as the plaintiffs claimed.[53]

Leon Panetta became Nixon's first director of the Office for Civil Rights under DHEW secretary Finch. Panetta's tenure lasted less than a year and he read about his own resignation in the newspaper before he knew (or the Secretary of DHEW knew) he was going to resign.[54] After Panetta's resignation, 125 OCR civil servants signed a letter to the president, widely circulated to the media, stating, "We earnestly hope that you may be prevailed upon to exercise the strong moral leadership that we feel is now essential to avoid a reversal of the Nation's longstanding commitment to equal opportunity."[55] Another eighteen hundred DHEW employees signed an open petition to Secretary Finch, asking him to explain the administration's civil rights policies in a meeting with them. Both the petition and letter were unprecedented aberrations in a low-profile bureaucratic culture. Finch himself was relieved of his duties as secretary three weeks later. Yet able leadership, at least from the perspective of OCR staffers, followed. Elliot Richardson took over as secretary, J. Stanley Potinger as director of the Office for Civil Rights.[56] OCR, consumed by the desegregation of public schools in the South, began to make some progress in education.

Health Planning and Civil Rights

The beginning of Medicare and the beginning of Medicaid a year later, in July 1967, produced a massive shift in the financing of health services. The federal share of health expenditures jumped from 8.3 percent in 1965 to 26.6 percent a decade later. By 1975 the federal government was pumping in more than thirty billion dollars, the cost of the Medicare and Medicaid programs was doubling approximately every five years, and 39 percent of all dollars spent on health care came from public sources.[57] The 1970s saw a series of federal legislative initiatives to ensure that these funds were spent in a way that best met the needs of individual citizens and taxpayers and that the costs to those citizens and taxpayers would be effectively controlled. An implicit corollary, at least from the perspective of civil rights advocacy groups and staff in the Office for Civil Rights, was that dispersion of these funds to local communities should not have a racially disparate impact. Here, they felt, was an opportunity finally to close the gaps. It would represent the next wave of Title VI enforcement. The orphaned agency now hoped for new sponsorship and advocates through a federally mandated health planning process.

The first health planning legislation in the United States had been Hill-Burton. Just as the "separate but equal" provisions in the Hill-Burton legislation in 1946 had haunted DHEW and the hospitals in the early 1960s, other long-ignored provisions in that bill now haunted DHEW and the hospitals in the early 1970s. According to the legislation, hospitals receiving Hill-Burton funds were required to (1) make their facilities available to "all persons residing in the territorial area of the applicant" (the community service requirement), and (2) provide "a reasonable volume of services to persons unable to pay" (the indigent care requirement).[58] The community service requirement was integral to the purpose of the legislation and to the reasoning embedded in the legislation as to how these funds would be distributed for such projects. The indigent care requirement had been added as a concession to Senate liberals that had been unsuccessful in including health insurance in the legislative package. No effort had been made by DHEW to promulgate regulations to enforce either of these requirements, and they had lain dormant for twenty years. Marilyn Rose described her recollections of their awakening.

> Sometime in 1967, while I was still with HEW, Frank Beddow, an OEHO staff member who worked out of the Charlottesville Office,

called me about problems that office was having with the Maria
Parham Hospital in a small town near the Raleigh-Durham area of
North Carolina. The reputation of the hospital in handling black people who came to the emergency room was notoriously bad. The parking lot was known sarcastically as the "black obstetrical unit." A
number of babies had been born in the parking lot, because the mothers did not have the deposit needed to get admitted. There was one
awful situation when a woman with an ectopic pregnancy had almost
died. Beddow told me that similar problems occur a lot with this hospital, which he understands was built with federal Hill-Burton
money. He further said that he had heard that Hill-Burton hospitals
were supposed to give some free care to the poor, but no poor blacks
appeared to be getting any of this free service.

   I very quickly found the language in both the statute and the
implementing regulation that grantees would be obligated to provide "a reasonable volume of care to persons unable to pay." I
requested a copy of the contract signed by the Maria Parham Hospital from the Hill-Burton office of the Public Health Service, and it
clearly contained that contractual provision. In the interim, Beddow
continued to investigate and developed facts which showed that, in
a number of cases, poor white people got "vouched for" and did not
have to pay an admission deposit, but poor black people did not
ever seem to get the same treatment. While Beddow was trying to
develop sufficient facts to establish a litigable discriminatory pattern, I sent a formal complaint to Harold Granning, the Director for
the Hill-Burton program in the Public Health Service, reporting that
the hospital did not honor its contractual obligations, and citing the
evidence we had developed. I never heard anything from that office,
nor did OEHO.[59]

Rose published two articles, one in the *Legal Services Newspaper* in
December 1969 and one in the *Clearinghouse Review* in February 1970 that
attracted the attention of local legal service program attorneys. Three suits
emerged out of this interest in 1970 and four the following year. The first
case, *Cook v. Ochsner,* was filed in federal court in New Orleans in July
1970. The class action suit was brought against ten Hill-Burton-funded
hospitals in New Orleans. HEW was later added as a defendant for its failure to enforce its governmental responsibilities. As originally drafted there
were nine plaintiffs, one black man and eight black women.

   The original first named plaintiff was Clifford Breaux, who died
shortly before the case was filed. While he could not be a plaintiff in

the case, allegations describing his case remained in the complaint, and were very dramatic. He died of congestive heart failure. A month before he died, he had appeared in the emergency room at Charity Hospital, but the hospital was over-crowded, and did not have beds for all the poor people coming to it, either directly or being dumped by the other hospitals in the community. He did not get admitted. During discovery we later uncovered the fact that prior to his rejection at Charity Hospital, he had appeared at the Ochsner emergency room. The physician's report of the emergency visit of Breaux in the Ochsner record documented that he needed hospitalization but lacked the $200 to get admitted, and the physician noted that he was referring him to Charity and hoped that he would be admitted there. Ironically, with borrowed money several weeks later he finally did get admitted to Ochsner, but died in Ochsner during the hospital stay.[60]

The suit alleged that the New Orleans hospitals were engaged in racially discriminatory practices violating Title VI and were not fulfilling their "community service" and "uncompensated services" obligations as recipients of Hill-Burton funding. In May 1971, DHEW was added as a defendant party. The appellants alleged that DHEW had failed to provide an enforcement program under Title VI and Hill-Burton and had allowed the defendant hospitals to violate their Title VI and Hill-Burton obligations. By agreement of the parties, the Hill-Burton and Title VI enforcement issues were severed and litigated in separate lawsuits. The Hill-Burton free service issue was settled by a consent decree in July 1972, on the eve of the trial and the community service obligation involving the failure of hospitals to participate in the Medicaid program was resolved by court order later that same year.[61] The federal district court rulings concluded that (1) the hospital recipients of Hill-Burton funds were required to admit Medical Assistance patients on the same basis as privately insured patients as a part of their community service requirement, and (2) DHEW was required to issue regulations in indigent care requirements.[62] These landmark rulings were largely responsible for producing the uncompensated-care and community service requirements for institutions receiving Hill-Burton funds that were subsequently promulgated by DHEW regulations and enforced nationally by OCR.[63] The person in charge of OCR enforcement activities recalled bureaucratic battles during this period.

> Hill-Burton had these two requirements, the community services and uncompensated-care requirements, that were really dormant. We waged an aggressive effort to have OCR become the primary enforce-

ment agency and to revise the regulations on what uncompensated-care requirements meant and what the community service requirement entailed. Neither, particularly the community service requirement, had been spelled out, and the department wasn't paying much attention to it. In conjunction with HRA and HCFA [Health Resources Administration and Health Care Financing Administration] we developed the formula for free indigent care. It was a mechanical formula. What was controversial was whether you could buy out of that requirement and what that might entail. On the community services side, where it had not been defined, the issues were much more contentious. We, of course, wanted the maximum. We wanted community services defined in a way that would give it real meaning: forcing facilities to provide access to Medicaid and uninsured populations. In the end, we got pretty much what we wanted on uncompensated care, and we got a lot of good language on community services, but virtually no enforcement. What we really lost out on was giving it any teeth.[64]

The *Cook v. Ochsner* litigation and the Title VI discrimination issues that were a part of the original case dragged on in separate litigation and administrative review through the rest of the 1970s.

While eventually inconclusive, the case may have had some clearly unintended consequences on the health care landscape in the United States. In 1969, partly in response to the passage of Medicare and Medicaid, the Internal Revenue Service, with some prompting by the American Hospital Association, had changed the interpretation of "charity" as it pertains to nonprofit or voluntary hospitals. For forty years the IRS required the provision of free care by a hospital as a test for a hospital to be eligible for 501(c)3 status for donors. In other words, in order for one's donations to a hospital to be tax exempt the hospital had to provide free service. In 1969 the IRS changed the standard to "community benefit." No one was clear about what this meant, but it certainly provided much more wiggle room for the hospitals. A suit, *Eastern Kentucky Rights v. Simon,* brought by one of the lawyers in the *Cook v. Ochsner* case had challenged the authority of the IRS to make such a sweeping change but was lost on appeal to the Supreme Court, which ruled that the plaintiffs did not have standing to sue. Members of the Senate Finance Committee were also disturbed by the IRS change and the apparent usurpation of their authority. According to Marilyn Rose, who had been the lead attorney in both the *Eastern Kentucky Rights v. Simon and the Cook v. Ochsner* cases, that caseload may have proved unfortunate.

Senator Long (LA) held hearings on this matter in 1969 and 1970 and was very concerned about the change. There was the clear implication that he wanted to restore the prior definition. A year or so after we brought the Cook case, Jay Constantine, Long's principal staff person on these matters, indicated very clearly to me that the bringing of the Cook case in New Orleans either infuriated Long, or resulted in pressure on Long, to let the IRS ruling stand.[65]

The IRS community benefit standard has, belatedly in the 1990s, served to produce a diverse variety of initiatives to (1) promulgate voluntary hospital standards to avoid legislative ones, (2) pass more precise state legislation defining the community benefit obligations of tax exempt hospitals, and (3) develop more collaborative and better organized community benefit initiatives between hospitals and other organizations in local communities.[66]

The efforts through federal legislation to create a system for planning for the needs of the population that had begun with Hill-Burton culminated in the passage of the Health Resources and Development Act of 1974. It provided federal funding for local planning agencies, known as Health Systems Agencies (HSAs), and state health planning agencies, known as State Health Planning and Development Agencies (SHPDAs). Health facility capital construction projects and new services meeting certain criteria would first need to receive approval in order for the services provided to receive federal funding. Requirements were developed to assure that the boards of local agencies not simply be the captives of local providers. In most urban areas, many scarred by riots in the 1960s, the predominantly white and affluent suburban flight accelerated in 1970s. Planning agencies served as potential arbiters of the flight of health services that would follow. The new civil rights battles would be fought in this arena. What role should the HSAs play in civil rights? What would a facility be required to do if it wanted a Certificate of Need (CON) or approval to relocate? An OCR staff person at the time recalled these battles.

The situation was always the same. You had an aging inner city facility. The parent organization wanted to move to the burgeoning suburban area, basically, leaving a black area for a wealthier and growing white area. What should be the civil rights responsibilities of the planning agency? In most states, those issues would not occur today because the planning apparatus has largely been dismantled. Now it occurs as a market transaction, not some transaction requiring governmental approval or consent.

OCR wanted the planning agencies to collect civil rights data and provide added leverage for civil rights compliance. They wanted facilities to submit as part of their CON application data on patterns of use by race. The federal planning program and the local planning agencies resisted. They viewed their responsibilities as health planners and not civil rights enforcers.

> Henry Foley, the director of the federal planning program, didn't want the planning agencies burdened with these responsibilities. We clashed. You have to remember that we were young, largely legal services lawyers who were very aggressive. We didn't always operate shrewdly politically. We were often arrogant, contemptuous of the opposition and, sometimes, unwilling to compromise. Henry may have respected us, but I doubt he liked us. The local HSAs were adamantly opposed. I can't remember any of the HSAs that took civil rights seriously.[67]

OCR, perhaps predictably, was politically and bureaucratically out-maneuvered, and the grand plans for expanding the civil rights monitoring and compliance responsibilities of local planning agencies died in 1978.

> We had shared the early draft with Henry's office. It was meant to be a discussion point. It was leaked in Texas, and that was the end of it. Secretary Califano killed it. The outcry was substantial. It was too burdensome. I'm sure if I read the draft now, I would be horrified at what I was trying to do. At the time, it seemed entirely reasonable, if aggressive. What it actually did is to allow opponents to say, "See, they want to transform planning agencies into civil rights enforcement agencies." We didn't succeed, and it was perhaps primarily because health planning collapsed anyway in the 1980s. We could have been more sophisticated about what we tried to do, but the result would have been the same. Health planning was not sustainable.[68]

The Courts, Civil Rights, and Health Planning

The *Ochsner* case, which had forced the promulgation of federal Hill-Burton regulations, had been separated from the original suit that also dealt with the Title VI enforcement issues related to New Orleans hospitals. The separate Title VI litigation absorbed most of the rest of the 1970s and proved far less fruitful.[69]

The Title VI issues in *Ochsner* were those that OEHO had struggled with in 1967 in the Mobile Infirmary case. They were also similar to the ones faced by the Committee to End Discrimination in Chicago Medical Institutions in the 1950s. The referral patterns of physicians in New Orleans perpetuated a high degree of racial segregation in its hospitals, even with the elimination of all Jim Crow laws from the books and any easily identifiable discriminatory admission practices on the part of its hospitals.

By the time the Title VI civil rights part of the case was addressed, the original judge who had ruled on the Hill-Burton issues had returned to private practice, and the new judge, who had been a member of a law firm that had represented one of the hospitals in the case, was more hostile to the plaintiffs. As a result, the plaintiffs' lawyers decided to let HEW-OCR pursue administrative remedies rather than force the issue in court. As a result of the previous consent decree, HEW had agreed to conduct a Title VI compliance review of eighteen New Orleans area hospitals.

Beginning in 1974 OCR faced for the *first time* the difficulty of formulating a way to systematically collect data from the hospitals to learn whether they met Title VI. The agency floundered badly. Relying heavily on approaches used in reviews of educational institutions, investigators first requested information on racial composition and privileges of staff physicians. Second, the investigators requested information from the hospitals on total inpatient and emergency room admissions, broken down by race, method of payment, and source of referral. There was no attempt to gather information broken down by services or service area, or in any way to assess the appropriateness or quality of treatment. The data was cumbersome to collect, and much of it was hand tallied from medical records by OCR staff.

The findings from this time-consuming effort were not released until 1977. It was the only systematic effort ever conducted to evaluate the impact of the Civil Rights Act and the enforcement of Title VI in the Medicare program on racial segregation in hospital care in a metropolitan area. The findings highlighted both patterns of use of services in a metropolitan area due to lingering patterns of segregation and the problems faced by OCR in developing defensible definitions and data to test compliance. In 1966 the hospitals in New Orleans all executed Title VI assurances and ended overt discriminatory practices, and most began admitting some black patients. Nevertheless, OCR's analysis of admission practices at these hospitals in from 1974 to 1977 showed clear patterns of de facto discrimination. Within the sixteen hospitals in the metropolitan area, 75 percent of blacks were admitted to Flint-Goodridge Hospital, built to accommodate black private patients, or to Charity Hospital, the public charity institution.[70] The end of hospital segregation in 1966 left the admitting practices of New Orleans physicians essentially untouched.

Charity Hospital, as the place for the poor, allowed private physicians to restrict the number of indigent patients that they saw and, consequently, the number they would admit to the city's other hospitals. Flint-Goodridge, whose staff had been predominantly white, adopted a policy to bring it into compliance with Title VI, prohibiting physicians from sending only their black patients to Flint-Goodrich. As a result, most white physicians dropped their staff privileges. De facto segregation, with some token black representation among medical staffs and patients, remained in the historically all-white facilities.

In July 1977, DHEW notified three of the hospitals (Hotel Dieu, Mercy, and Southern Baptist) that they were not in compliance with Title VI. Protracted negotiations, in which the hospitals denied any discrimination, followed. DHEW requested, as a part of a plan of a corrective action, that the hospitals (1) set up outpatient primary-care clinics that would result in inpatient admissions, (2) develop a referral system from outside clinics, (3) require as a condition of staff privileges that physicians treat Medicaid patients, (4) find out which physicians provided care for the black community and encourage them to apply for staff privileges, and (6) appoint leaders of the black community to the hospitals' boards.

In May 1978, OCR concluded that further negotiations would be futile and referred the cases to DHEW's general counsel for fund termination proceedings. An administrative law judge held hearings on the matter from April through June 1979. The judge took a sympathetic view toward the hospitals, narrowly defining the grounds of Title VI and largely dismissing the need to take action to correct the legacy of a period of legal discrimination for which the hospitals were not directly responsible. Some limited corrective actions were agreed to by the hospitals, but the implications of this decade-long struggle were clear. Discrimination would be based on the more narrow and difficult-to-prove ground of intent rather than actual disparity. There would be no further effort to correct patterns of segregation and discrimination that had their roots in Jim Crow.

Even more discouraging, the Legal Defense Fund and other advocates now found themselves trying to restrain new forms of discrimination. The great migration of blacks to northern urban centers in search of employment accelerated in the 1960s. A downward cycle involving loss of blue-collar employment, urban decay, and riots accelerated white flight to the suburbs in the 1970s. That flight left behind increasingly black urban areas and a declining infrastructure. Private doctors' offices, local pharmacies, and related services led the flight. In many areas the hospitals remained as the only anchor in their communities: a source of employment, a provider of last resort, and a center of the only remaining resources available to mount a struggle against a spreading plague of poverty and despair. Did the move of hospitals to the suburbs, a move that would clearly have a disparate impact on blacks, violate Title VI? Could a hospital survive in the face of this urban transformation if it didn't relocate? Analyses of hospital closings and relocations in large cities in the Midwest and Northeast during this period revealed a disturbing pattern. The rate of closings and relocations went up directly in proportion to the percent of the population that was black.[71]

The Struggle over Hospital Relocation in Gary, Indiana

Gary is a microcosm of the rise and fall of an industrial northern city in the twentieth century, mirroring most northern industrial centers whose industrial bases had been a magnet for almost three decades for blacks uprooted by the mechanization of agriculture in the South. In the 1960s Gary began to feel the impact of major structural changes in the U.S. economy and the decline of heavy industry. Gary's population, from a high of 178,312 in 1960, began to decline, propelled by a white exodus to the suburbs and declining employment. By 1970, blacks had become the majority of Gary's population.

A blue-collar steel town, Gary had adapted uncomfortably to its growing black population. Waves of eastern European immigrants had worked the steel mills and learned the racial structure from United States Steel and the business elite of Gary. Jim Crow practices were well entrenched. Neither of Gary's major hospitals began admitting blacks until the 1930s. Black physicians could not practice in either institution until 1947. Two small, substandard hospitals on the south side served blacks until the relaxation of policies. The schools remained segregated until the 1960s, and Methodist Hospital did not begin to integrate room accommodation of patients until 1963. As late as 1963, a local cemetery refused to accept for burial the body of a black soldier killed in Vietnam.[72]

Everett Johnson, CEO of Methodist Hospital at the time, describes the issues of integration and population shifts.

> The only thing that was not integrated until the 1960s were the patient rooms. The registrars would put blacks and whites in separate rooms. We dropped this kind of assignment. If a patient objected, we would move the patient that objected. We didn't ask the reason. It happened, but it was not a frequent occurrence.

Early in 1960 it was clear that the population was headed south. In 1970 land was purchased [for a new hospital]. However, the board procrastinated. There were thirty-six seats on the board, twelve held by Methodist ministers. The Methodists didn't control the institution directly but could swing the vote. The Methodist bishop would show up maybe once a year for important votes, such as ones related to abortion. He would, on these occasions, give the invocation, and in it, subtly tell the Methodist ministers how they should vote.[73]

While in the process of planning a new hospital in the southern suburbs,[74] Methodist Hospital was negotiating policies of nondiscrimination with the local NAACP chapter, supported by the Gary Community Council Human Relations Committee. The issue of room assignments had not been resolved to everyone's satisfaction. A board member expressed his concerns at the October 1963 meeting.

He stated the primary purpose of the hospital is to promote healing. Whenever the hospital strays from the primary job of operating a hospital and practicing the finest concept of the Christian religion difficulties result. The hospital has given its word that we are going to do this job. There is already a radical change. Administration has worked very hard with employees to accept integration and to do so with good faith. He mentioned the statement made by Civil Rights groups that if a person is brought into the hospital and does not wish to be integrated, then he must go home. This is certainly forcing integration. Prejudice exists and the hospital must operate around it, and it takes time.[75]

In March 1964, a special meeting of the board dealt with the issue of room assignments and black representation on the hospital board. The hospital had, apparently, adopted the practice of asking patients whether they were willing to share a racially mixed room during the admission process. The Human Relations Committee argued that the hospital had no right to ask questions about a patient's racial preferences in room accommodations. The administration, anxious to avoid patients' objections that might disrupt hospital routines, maintained that the question should be asked. As was his pattern on such occasions, the bishop spoke to the board first, urging a consideration of the Human Relations Committee's position on admissions and the appointment of black board members. Johnson asserted that the hospital lacked sufficient rooms to provide single accommodations to all patients, and that arrangements that did not accommodate patients' wishes could create chaos on the nursing floors.

> Mr. E. A. Johnson . . . stated that at least 90% would object and the great problem of integration is we do not have enough beds. We have many surgical cases and all must go to a special place in the hospital. We must notify 14 departments as people come into the hospital. Dismissals come at unanticipated hours. In reality we send a patient upstairs and oftentimes any other bed available to them will not be available later on. When we have to cancel, the work situation is confused, families upset, so that we have a condition of chaos and lowered level of nursing care for the patients in the hospital. If we do have confusion, we cannot continue this. Even though they were not asked, over half asked that they not be placed with a Negro. Women patients are more prejudiced and concerned about this than male patients. . . . It runs two to 3% of Negroes object and about 90% white.[76]

By September 1964, however, whether it was through the *Simkins* decision, revision of the Hill-Burton regulations, the passage of the Civil Rights Act that summer, the local pressures of activists, the initiative of the board and administration, or the persuasive powers of the bishop, the hospital was now able to assign rooms without asking about racial preferences. The board now found itself insisting on the hospital's prerogative to respect a patient's request to be changed to another room.[77]

The originally proposed annex hospital, Broadway Methodist, was completed in a southern suburb of Gary, in 1975. The approval by DHEW of a request from Methodist for $8.143 million in Hill-Burton funds earmarked largely for the expansion of this facility triggered a class action lawsuit. The plaintiffs contended that the construction and expansion discriminated against the black citizens of Gary in the provision of health services. A consent decree in 1979 provided some protection from the feared cannibalization of the Gary facility. The larger question of the role of federal planning efforts in dealing with such issues was never answered.

The Wilmington Hospitals Consolidate and Relocate

A similar pattern repeated itself in Wilmington, Delaware. The Wilmington Medical Center (WMC) was organized through a merger in 1965 of three nonprofit hospitals, General, Memorial, and Delaware, that served different parts of the city. WMC supplied 1,104 of the total 1,471 acute general hospital beds in the county. Two other not-for-profit hospitals, St. Francis with 290 beds and Riverside Osteopathic with 100 beds, made up the remaining acute inpatient resources. WMC faced the problem of aging physical plants and $8 million annually in free care. As with Methodist Hospital in Gary, the population shift to the southwestern suburbs represented both a threat and an opportunity. If WMC did not move, another hospital probably would, siphoning off its medical staff and much of its privately insured patient population, essential for cross-subsidizing indigent care. After a review of many options, the hospital's board adopted what was to be called Plan Omega. General and Memorial would be closed and Delaware renovated, reducing the number of beds in downtown Wilmington to 250. A new 780-bed facility would be built in a suburban area about nine miles southwest of Delaware Hospital. A division of labor would assign the suburban facility the responsibility for obstetric, high-risk prenatal and specialty pediatric, gynecology, and hemodialysis, among other services. The primary-care clinics would be consolidated at Delaware Hospital, as would be psychiatry, dentistry, and some other services.

In the summer of 1976, a community organization, Wilmington United Neighborhoods, sought out the legal assistance of the Center for Law and Social Policy (CLASP) in Washington, D.C. Hospital protestations to the contrary, the message seemed to be that "other peoples lives and welfare are more important than ours." The local chapter of the NAACP joined this group in initiating a lawsuit against WMC, charging that the plan violated Title VI. At WMC, as at other hospitals involved in similar relocation efforts in the 1970s, the suit was greeted with genuine shock and indignation.

The district court ordered that DHEW conduct a civil rights investigation.[78] That investigation led to a finding that the plan did indeed have a discriminatory impact upon minorities and the handicapped.

> The Office for Civil Rights concludes that, as presently formulated and explained, Plan Omega would, if effectuated, violate Title VI of the Civil Rights Act of 1964 and Section 504 of the Rehabilitation Act of 1973. The shifting explanations of the Plan's provisions minimizing duplication of services subject to "physician option" at the two sites had been particularly troubling.[79]

The subsequent negotiated settlement between DHEW and WMC, which provided for free shuttle bus transportation between the two centers and assurances of integrated programs, was challenged by the plaintiffs. The district court rejected the challenge, as did the Court of Appeals for the Third Circuit.[80]

The five-year lawsuit had cost WMC more than a million dollars in direct costs. The five-year delay had increased the cost of Plan Omega from $87 million to $165 million in construction cost inflation.[81] The plaintiffs had extracted a cost on the WMC but had little else to show for

180   Health Care Divided

their efforts. DHEW by their prodding had extracted some concessions
such as transportation and investment in the Wilmington physical plant.
From the perspective of the Wilmington Medical Center, it was a reasonable outcome, and they felt fully vindicated. As a member of its medical
staff concluded,

> Marilyn Rose has departed from the Center for Law and Social Pol-
> icy (CLASP) and the Christiana Hospital has been built. The poor,
> the elderly, the handicapped, the blacks and the Hispanics are being
> cared for in both hospitals of the Medical Center; mothers are having
> babies in large numbers daily at the Christiana Hospital, and the clin-
> ics at Wilmington Hospital (formerly the Delaware Division) have
> been upgraded, modernized and continue to serve that portion of the
> city's population in need of its services. The transport system is work-
> ing with new busses on a regular schedule as agreed with HEW and an
> Ombudsperson has been designated and is available. The sky has not
> fallen, and the judicial system has been vindicated as a peaceful means
> of settling disputes with both sides putting their disagreements behind
> them and moving on after a decision has been rendered. It is a good
> system; it is slow, but it works.[82]

A subsequent anecdote told by Rose suggests perhaps a less comfort-
ing conclusion about the "system,"

> I got a telephone call from the staff member of the Ford Foundation,
> who reviewed our activities usually on an annual basis. I was asked
> how we got to file the lawsuit, and who was on the Board which
> approved it. I wondered about the call as no one had remembered this
> happening before and CLASP had been in existence since 1969. A
> couple of weeks later I was shown an article reporting new members
> of the Ford Foundation Board, one of whom was Irving Shapiro.
> [Chairman of the Board of Dupont and an active supporter of
> WMC.] Shortly thereafter, at a party at CLASP, the Ford Founda-
> tion staff person was present and I told him on reflection that I had
> wondered about his call and asked whether it had anything to do with
> Shapiro having become a member of the Ford Foundation board. He
> made some comment to the effect that I was very perceptive. A sequel
> to the story perhaps is that the Ford Foundation got out of public
> interest law firm funding, gave CLASP a "buy-out" in early 1980 or
> 1981, and was gone from the scene. From a legal staff of 18–20 attor-
> neys, positions were available to only 4–5.[83]

As far as establishing national precedents or changing the behavior of federal planning and civil rights agencies, the results from the hospital relocation lawsuits were abysmal from the perspective of the civil rights advocacy groups. The real cost for them, however, was the loss of the resources to mount effective legal opposition to health care transformations in the future.

The Relocation Cases, with the Courts as Increasingly Unwilling Partners

The dance of regulation, if it is to be effective in changing the behavior of an industry, requires the courts to be an active partner. They must prod the executive branch to do what it has been instructed to do in laws passed by Congress. Increasingly, however, the federal courts became reluctant to be drawn into disputes about the lack of aggressiveness of the Department of Health and Human Services (DHHS, or DHEW as reorganized under the Carter administration) in enforcing Title VI. Several court decisions, *Adams v. Richardson* and *Women's Equity Action League v. Cavazoz* among them, have restricted the right to sue DHHS for its *failure* to enforce Title VI.[84] According to the more recent *Women's Equity Action League* decision, the procedures DHHS uses to enforce a law are the exclusive discretion of the agency and are not reviewable by the courts. Of course, any actions an agency *does* take to enforce Title VI against a provider are reviewable, and providers can seek relief in the courts. Consumer and community groups can, however, only sue a specific provider who allegedly discriminates. Bringing such legal suits against individual providers basically attempts to do what the federal agency should have been doing in the first place.

Civil rights litigation, whether initiated by private parties or by the OCR, struggled in the 1970s period with two contradictory standards of proof. If a facially neutral policy, such as a hospital relocation, had a disparate racial impact, did one have to prove "intent," or just disparate impact? Under Title VII (discrimination in employment) of the 1964 Civil Rights Act, a "discriminatory effects" test emerged. That is, one must first show that a "facially neutral" policy causes a statistically significant disparate impact on a protected group. Once this impact has been established, the burden of proof then shifts to the defendant, who must prove that the challenged practice has a "manifest relationship" to the organization (e.g., is a business necessity or vitally necessary). Finally, if the defendant succeeds in showing such a relationship, the burden of proof then shifts back to the plaintiff, who must show that the same objectives can be achieved through means that have a less discriminatory impact.[85] The regulations established with Title VI incorporated such an effects test.[86] However, in *Washington v. Davis* in 1976, the Supreme Court ruled that a statistically disproportionate impact was not sufficient to violate the Fourteenth Amendment's equal protection clause without showing intent to discriminate.[87] The intent standard means that (1) the plaintiff must make a prima facie case showing discriminatory intent, and (2) should such a case be made, the defendant must then prove there was no discriminatory intent. Usually this requirement represented an almost impossible burden for the plaintiff. Only rarely in the era after the 1964 civil rights law have organizations been careless enough to have such motives captured in writing or otherwise recorded. *Washington v. Davis* left it unclear whether the courts viewed Title VI standards as the same as those for the Fourteenth Amendment. Specifically, it was unclear whether DHHS had the authority to apply the more stringent disparate-impact standard. Some of the Title VI health care discrimination cases have been litigated in this atmosphere of uncertainty.[88]

The courts have subsequently provided some clarification, apparently acknowledging the appropriateness of disparate-impact standards.[89] However, Title VII has been perhaps inappropriately used as the model to guide the approach to impact-based standards of discrimination in Title VI cases.[90] Title VII deals with private employment decisions, and the courts have been increasingly reluctant to scrutinize private employment practices that impact protected groups disproportionately. As a result, the courts have given increasingly wide latitude to defendants. They can show that the challenged practice has a "manifest relationship" to the operation of the business. The plaintiffs have more narrow latitude in showing that alternative approaches can achieve the same objectives with less discriminatory impact. In effect, in Title VI cases the use of public program funds with a discriminatory impact seems to need to be justified only in the same way it would be in an employment case in a private business involving no public funds and no contractual relationship with a public agency.

Most of the health-related civil rights cases after 1970 have involved the physical relocations of hospitals and services, reflecting the increasingly limited nature of civil rights monitoring.[91] A hospital relocation is (1) a highly visible public act, and (2) an action whose impact on care is easily interpretable by community members. Knowledge of such events and their impact does not require the existence of any civil rights monitoring.

Furthermore, with the exception of *United States v. Bexar County,* dealing with the relocation of maternity services in Texas, all these cases included as defendants the Office for Civil Rights as well as health care providers. The remedies sought included requiring OCR to promulgate regulations, conduct investigations, and hold administrative hearings.

Finally, the federal court outcomes from the perspective of the plaintiffs were generally abysmal.[92] In *Terry v. Methodist Hospital* a compromise through a consent decree was achieved that preserved programs at the urban hospital site, and, as we have seen, in *NAACP v. Wilmington Medical Center* a negotiated settlement enhanced hospital-subsidized transportation to the new site. Yet, in *United States v. Bexar County* and *Bryan v. Koch,* involving a relocation to a suburban campus and a closing of a municipal hospital, respectively, the plaintiffs failed according to the courts even to convincingly meet the first threshold of proving a disproportionate and adverse impact on minorities. In addition, the courts interpreted "necessity" in favor of the defendants, interpreted the second threshold broadly, and limited the review of "alternatives," the plaintiffs' last possibility of seeking remedial action. The precedents set in some hospital relocation cases represented an "imposing hurdle" to such litigation.[93] The courts often dismissed the hardships of travel to a distant location as mere inconveniences. The massive federally subsidized capital construction supported by Medicare and Medicaid dollars continued largely unchecked by anything but small local firefights. No coherent policy that would shape the flow of these funds toward reducing racial inequities emerged.

Reorganizing the Office for Civil Rights

Organizationally, civil rights activities related to health care in DHEW faced two difficulties in the first decade of the centralized Office for Civil Rights. First, the shift to a centralized Office for Civil Rights in DHEW at the end of 1967 resulted in a preoccupation with the more visible public crisis of school desegregation.[94] The Health and Social Services Branch (HSSB) was a small part of OCR. Most of the compliance staff in HSSB were detailed to education to deal with the load of court-mandated reviews. The director of the Office for Civil Rights acknowledged at the end of the decade that "the record of achievement in elimination of discrimination in health is bleak in comparison to what has been accomplished in the schools."[95] In this vacuum, isolated from the operational health agencies and isolated in the main preoccupations of the OCR, the Health and Social Services Branch, quite understandably, had to be quite circumspect in what it would undertake. Health care was put on the back burner as energy and staff were diverted.

Second, OCR was isolated from the operational divisions of DHEW essential for the effective performance of its mission. Initially, Title VI was the responsibility of the assistant secretary of DHEW, with each operating division (Public Health Services, Office of Education, Social Security, Welfare/Vocational Rehabilitation) responsible for carrying out day-to-day enforcement. OEHO was charged with responsibility for the initial Medicare certification and Title VI efforts. In October 1967, as we have seen, DHEW reluctantly responded to pressures from these appropriations committees and reorganized the Title VI program, centralizing it into a single unit. Each region was given a separate civil rights office and staff to carry out its programs. However, unlike other regional functions, the regional OCR staff reported directly to OCR in Washington, rather than to the regional director. One consequence of this reorganization was an increased isolation, even an adversarial relationship, between OCR and the Medicare program and the Public Health Service. During the 1970s the adversarial relationship between the Health Resources Administration, which was responsible for overseeing local health planing agencies, and OCR was particularly pronounced. The Health Resources Administration through local Health Systems Agencies worked to reduce excess hospital bed capacity through hospital closings and was unwilling to press for the analysis of racial segregation in patterns of local use of hospitals. The agencies were concerned that such analysis would impede local acceptance of health-planning activities and the collection of data for local planning purposes.[96] Thus, in a period when access to data and an understanding of the operational complexities and subtleties of how discrimination might take place became increasingly important, civil rights enforcement was bureaucratically isolated. The operational agencies saw OCR as an impediment and bottleneck. As Rose described the transformation, "After 18 months the blinds were pulled down on the window when we wanted to get beyond the issue of simple segregation."[97] Another critic put it perhaps more diplomatically, observing in 1978 that "the integration of Title VI responsibilities into normal program operations and the communication between OCR and the rest of the DHEW bureaucracy . . . are problems that have never been fully resolved."[98]

Reorganization of DHEW during the Carter administration had the potential to address both problems. In 1977 the Health Care Financing Administration (HCFA) was created, extracting the Medicare program from the Social Security Administration and the Medical Assistance program from the Social and Rehabilitation Service. The logic seemed sound, combining all the agencies involved in paying providers into a single agency where greater uniformity and economies of scale could be achieved and the federal government would gain more leverage over service providers. These financing mechanisms had proved effective in encouraging civil rights compliance in hospitals. However, the reorganization appears to have strengthened the influence of the provider constituency of the agency at the expense of its beneficiary constituencies. The staff person in charge of enforcement activities in OCR during this period felt frustrated.

> We tried for years to get HCFA to include race data. They were obdurate. HCFA was a captive of the industry in the late 1970s. The department never took it on, and we never got anywhere. The data people said, "We can't do it." The reality was they didn't want to do it. There were some committees, but it was never seriously considered.[99]

OCR became as isolated an adversary of HCFA in the 1980s as it had been of the Health Planning Program in the 1970s. However, the creation of a separate Department of Education seemed, at least initially, to directly address OCR's other organizational problem by forcing the office to focus only on health issues. Health-related civil rights issues had been submerged under the more visible pressures involved in education. Now the newly constituted OCR in the Department of Health and Human Services, including about a third of the staff of the old OCR of DHEW, could concentrate on them.

A new Department of Health and Human Services, with its separate Office for Civil Rights, was established in May 1980. There was a brief resurgence of energy focused on health care civil rights issues. Sylvia Drew Ivie was appointed director on August 4, 1980, OCR staff generally felt that they finally had one of their own in charge. Ivie had served as law student intern in the Office for Equal Educational Opportunity during the summers of 1966 and 1967, as a lawyer for the Legal Defense Fund, and then as director of National Health Law Program in Los Angeles. As Ivie described her intent, "We set guidelines for what we would do and tried to stem the loss of staff to Education, which was going to take all of them."[100] Through negotiations, responsibilities for enforcement of the Hill-Burton community service obligations was reassigned to the OCR. Some headway was also made in collecting data through the operating components of DHHS. HCFA and several other agencies agreed to assist in collecting admission data on race and disability. There was hope that the new office could make headway with health care. That period, according to critics of the office, ended in November 1980 with the election of Ronald Reagan. William Bradford Reynolds, Reagan's appointee to assistant attorney general for civil rights, was symbolic of the shift. Widely regarded by conservatives as one of the heroes of the Reagan Revolution, he had no connection to the civil rights community and shifted the focus of that office away from advocacy for that community to concern about discrimination against whites.[101] As one staff member in OCR at the time observed:

> Once Reagan came in, the health planning apparatus was disman-
> tled. The change after Reagan was incredible. Before the election we
> had agreement on language going to HSAs on what their civil rights
> responsibilities were. Once the election came, that was it. Then OCR
> was downsized, and the planning apparatus was eliminated. Betty
> Lou Dobson became OCR director. Her organizing principle was
> called "Preventive Civil Rights." I cynically interpreted it as prevent-
> ing civil rights compliance. What she really meant was voluntary
> compliance.[102]

During the Clinton administration's first term there was an effort, in the midst of major changes in the organization and financing of health ser-vices, to "reinvigorate and reinvent" the civil rights function. House over-sight hearings in 1986 had portrayed OCR as a rudderless agency and crit-icized it for its management of complaints and compliance reviews.[103] The Clinton administration's completed Health and Human Services Civil Rights Strategic Plan acknowledged the organizational limitations and identified strategies for improving links to the operating divisions, state agencies, provider, and advocacy communities.[104] Part of that strategy involved getting a better handle on the existing data resources. It also acknowledged that "there is a general sense in OCR that OCR's best days were its earliest days" and that there exists a need to build staff morale. None of this effort suggests, however, that these organizational limitations are close to being overcome. Of all the federal agencies involved in civil rights enforcement, OCR has received the severest budget cuts. While complaints to the office were 44 percent higher in fiscal year 1996 than in 1981, staffing was half that of 1981.[105]

A report by the U.S. Commission on Civil Rights on federal Title VI enforcement was completed in June 1996.[106] It was the first reassessment of Title VI by the commission in two decades and a balanced but scathing indictment. The assessment of OCR was among the more discouraging ones. At the time of the creation of the Department of Education in 1979, OCR in the newly formed office in DHHS was assigned only one-third of the staff of the old office. Such a staffing allocation had no relationship to the funds that these two offices were responsible for Title VI oversight. DHHS financial assistance subject to Title VI reviews in 1993 was esti-mated at 225 billion dollars, approximately eight times that of the assis-tance provided by the Department of Education. "OCR," the report concluded, "has little contact with and no authority over the operating divisions."[107] Its regulations have not been revised since its split with the Department of Education. OCR, according to the commission report, allocates a disproportionate share of its limited resources to complaint investigations and exercises almost no oversight of state-funded programs. While the report viewed OCR's new strategic plan and efforts to work out new collaborative arrangements with the operating divisions positively, the report did not suggest that OCR had an aggressive future in civil rights enforcement. In its three decades of operation, an agency that had originally defined its role as an advocate and prosecutor had been transformed largely into a passive arbiter of disputes that avoided taking sides. In the process, it was transformed from a central, driving force into an increasingly isolated, decaying part of the federal bureaucracy.

Health care, however, is today a far different world than the private, fragmented, insulated one the civil servant "volunteers" to OEHO entered in 1966. The computer-information revolution, the explosive growth of managed care, the massive consolidation and integration of health-related services, and the growing purchaser-driven demand for accountability suggest both new threats and opportunities. The next section of this book assesses those threats and opportunities. It will assess the legacy of a divided health care system and the unfinished agenda of the civil rights struggle.

PART 2

The Legacy of a Divided Health Care System

CHAPTER 6

What Happened and What Didn't?

I went to the walk-in medical center. When I got there, there were about ten names on the list, and I waited my turn. They skipped me. They went all the way down to the bottom of the list! I got up and walked out. It was because I was black and the other people were white. (A patient at a medical office in a northern New Jersey suburb)[1]

With my third little boy he was supposed to be on my insurance. He was very ill. Eventually the doctors sued me for $300 they didn't receive from my insurance. They picked me up at my job and arrested me for the $300 . . . in a paddy wagon and everything! I don't know how . . . they had a warrant for my arrest. I had moved and they had sent letters that I hadn't received. (A South Florida mother with private insurance)[2]

I went through five interviews there. Got a job as a dietician to work in the kitchen. People came there after I did, had the same job, and never had to interview. I worked the job till I became good at it. The people I worked for thought I was a little *too* good and they started tearing me down. There were false accusations. I was placed on an attrition list. Luckily the hospital president and some people who had confidence in me found me another position. This goes on in a lot of suburban hospitals. (A hospital worker in a suburban Philadelphia hospital)[3]

When I first came to the hospital, the chairman of the department would ask me how things were going. I'd say, "My day is made very long for the simple reason that the ward clerks (all white) won't speak to me, won't answer any questions about my patients. It makes my days very long when I can't get information from them about a patient. What happens to the family that comes to find out about their relative who is a patient? . . . It slowly happened. It was subtle. Suddenly I caught myself. All the ward clerks were now black. I didn't ask for that, I just wanted someone who would answer my questions. (A medical school faculty member in North Carolina)[4]

"Thirty-two-year-old black man presents with . . . 63-year-old white male complains of . . . 40-year-old Hispanic female presents with . . ." Age, race or ethnicity, and sex are the leadoff patient identifiers in most medical presentations and written medical records. Race or ethnicity is the second or third piece of data health care practitioners hear or read before processing any information about the patient. Health care practitioners use ethnic and racial identification because they conclude that these identifiers assist them in formulating a medical diagnosis. Additionally, they believe that racial and ethnic categories have a scientific basis and they have not considered that these categories are social constructions that have been designed to maintain, preserve, and reinforce racial and ethnic assumptions practitioners may have about their patients. (A nurse practitioner at a New York City teaching hospital)[5]

Blacks sometimes have painful stories to tell about their experiences in health care settings. Some persons dismiss such stories as aberrations, flickering shadows of a distant past. For others, though, they are an indictment of a system, which has yet to attain true equality in its treatment of either patients or practitioners. How does one write the conclusion to the story of a divided health care system?

One could be triumphal. A shameful past has been overcome. Race is no longer officially an issue, and access to care has been expanded. All the Jim Crow signs have been torn down. The racial discrepancies that persist reflect discrepancies in income and insurance coverage, and that's a *different* problem. End of story.

On the other hand, one could also be angry and despairing. Not much has happened to close persistent racial discrepancies in health care. The paper civil rights compliance process described in the last chapter assures nothing. Blacks have become increasingly divided along class lines. The common institutions that they once shared, the black hospital and a network of related services, have been dismantled. The protective buffers provided by these institutions have been removed. Racism remains, and indifference has grown. The story has been about empty promises and blacks being short-changed once again.

The question, however, is both too interesting and too important to dismiss so quickly with either response. It begs for at least a temporary suspension of final judgment. The "real" answer about what happened and what didn't is more complex. So much that is distinctive about health care in the United States was shaped by racial histories. So much of what is involved in addressing the contradictions evident in the current critical period of transformation of health care in the United States is tied up in the lessons of this story.

Part of the more complex "real" answer to this question is presented in this chapter through a review of existing data and published research that can frame more objective answers. The numbers provide a partial antidote to the more common responses driven by emotion and ideology. It would be helpful if such "objective" evidence could resolve the question, but it doesn't. The evidence is often ambiguous and sometimes contradictory. As a result, there are fragmentary pieces of a puzzle that must somehow be put together to create a coherent whole. Figure 6.1 summarizes how this chapter will fit these different pieces together. It envisions a set of three nested Chinese boxes. The outer box deals with changes at the *national* level. The next box addresses the dynamics of *state and local communities.* The innermost box deals with the *institutional* behavior of local health professionals and their organizations. What happens inside each of these boxes is governed by rules and dynamics shaped by distinctive histories, politics, economies, institutions, and individual leaders, but it is also formed by what happens inside the other boxes.

To examine the "dimensions" of each of these three nested boxes, three distinctive questions could be asked. That is, how did the efforts to end a divided health care system affect (1) racial differences in access to health care and health outcomes, (2) the degree of racial integration achieved, and (3) the way health services organizations changed? Only in triangulating the answers to these three different sets of questions is it possible to begin to get a three-dimensional answer to the more basic question.

The first part of this chapter focuses on the most commonly asked questions concerning changes in access to care and the health of blacks as compared to whites. Such a *health care assessment* of what happened and what didn't focuses on structure, process, and outcomes.[6] *Structure* refers to the characteristics of the organizations providing services. *Process* describes the patterns of use of those services. *Outcomes* describe the resulting consequences of an episode of care for both individual patients and the overall health of a population. This is ground covered extensively by studies and literature reviews and only briefly summarized here. The "process" statistics about use of medical services come from national household health surveys and Medicare program information. The "outcome" statistics about the health of blacks and whites come from the statistics on births and deaths in the United States.

The second part of the chapter addresses the traditional civil rights

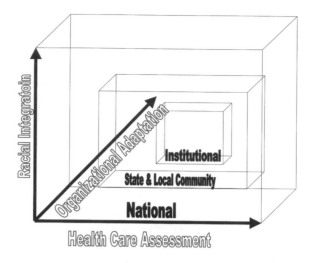

Fig. 6.1. What happened and what didn't

questions. What degree of *racial integration* has actually been achieved in the provision of health services and in health care occupations? Is health care still divided? Much information is regularly reported about the racial integration achieved in education, employment, and housing in the United States. This information is often summarized by measures that describe the degree of inequality or segregation that persists. The most commonly used of such measures is the index of dissimilarity. A value of 1 on this index would indicate complete inequality or segregation between the races. A value of zero would indicate full equality or integration. The value of the index indicates the proportion of the black or white population that would need to be reassigned (to schools, income categories, or residential areas) in order to achieve full integration. Such measures have never been regularly reported about health care. We will use information from the Medicare program about hospital discharges to construct an index of dissimilarity for the nation's hospitals and to describe the factors that might explain differences in the degree of hospital racial segregation in different service areas.

Finally, the chapter will explore the *organizational adaptation* question. How did health care organizations and the health care system as a whole adapt to federal pressures imposed on providers in the face of sometimes conflicting pressures of local constituencies? How did these dynamics help shape the evolution of health care in the United States and its distinctive characteristics and problems? This is unexplored territory, but essential in developing a realistic picture of the failures and accomplishments.

A Health Care Assessment: Changes in Structure, Process, and Outcomes

Structure: The Demise of Black Hospitals and the Marginalization of Public Institutions

Whatever the final assessment, the civil rights movement brought about one of the most profound structural changes in health care in the in the twentieth century. As a watershed, it rivals the Flexner-related reforms in medical education in 1910, the American College's Hospital Standardization program that began in the 1920s, and the Voluntary Hospital Insurance programs that began in the 1930s. It changed the institutional landscape and access to health care.

The most obvious change was the disappearance of the black hospitals. "The Negro Hospital is dead. The Civil Rights Act killed it," observed Hiram Sibley, executive director of the Hospital Planning Council of Metropolitan Chicago, in 1967.[7] Most black medical leaders, even those who had helped lead the long fight for integration, were ambivalent about this passing. Montague Cobb observed, "Inherent in the situation is the feeling on the part of the Negroes involved that the product of their sweat and toil over the years will be dashed away in the name of progress and that they will find themselves again at the bottom of the ladder where they started."[8] An editorial in the *Journal of the National Medical Association* in 1974 addressed the problem of the flight of physicians and their black patients to previously white facilities, which was having a devastating impact on the census and financial viability of many historically black hospitals.

> It will be a sad commentary and a blight on all black pioneers in medicine if we allow our black community hospitals to succumb to inaction and expediency. If the trend continues, the black community hospital, as we know it, will become extinct.[9]

Nevertheless, nothing stemmed the tide. Between 1961 and 1988 seventy black hospitals closed or merged with historically white facilities. As indicated in table 6.1, the peaks in such closings or mergers took place in 1967, in the middle of the 1970s, and in 1983. These peaks corresponded to the final year of operation of the Office of Equal Health Opportunity in 1967, the height of regional planning efforts in the mid-1970s, and the passage of Medicare Prospective Payment System in 1983.

The conventional wisdom is that a hospital is almost impossible to kill. Such deaths are traumatic events for local communities, conditioned to the geographic convenience and sense of safety that such a facility provides. The hospital is also typically one of the largest sources of employ-

TABLE 6.1.   Black Hospital Closings, 1961–88

Year	Closings	Cumulative Closings
1961	2	2
1962	0	2
1963	2	4
1964	1	5
1965	3	8
1966	2	10
1967	8	18
1968	1	19
1969	1	20
1970	1	21
1971	1	22
1972	1	23
1973	1	24
1974	5	29
1975	4	33
1976	4	37
1977	5	42
1978	2	44
1979	2	46
1980	3	49
1981	3	52
1982	0	52
1983	9	61
1984	0	61
1985	3	64
1986	1	65
1987	3	68
1988	2	70

Source: Data from Nathaniel Wesley, "Struggle for Survival: Black Community Hospitals, 1961 to 1988," thesis prepared for Fellowship of the American College of Healthcare Executives, 1989, 68–72.

ment in a local community. Yet the black hospitals died, even in the midst of a period that was, for historically white hospitals, a time of unprecedented growth and financial health. Black hospitals had existed in more than thirty states. More than three hundred and fifty historically black hospitals served local communities at some point in this century.[10] Most faced difficult uphill struggles, many living brief, tenuous existences. Efforts at hospital standardization in the 1920s, followed later by accreditation requirements for internships and residency programs, and the rising complexity and cost of hospital care exacted a continuing toll on these institutions.

Only a handful of survivors remain. They include those (George Hubbard Hospital and Howard University Hospital) that support the two historically black medical schools, Meharry and Howard, about four voluntary hospitals with fewer than one hundred beds, and a small contingent of larger public municipal hospitals that have historically served the black communities (Harlem and Kings County in New York, Cook County in Chicago, DC General in Washington, Grady in Atlanta, etc.). The rest are gone, testimony to the ability to erase the past.

Many of these disappearing hospitals were key landmarks in the story presented in the first section of this book. Mercy-Douglas Hospital in Philadelphia, founded in 1895 and essentially the only hospital in Philadelphia where black physicians could receive training or obtain staff privileges until the mid-1960s, closed in 1973. The facility was converted to a nursing home and continues to serve the black community of West Philadelphia with a strong reputation among knowledgeable providers.

Mound Bayou Hospital in Mississippi (formerly Tabourian Hospital), established by the Knights and Daughters of Tabor in the 1940s and a monument to the strength of black benevolent societies in the face of adversity (see chap. 2), finally closed in 1983.

Hughes Spalding, the Atlanta public hospital constructed in 1952 so that physicians would have a place to send their black private patients, added an $8.3 million wing in 1984, designed to reverse a trend that resulted in the plummeting of occupancy rates to 40 percent.[11] The hospital finally closed in 1989.

L. Richardson Hospital in Greensboro (see chap. 3) went through even more protracted death throes. Dr. Blount's—he had been one of the plaintiffs in *Simkins*—surgical patients had accounted for as much a third of the hospital's census, and his practice was winding down. Ownership of the facility changed hands. Faced with the loss of jobs for its predominantly black employees, many struggled to keep the facility afloat. The hospital was finally sold to Vencor, a for-profit specialty nursing-home chain, in 1993.

The transformation in Durham, North Carolina, illustrates many of the ambiguities in assessing the structural changes that swept across the nation. Two hospitals, Lincoln for blacks (see chap. 1) and Watts for whites, had served the community since the beginning of the twentieth century. Lincoln provided one of the few places in the nation where black physicians could receive residency training. Paul Cornely, M.D., who had worked with Dr. Cobb at Howard in organizing the Imhotep Conferences against discrimination in the 1950s, for example, interned at Lincoln. In 1976, a single regional facility replaced the older hospitals. For some of Durham's black community, there was bitterness about this transition.

> Durham Regional opened. Lincoln closed down. They tore it down and built a new clinic building on the site. Why not maintain the old hospital as a landmark? It was erased. . . . it had historical significance in people's lives. Most things black are torn down. I suspect some people don't want blacks to know their history and some people don't want to be reminded. . . . maybe it was just not important to the person making the decision.[12]

Others saw advantages in a fresh start.

> For sixty years Watts had not served or employed any blacks and wouldn't cooperate with Lincoln. They wouldn't even give us any O-negative blood when we needed it. After integration, I practiced at Watts before the merger. The nurses had never worked with black physicians and made it known they didn't like it. It was interesting to see what happened at Regional. Some of them became very good friends. I ran into one of them on the street the other day, and I couldn't get away with the hugging and stuff. In the atmosphere of Watts, I doubt they would have.[13]

Many black facilities, of course, didn't disappear. Most frequently, they were converted to nursing homes. The legacy of Detroit's system of black physician-owned hospitals is a relatively plentiful supply of nursing homes in which blacks feel welcome. In contrast to more slowly changing national patterns and a research literature that has often ascribed the substantially lower use of nursing homes by blacks to "cultural preferences," black elderly in Detroit had *a higher* rate of nursing-home use than white elderly.[14]

Public hospitals had played a key historic role in providing access to care for blacks and in removing training and practice barriers for black physicians. Coinciding with the death of the black hospitals was the death of many such public facilities. They had been key targets in the early integration efforts of the 1940s and 1950s. The staff privileges and training opportunities provided by these institutions were less insulated from the pressures of local politics and the needs of local politicians for black votes. The color lines fell first in the urban public hospitals.

Philadelphia General Hospital (PGH), the oldest hospital in the nation, closed in 1977. Like many of the nation's larger municipal hospitals, PGH was considered one of the more desirable places for postgraduate medical training during the 1930s and 1940s.[15] PGH had served the growing Philadelphia black population in the years between World War I and World War II. It also served as the "foot in the door" for the integration of professional staffs and training programs in the Philadelphia area, admitting its first black resident, after considerable political pressure, in 1947. However, a single-affiliation agreement with the University of Pennsylvania Medical School in the mid-1950s and Medicare and Medicaid legislation in 1965 sealed the fate of PGH.[16]

The implementation of the Medicare and Medicaid program had a similar dramatic effect on public hospitals in many large cities. New options opened, and many patients and their physicians voted with their feet. In New York City, for example, five of the municipal hospitals closed inpatient services. The New York municipal hospitals had begun the integration of their medical staffs before World War II. These hospitals accounted for about a third of the hospitalizations of the elderly prior to the implementation of the Medicare program. By 1975 that share had dropped to 13 percent.[17] The short supply of private physicians in many poor neighborhoods and the general unwillingness of private physicians to accept Medicaid prevented an even more dramatic loss in volume. The census in the New York municipal hospitals, however, rebounded somewhat after subsequent Medicaid cutbacks in eligibility. Partly in response to the New York City fiscal crisis in 1975, inpatient general care services were closed at five hospitals in the city's municipal hospital system between 1975 and 1980. Sydenham Hospital, a 132-bed public hospital in Harlem, closed finally in 1980. In 1943 Sydenham had become the first fully racially integrated (medical staff and board), historically white voluntary hospital in the nation. In 1949 it became part of the municipal hospital system.[18] Elsewhere, similar closings and downsizing of public hospitals took place. In 1979, St. Louis's black public hospital, Homer G. Phillips, closed. It had been an important source of post-graduate training for black physicians. Sixty-eight demonstrators who were protesting the closing, including comedian Dick Gregory, were arrested in August.[19]

The pressures on public hospitals continued after shocks of the Medicare program's shift to a new form of payment for hospitals in 1983, subsequent inroads of managed care in the Medicare program, and the rapid transformation of Medical Assistance to managed care. These events further altered the landscape in most medical-service markets, generating declining occupancy rates and, most believe, further downsizing of the larger urban public hospitals that had historically served blacks.[20]

Little effort has been devoted to assessing the effects of the closing of public hospitals on access and the health status of populations. One of the few published studies evaluated the impact of the closing of a small public northern California hospital. In a follow-up of patients of the closed facility, in contrast to patients of a public hospital that had not closed, a significant decline in access and health status was reported.[21]

Whether under public or voluntary auspices, however, hospital closings in urban areas have had a disparate impact on blacks. A study of hospitals in eighteen cities between 1937 and 1977 found that hospital closings and relocations were directly related to the proportion of the population in the service area that was black. In those neighborhoods where more than 50 percent of the population was black, almost half of the hospitals either closed or relocated.[22] A more recent analysis of 190 urban community hospitals that closed during the period 1980–87 found that by far the most significant factor associated with closure was the percentage of black residents in the community.[23]

Process: Narrowed Gaps in Access, but with Persistent Discrepancies

However troubling the loss of these landmarks in the institutional landscape, their disappearance coincided with a well-documented improvement in access to health care for the poor and for blacks. Both national health interview surveys and Medicare statistics on the use of services document a remarkable transformation. The gaps in access found in health interview surveys had helped fuel the passage of the Medicare and Medicaid legislation in 1965. The earlier debate over health insurance in the 1930s and 1940s had been hindered by lack of reliable information on use of services. Opponents of the development of national health insurance insisted that no drastic measures were required, that anyone who needed medical care received it. (No one in the United States has ever advocated that essential health care should be denied those who can't afford to pay for it.) Yet, early proponents of national health insurance lacked the evidence to show that medical care was *not* always available to those in need. The few surveys that had been done ignored the access problems of blacks. For example, the Committee on the Cost of Medical Care, in the first comprehensive study of medical care in the United States, completed in 1931, chose to restrict its survey to white families. It argued that "the procedure adopted could not procure satisfactory information from Negro families."[24] National estimates on black use of health services did not begin to be collected until the introduction of the National Health Interview Survey in fiscal year 1958. Attention to this information reflected the changed environment produced by civil rights efforts. The National Health Interview Survey and other data collection efforts not only added to the pressure to address the problem of a gap in care, leading to the passage of the Medicare and Medicaid legislation in 1965, but also documented the subsequent dramatic closing of that gap over the next three decades.

Black-white disparities in the number of physician contacts per year began to shrink. In 1964, as indicated in table 6.2, age-adjusted contacts with a physician averaged 3.6 contacts for blacks and 4.7 for whites. The number of contacts per person has since narrowed to the point where they are roughly comparable. In 1964 whites were 47 percent more likely than blacks to have seen a physician in the two preceding years. In 1994 this difference was reversed, and blacks were about 12 percent more likely than whites to have seen a physician in the two preceding years.[25] Nevertheless, racial differences have persisted in regard to where individuals received care. Blacks continue to be almost twice as likely to use hospital outpatient departments for care, and whites are substantially more likely to use private physician offices.

This convergence in black and white use of physicians resonated from the powerful impact Medicare and Medicaid programs had on reducing income barriers to use. The convergence in physician contact rates between rich and poor was far more dramatic than the convergence between whites and blacks and is widely acknowledged as one of the major accomplishments of Medicare and Medicaid. In 1964, the number of physician contacts for the lowest income group was 3.9, as opposed to 5.2 for the highest income group, and by 1994, the average number of physician contacts per year for the lowest income group was 7.6, as opposed to 6.0 for the highest income group. In other words, the lowest income group used physicians at a rate of only 75 percent of the highest income group in 1964; by 1994 that pattern had reversed itself, with the lowest income group having 26 percent more contacts with physicians than the highest income group.

The impact of Medicare and Medicaid on racial and income patterns of hospital use was even more dramatic. As indicated in table 6.3, age-adjusted discharge rates from hospitals for blacks were only 75 percent of those of whites in 1964. By 1994 black discharge rates were 31 percent higher than white and the number of hospital days per one thousand was 44 percent higher. Just as with physician contacts, these changes were overshadowed by even more dramatic changes in disparity of hospital use between the lowest and highest income groups. Reflecting the historic pattern of substituting inpatient hospital care for private physician use for the poor, hospital days for the lowest income group in 1964 were 14 percent higher than the highest income group. However, by 1994 the number of age-adjusted hospital days per one thousand for the lowest income group had jumped to more than three times the rate of the highest income group.

Far larger and far slower to change have been the disparities between black and white use of nursing homes. As indicated in table 6.4, white elderly persons in 1963 were more than 2.5 times as likely to be residents in a nursing home than were blacks. By 1985, white elderly were only 1.34 times as likely as blacks to be residents in nursing homes. However, by 1995 the gap in gross measures of nursing-home use had closed. Nursing-home use by those over 65 was 6 percent higher for blacks than whites.

One of the basic aims of the Medicare program was to eliminate the income and racial barriers that prevented elderly persons from receiving care on the basis of need. Much early concern was focused on the ability of the program to achieve this goal.[26] As indicated in tables 6.5 and 6.6, significant racial disparities did exist in the first several years but progressively narrowed. In 1995 expenditures per beneficiary for elderly nonwhites were 21 percent higher for inpatient hospital care, 13 percent higher for Supplemental Medical Insurance, and 2 percent lower for skilled nursing care than those for whites.

TABLE 6.2.   Age-Adjusted Physician Contacts per Year, by Race and Income

	Race			Income		
	White	Black	Odds Ratio	High	Low	Odds Ratio
1964	4.7	3.6	0.77	5.2	3.9	0.75
1970	4.8	3.8	0.79	4.9	5.3	1.08
1975	5.1	4.9	0.96	5.0	5.9	1.18
1980	4.8	4.6	0.96	4.6	5.5	1.20
1985	5.3	4.9	0.92	5.5	5.8	1.05
1990	5.6	5.1	0.91	5.6	6.3	1.13
1994	6.1	5.7	0.93	6.0	7.6	1.27

Source: Data from National Center for Health Statistics, *Health in the United States, 1996–97, and Injury Chart Book* (Hyattsville, Md.: Public Health Service, 1997), table 76, p. 197; Health Resources and Services Administration, *Health Status of Minorities and Low-Income Groups,* 3d ed. (Washington, D.C.: U.S. Government Printing Office, 1991), 332; Health Resources Administration, *Health Status of Minorities and Low-Income Groups,* DHEW Publication No. (HRA) 79–627 (Washington, D.C.: U.S. Government Printing Office, 1979), table 3, p. 239.

Note: Income categories and definitions of race vary year by year and are not completely comparable.

Thus, in terms of gross household survey and program statistics, a remarkable transformation has taken place. The gaps between black and white use rates and expenditures for care have closed significantly. Even more significantly, the gaps between patterns of use by the poor and by the affluent have reversed themselves. Two "iron laws" of the health care market had been formulated from the health surveys before the civil rights era:

1. The use of health services in the United States is directly related to income.
2. The prevalence of illness and, consequently, the need for health care is inversely related to income.

TABLE 6.3.   Age-Adjusted Hospital Discharge Rates by Race and Income

	Hospital Discharges			Days of Care		
	White	Black	Black/White Ratio	White	Black	Black/White Ratio
1964	112.4	84.0	0.75	961.4	1062.9	1.11
1972	124.5	118.2	0.95	1061.4	1409.7	1.33
1975	124.5	129.3	1.04	1016.3	1359.3	1.34
1980	119.4	130.4	1.09	921.0	1365.7	1.48
1985	105.1	115.2	1.10	729.5	983.1	1.35
1990	89.5	112.0	1.25	580.9	875.9	1.51
1994	85.1	111.6	1.31	518.7	746.5	1.44

	Income			Income		
	High	Low	Low/High Ratio	High	Low	Low/High Ratio
1964	110.7	102.4	0.93	918.9	1051.2	1.14
1972	98.4	142.5	1.45	725.6	1444.2	1.99
1975	106.5	161.2	1.51	808.3	1674.6	2.07
1980	102.4	157.5	1.54	714.1	1457.8	2.04
1985	81.0	139.1	1.72	489.1	1191.9	2.44
1990	72.5	142.2	1.96	446.2	1141.2	2.56
1994	60.6	134.6	2.22	320.4	969.9	3.03

Source: Data from National Center for Health Statistics, *Health in the United States, 1991* (Hyattsville, Md.: Public Health Service, 1992), table 81, p. 224 (for years 1964, 1985, 1990); National Center for Health Statistics, *Health in the United States, 1996–97, and Injury Chart Book* (Hyattsville, Md.: Public Health Service, 1997), table 85, p. 208 (for years 1990, 1994); National Center for Health Statistics, *Health in the United States, 1979* (Hyattsville, Md., 1980), 199 (for year 1972).

Note: Data based on household interviews of noninstitutionalized civilian population.

The Medicare and Medicaid programs had succeeded in breaking the first of these two laws.

None of the crude statistical comparisons by race and income presented above, however, adjust for need. Racial and income group equivalence in use and expenditures, of course, doesn't imply equivalence in need. At the time of the introduction of the Medicare and Medicaid programs, white rates of use and expenditures relative to nonwhite use tended to be higher in the South, reflecting income disparities, rural versus urban disparities in use, and the lingering legacy of Jim Crow. These regional differences have, however become progressively less pronounced over time.[27]

Beneath these household survey and Medicare program indicators, however, many more subtle but troubling racial disparities remain. Large

TABLE 6.4.   Nursing Home and Personal-Care Home Residents 65 Years of Age and Older per 1,000 Population, by Race and Age

	Age			
Race	65 Years and Older	65–74 Years	75–84 Years	85+ Years
White				
1963	26.6	8.1	41.7	157.7
1973–74	46.9	12.5	60.3	270.8
1985	47.7	12.3	59.1	228.7
1995	42.3	9.3	44.9	200.7
Black				
1963[a]	10.3	5.9	13.8	41.8
1973–74	22.0	11.1	26.7	105.7
1985	35.0	15.4	45.3	141.5
1995	45.2	18.4	57.2	167.1
Black/white Ratio				
1963[a]	0.39	0.73	0.33	0.27
1973–74	0.47	0.89	0.44	0.39
1985	0.73	1.25	0.77	0.62
1995	1.07	1.98	1.27	0.83

Source: Data from National Center for Health Statistics, *Health in the United States, 1996–97 and Injury Chart Book* (Hyattsville, Md.: Public Health Service, 1997), table 93, p. 223.

Note: Data are based on a survey of nursing homes. Residents in personal-care and domiciliary homes were included in 1963 survey but excluded in subsequent years.

[a]Blacks includes all nonwhites.

TABLE 6.5. Use of Medicare Services by the Aged, Persons Served per 1,000 Enrolled

	Inpatient Hospital			Skilled Nursing			Supplementary Medical Insurance		
	Race			Race			Race		
	White	Nonwhite	NW/W Ratio	White	Nonwhite	NW/W Ratio	White	Nonwhite	NW/W Ratio
1967	189	138	0.73	19	7	0.37	372	263	0.71
1968	201	154	0.77	21	9	0.43	403	304	0.75
1969	208	165	0.79	20	9	0.45	434	341	0.79
1971	215	173	0.80	12	6	0.50	460	388	0.84
1973	216	178	0.82	12	6	0.50	474	412	0.87
1974	216	180	0.83	12	7	0.58	505	448	0.89
1975	222	185	0.83	12	7	0.58	541	488	0.90
1976	261	193	0.74	13	8	0.62	569	518	0.91
1980	239.8	214.7	0.90	10.2	6.9	0.68	639.6	576.2	0.90
1981	240.2	213.4	0.89	9.9	6.3	0.64	656.8	588.7	0.90
1982	245.7	218.5	0.89	9.7	5.9	0.61	642.7	573.7	0.89
1983	244.2	219.9	0.90	10	6.5	0.65	676.5	635.2	0.94
1984	241.3	227.6	0.94	11.1	7.4	0.67	703.1	663.2	0.94
1994	335	365	1.09	40	30	0.75	883.9	743.8	0.84

Source: Data from M. Ruther and A. Dobson, "Unequal Treatment and Unequal Benefits: A Re-examination of the Use of Medicare Services by Race, 1967–1976," Health Care Financing Review 2, no. 3 (1981): 55–83; Bureau of Data Management and Strategy, Health Care Financing Administration; Karen Davis, "Equal Treatment and Unequal Benefits: The Medicare Program," Milbank Quarterly 53, no. 4 (1975): 449–88; C. Link, S. Long, and R. Settle, "Access to Medical Care under Medicaid: Differentials by Race," Journal of Health Policy Politics and Law 7, no. 2 (1982): 345–65.

TABLE 6.6. Use of Medicare Services by the Aged, Reimbursement per Enrollee by Type of Service

| | Inpatient Hospital | | | Skilled Nursing | | | Supplementary Medical Insurance | | |
| | Race | | | Race | | | Race | | |
	White	Nonwhite	NW/W Ratio	White	Nonwhite	NW/W Ratio	White	Nonwhite	NW/W Ratio
1967	$139	$102	0.74	$14	$5	0.33	$73	$44	0.60
1968	$175	$137	0.78	$17	$8	0.46	$83	$54	0.66
1969	$198	$160	0.81	$16	$8	0.49	$91	$62	0.68
1971	$251	$215	0.86	$8	$4	0.54	$102	$73	0.71
1973	$286	$260	0.91	$9	$5	0.57	$113	$88	0.79
1974	$320	$302	0.95	$10	$6	0.57	$134	$110	0.82
1975	$396	$373	0.94	$11	$7	0.71	$161	$140	0.87
1976	$482	$460	0.96	$13	$8	0.65	$190	$169	0.89
1980	$777	$832	1.07	$13	$11	0.85	$303	$261	0.86
1984	$1,253	$1,328	1.06	$17	$13	0.76	$497	$465	0.94
1994	$2,101	$2,579	1.23	$180	$143	0.80	$2,489	$2,456	0.99
1995	$2,044	$2,480	1.21	$230	$225	0.98	$1,530	$1,726	1.13

Source: Data from M. Ruther and A. Dobson, "Unequal Treatment and Unequal Benefits: A Re-examination of the Use of Medicare Services by Race, 1967–1976," *Health Care Financing Review* 2, no. 3 (1981): 55–83; Bureau of Data Management and Strategy, Health Care Financing Administration; Karen Davis, "Equal Treatment and Unequal Benefits: The Medicare Program," *Milbank Quarterly* 53, no. 4 (1975): 449–88; C. Link, S. Long, and R. Settle, "Access to Medical Care under Medicaid: Differentials by Race," *Journal of Health Policy Politics and Law* 7, no. 2 (1982): 345–65.

inequities in the use of specific types of services continue to be reported.[28] Household surveys have documented the discrepancies in access to primary care.[29] The proportion of blacks receiving adequate prenatal care, up-to-date childhood immunizations, flu shots as seniors, and cancer screening lags significantly behind whites, even though most of the financial barriers to such preventive services have been eliminated.[30] Once into the medical-care system, where the decisions of providers shape patterns of use of more specialized, costly, state-of-the-art procedures, the large differences in rates of use continue. Nationally, age-adjusted white rates of many costly procedures such as hip replacement, arthroscopy, and coronary artery bypass grafts are more than twice those of nonwhites.[31] Even where the effects of differences in insurance coverage are muted, wide differences have been found in rates of cardiovascular procedures.[32] Significant variations in use have been reported in the Medicare population with lower rates of use for specialized procedures.[33] In spite of a national computerized point system for allocating organs and universal coverage under the Medicare program, black dialysis patients are less likely to receive a kidney and less likely to survive a transplant.[34]

The effects of income and race are difficult to untangle, even in the Medicare program, which provides uniform entitlement to those over 65. The out-of-pocket costs are substantial and will shape beneficiary decisions about care. As indicated in table 6.7, the median household income of persons over 65 differs dramatically by race. The lowest income category includes 73 percent of black Medicare beneficiaries but only 19 per-

TABLE 6.7.   Medicare Beneficiaries by Race and Income 1993

Income	Whites		Blacks	
	Number	Percent	Number	Percent
Less than $13,100	4,640,929	19	1,497,441	73
$13,101 to 16,300	6,296,521	26	278,303	14
$16,301 to 20,500	6,576,610	27	151,430	7
Greater than $20,500	6,688,976	28	128,056	6
Total	24,203,036	100	2,055,230	100
Index of Dissimilarity:		0.58		

Source: Data from M. Gornick et al., "Effects of Race and Income on Mortality and Use of Services among Medicare Beneficiaries," *New England Journal of Medicine* 355, no. 11 (1996): 793.

Note: Median household income for persons 65 or older by race for beneficiaries by zip code of residence based on 1990 U.S. census.

cent of whites. Such statistics understate the gaps in resources since there are even greater racial disparities in wealth than there are in income. Thus, how much of the differences in use are simply a reflection of this disparity in resources?

As indicated in table 6.8, however, racial discrepancies in the Medicare program persist even when controlling for income. The black/white differences are actually larger, in terms of physician visits (higher for whites) and hospital discharges (higher for blacks) in the highest income category. Gaps in rates of mammography and hip fracture repair by race do not close as one controls for income. Rates of amputation of lower limbs, typically done as a result of complications of diabetes, are more than three times higher for blacks in all income categories. Similarly, bilateral orchiectomy, a procedure primarily performed to treat metastatic prostate cancer, are more than twice as high for blacks in all

TABLE 6.8.   Differences between Black and White Beneficiaries in Use of Services, Adjusted for Income

	Per 1,000 Beneficiaries		Age-Sex Income Adjusted	
	White	Black	Black-White Rate Ratio	Standard Error (+/–)
Visits to Physicians for				
Ambulatory Care	8.1	7.2	0.93	0.003
Mammography	26.0	17.1	0.75	0.001
Hospital discharges				
All discharges	329.1	375.6	1.15	0.001
Ischemic heart disease				
discharges	33.8	25.0	0.78	0.003
Inpatient procedures				
Percutaneous transluminal				
coronary angioplasty	4.8	1.9	0.51	0.007
Coronary-artery bypass				
surgery			0.43	0.007
Reduction of hip fracture	7.0	2.9	0.43	0.007
Bilateral orchiectomy	0.8	2.0	2.32	0.062
Amputation of all or part				
of lower limbs	1.9	6.7	3.30	0.032

Source: Data from M. Gornick et al., "Effects of Race and Income on Mortality and Use of Services among Medicare Beneficiaries," *New England Journal of Medicine* 355, no. 11 (1996): 793–97.

income categories. While these two conditions occur at somewhat higher rates in blacks than in whites, this doesn't account for these disparities in treatment. In the case of bilateral orchiectomy, the rates for blacks increase by income, while declining by income for whites. Adjusting for age, sex, and income for use of services by Medicare beneficiaries, black use rates are significantly higher for hospital discharges, amputations, and bilateral orchiectomy, but rates are lower for ambulatory care visits, reduction of hip fracture, mammography, percutaneous transluminal coronary angioplasty, and coronary artery bypass surgery. In other words, white Medicare beneficiaries are more likely to receive preventive and complex restorative services, and black beneficiaries are more likely to receive services for conditions that are partially preventable through adequate screening and primary care.

Many factors, of course, play a role in producing racial inequities in use of services. The most commonly offered explanations include (1) inequities in insurance coverage and the wealthier individual's ability to pay out-of-pocket costs for services, (2) the lower payments and increased administrative red tape that discourage provider participation in the Medical Assistance programs that many minorities must rely on for care, (3) the geographic maldistribution of health resources, and (4) the lack of trust in and familiarity with resources that inhibits blacks from seeking early intervention and treatment. All of these explanations may influence the character of patient-physician interactions during the discussion of treatment options.[35]

Some studies reporting inequities, however, also identify racial discrimination by providers as a possible explanation. This possibility is typically alluded to only in the discussion section of these studies. For example, a study analyzing the factors affecting delays in placement of patients from hospitals to nursing homes in North Carolina showed that race, adjusting for payment status and medical condition, was the strongest independent predictor and suggested that it was related to the apparent practice of racially matching semiprivate room occupants.[36] Falcone and Broyles, identifying similar race-related delays in nursing-home placement, suggest that discrimination in room assignments may take a variety of forms—from passively accession to the wishes of patients and family members, to active adoption as a business strategy.[37] Other researchers, reviewing large differences by race in the rates of procedures performed in hospitals for Medicare beneficiaries, note that "while difference in economic status and health care delivery may explain some of the differences by race, patient preferences, as well as provider opinion and selection, may also contribute."[38] The American Medical Association's Council on Ethical and Judicial Affairs, in its own review of the black-white disparities in medical treatment, was less circumspect.

Such treatment decisions may reflect the existence of subconscious bias. This is a serious and troubling problem. Despite the progress of the past 25 years, racial prejudice has not been entirely eliminated in this country.[39]

The council went on to suggest that practice parameters should include criteria that would preclude or diminish racial disparities. Similarly, in discussing the discrepancies in cardiovascular procedures, one group of researchers concluded,

We believe that inadequate health education, differences in patients' preferences for invasive management, delivery systems that are unfriendly to members of certain cultures, and overt racism may all play a part. Allocating responsibility more precisely will require studies that control for angiographic data and directly examine interactions between patients and medical professionals. Debating how much "blame" should be allocated to which factor should not delay efforts to clarify and remedy each of these deficiencies within our medical care system.[40]

Outcomes: Improvements in Health, but with Persistent Gaps

Beyond the elusive goal of eliminating racial disparities in appropriate use of services is the even more elusive one of eliminating disparities in health. Most racial differences in use of health services understate these disparities, since they fail to correct for the generally higher need for services in the black population. As indicated in table 6.9, between 1950 and 1995 age-adjusted mortality rates declined 40 percent for whites and 38 percent for blacks. In 1995, however, black age-adjusted mortality rates were still 1.61 times that of whites, a disparity essentially unchanged since 1950. In terms of years of life lost before the age of seventy-five per 100,000 population, blacks continue to have rates more than twice those of whites.[41]

Researchers have struggled to untangle the complex relationships between race, income, social class, and health outcomes, just as they have struggled to untangle the same relationship between these factors and use of health services. As indicated in table 6.10, The age-adjusted odds that a twenty-five- to sixty-four-year-old person in the United States will die in any given year are higher for a black than for a white, and are not eliminated by either education or income.[42] Indeed, for adult males under sixty-five, the discrepancies between black and white mortality rates is most pronounced in the highest educational category, while for adult females it occurs in the highest income category. However, studies are fairly equally divided between those that conclude that, once adjusted for social class, there are no significant race effects, and those that report attenuated but still significant race effects. For example, one study developed models that progressively adjust for family status, income, and then both family status and income, using the same national data sources. The models progressively reduced the odds ratio between black and white infant mortality rates from 1.48 to 1.29 to 1.17 and, finally, to 1.01.[43]

The most convincing evidence for the persistence of racial differences, controlling for socioeconomic factors, appears to be in infant mortality and hypertension. Several studies have shown that racial differences in the rates of low-birth-weight babies actually increase rather than diminish at higher levels of social-economic status.[44] The racial differences in hypertension are well documented and appear to persist across socioeconomic levels. Hypertension is stress related, and many researchers hypothesize a similar connection with low birth weight and infant mortality.[45]

Racial discrepancies in outcomes are often attributed to differences in risk behaviors and "lifestyles" as well as to education levels. However, differences in lifestyle patterns such as alcohol, tobacco, and illicit drug use, which might shape health outcomes between whites and blacks, are also significantly altered by adjusting for socioeconomic status. As indicated in table 6.11, once such adjustments are made, most of the disparities disappear.[46]

Thus, in the complex equation that determines not only access to specific services but also to life chances, an individual's race, mediated by income and other measures of socioeconomic status, continues to play a role that is not fully understood. Blacks receive fewer preventative and technologically sophisticated services. They have shorter life expectancies and suffer from more chronic illnesses. Income differences and insurance status do not explain all of these differences in use and outcomes.

Racial Integration: The Persistence of a Divided Health System

A major focus of the civil rights movement in the 1960s was ending segregation. To be separate was, by definition, to be unequal. The restrictions blacks encountered in access to education as health professionals, the castelike employment structure that relegated blacks to lower-status positions, and the separate institutions and services for blacks and whites had to be eliminated. This meant (1) opening up paths to education, (2) equalizing employment opportunities, and (3) ending the pattern of providing services in racially separate settings. What happened and what didn't?

TABLE 6.9. Age-Adjusted Death Rates for Selected Causes of Death, According to Race, Selected Years 1950–95

	Deaths per 100,000 Resident Population							Percentage change 1950–95
	1950	1960	1970	1980	1985	1990	1995	
White								
All causes	800.4	727.0	679.6	559.4	524.9	492.8	476.9	−40.4
Natural causes								
Diseases of heart	—	—	—	497.7	471.9	442.0	428.5	—
Ischemic heart disease	300.5	281.5	249.1	197.6	176.6	146.9	133.1	−55.7
Cerebrovascular diseases	—	—	—	150.6	126.6	102.5	89.0	—
Malignant neoplasms	83.2	74.2	61.8	38.0	30.1	25.5	24.7	−70.3
Respiratory system	124.7	124.2	127.8	129.6	131.2	131.5	127.0	1.8
Colorectal	13.0	19.1	28.0	35.6	38.4	40.6	39.3	202.3
Prostate	—	17.9	16.9	15.4	14.7	13.3	12.3	—
Breast	13.1	12.4	12.3	13.2	13.4	15.3	14.0	6.9
Chronic obstructive pulmonary diseases	22.5	22.4	23.4	22.8	23.4	22.9	20.5	−8.9
Pneumonia and influerza	4.3	8.2	13.4	16.3	19.2	20.1	21.3	395.3
Chronic liver disease and cirrhosis	22.9	24.6	19.8	12.2	12.9	13.4	12.4	−45.9
Diabetes mellitus	8.6	10.3	13.4	11.0	8.9	8.0	7.4	−14.0
Human immunodeficiency virus infection	13.9	12.8	12.9	9.1	8.6	10.4	11.7	−15.8
External causes	—	—	—	—	—	8.0	11.1	—
Unintentional injuries	55.7	47.6	51.0	61.9	53.0	50.8	48.4	−46.3
Motor vehicle-related injuries	23.1	22.3	26.9	41.5	34.2	31.8	29.9	−29.0
Suicide	11.6	11.1	12.4	23.4	19.1	18.6	16.4	2.6
Homicide and legal intervention	2.6	2.7	4.7	12.1	12.3	12.2	11.9	111.5
				6.9	5.4	5.9	5.5	

Black								
All causes	1,236.7	1,073.3	1,043.9	842.5	793.6	789.2	765.7	−38.1
Natural causes				740.2	713.5	701.3	685.8	—
Diseases of heart	379.6	334.4	307.6	255.7	240.6	213.5	198.8	−47.6
Ischemic heart disease	—	—	—	150.5	130.9	113.2	103.4	—
Cerebrovascular diseases	150.9	140.3	114.5	68.5	55.8	48.4	45.0	−70.2
Malignant neoplasms	129.1	142.3	156.7	172.1	176.6	182.0	171.6	32.9
Respiratory system	10.4	20.3	33.5	46.5	50.3	54.0	49.9	379.8
Colorectal	—	15.2	16.6	16.9	17.9	17.9	17.3	—
Prostate	16.9	22.2	25.4	29.1	31.2	35.3	34.0	101.2
Breast	19.3	21.3	21.5	23.3	25.5	27.5	27.5	42.5
Chronic obstructive pulmonary diseases	—	—	—	12.5	15.3	16.9	17.6	—
Pneumonia and influenza	57.0	56.4	40.4	19.2	18.8	19.8	17.8	−68.8
Chronic liver disease and cirrhosis	7.2	11.7	24.8	21.6	16.3	13.7	9.9	37.5
Diabetes mellitus	17.2	22.0	26.5	20.3	20.1	24.8	28.5	65.7
Human immunodeficiency virus infection	—	—	—	—	—	25.7	51.8	—
External causes	—	—	—	101.2	80.1	87.8	79.8	—
Unintentional injuries	70.9	66.4	74.4	51.2	42.3	39.7	37.4	−47.2
Motor vehicle-related injuries	24.7	23.4	30.6	19.7	17.4	18.4	16.6	−32.8
Suicide	4.2	4.7	6.1	6.4	6.4	7.0	6.9	64.3
Homicide and legal intervention	30.5	27.4	46.1	40.6	29.2	39.5	33.4	9.5

(continued)

TABLE 6.9—Continued

	Deaths per 100,000 Resident Population							
	1950	1960	1970	1980	1985	1990	1995	Percentage change 1950–95
Black/White Ratio								
All causes	1.55	1.48	1.54	1.51	1.51	1.60	1.61	3.9
Natural causes								
Diseases of heart	—	—	—	1.49	1.51	1.59	1.60	—
Ischemic heart disease	1.26	1.19	1.23	1.29	1.36	1.45	1.49	18.2
Cerebrovascular diseases	—	—	—	1.00	1.03	1.10	1.16	0.4
Malignant neoplasms	1.81	1.89	1.85	1.80	1.85	1.90	1.82	0.4
Respiratory system	1.04	1.15	1.23	1.33	1.35	1.38	1.35	30.5
Colorectal	0.80	1.06	1.20	1.31	1.31	1.33	1.27	58.7
Prostate	—	0.85	0.98	1.10	1.22	1.35	1.41	—
Breast	1.29	1.79	2.07	2.20	2.33	2.31	2.43	88.3
Chronic obstructive pulmonary diseases	0.86	0.95	0.92	1.02	1.09	1.20	1.34	56.4
Pneumonia and influenza	—	—	—	0.77	0.80	0.84	0.83	—
Chronic liver disease and cirrhosis	2.49	2.29	2.04	1.57	1.46	1.48	1.44	-42.3
Diabetes mellitus	0.84	1.14	1.85	1.96	1.83	1.71	1.34	59.8
Human immunodeficiency virus infection	1.24	1.72	2.05	2.23	2.34	2.38	2.44	96.9
External causes	—	—	—	—	—	3.21	4.67	—
Unintentional injuries	—	—	—	1.63	1.51	1.73	1.65	—
Motor vehicle-related injuries	1.27	1.39	1.46	1.23	1.24	1.25	1.25	-1.7
Suicide	1.07	1.05	1.14	0.84	0.91	0.99	1.01	-5.3
Homicide and legal intervention	11.73	10.15	9.81	5.88	5.41	6.69	6.07	-48.2

Source: Data from National Center for Health Statistics, *Health in the United States, 1996–97, and Injury Chart Book* (Hyattsville, Md.: Public Health Service, 1997), 112.

Note: Dashes indicate data not available.

Education

Marked improvement in enrollment patterns in health professional schools has taken place since the 1960s. As indicated in table 6.12, black enrollment as a percent of total enrollment has more than doubled in medical schools and has increased significantly in dentistry and pharmacy. In 1947, only about 145 black physicians were graduated each year, with the two historically black medical schools, Howard and Meharry, producing more than 70 percent of this total. Blacks in 1947 represented only 3 percent of all medical graduates.[47] By 1994, blacks composed 9.6 percent of the students enrolled in medical schools, with more than twelve hundred of those graduating, roughly 70 percent at white-majority schools. The proportion of blacks in health professional schools of all kinds, however, still lags behind their representation in the population (12.6 percent).

Employment

The civil rights effort had set as one of its goals the elimination of a social and economic caste system that assigned jobs and socioeconomic status by race. Real equality in access and health outcomes, it was assumed, could

TABLE 6.10.   Age-Adjusted Ratio of Mortality Rates, by Education and Income, Ages 25–64, for 1986

	Ratio B/W	
	Women	Men
Education (years)		
0–11	1.82	1.76
12	1.56	1.86
13–15	1.52	1.16
16 or more	1.22	2.14
Income ($)		
<$9,000	1.17	1.22
9,000–14,999	1.32	1.06
15,000–18,999	1.12	1.72
19,000–24,999	0.93	1.02
25,000+	1.44	1.5

Source: Data from G. Pappas, S. Queen, W. Hadden, and G. Fisher, "The Increasing Disparity in Mortality between Socioeconomic Groups in the United States, 1960 and 1986," *New England Journal of Medicine* 329 (1993): 103–9.

TABLE 6.11. Relative Likelihood of Using Alcohol,
Cigarettes, or Illicit Drugs by Blacks and Whites, Age
18–49, 1991

	Odds Ratio
Alcohol	
Nonheavy	0.72
Heavy	0.55
Cigarettes	
Nonheavy	1.21
Heavy	0.36
Marijuana	
Nonheavy	0.68
Heavy	1.29
Cocaine	
Nonheavy	0.55
Heavy	1.87
Crack	1.87
Poly-illicit drugs[a]	0.43

Source: Data from R. Flewelling, *National Household Survey on Drug Abuse: Race/Ethnicity, Socioeconomic Status, and Drug Abuse, 1991* (Washington, D.C.: U.S. Dept of Health and Human Services, 1993).

Note: Adjusted for socioeconomic characteristics.

[a]Use of 3 or more illicit drugs in the past year.

TABLE 6.12. Black Enrollment as a Percentage of Total Enrollment in Schools for Health Professions, 1970–94

	1970–71	1980–81	1990–91	1993–94
Allopathic medicine	3.8	5.7	6.5	10.7
	(1,509)	(3,708)	(4,241)	(4,900)
Osteopathic medicine	1.2	1.9	3.2	3.3
	(27)	(94)	(217)	(256)
Dentistry	4.5	4.5	6.0	6.0
	(872)	(1,022)	(940)	(972)
Pharmacy	3.7	4.4	5.7	7.3
	(659)	(945)	(1,301)	(2,380)
Registered nursing			10.4	8.7
			(23,094)	(23,501)

Source: Data from National Center for Health Statistics, 1997, *National Center for Health Statistics Health in the United States 1996–97 and Injury Chart Book* (Hyattsville, Md.: Public Health Service, 1997), table 108, 240.

Note: Numbers in parentheses are *N*s.

not be achieved without the elimination of such boundaries. A distribution of jobs across various economic and occupational categories that reflected the racial composition of the population would signal the accomplishment of this goal. However, as indicated in table 6.13, marked gaps remain. Blacks continue to be underrepresented in higher-status employment categories and overrepresented in lower ones. For example, while blacks accounted for 10.7 percent of the workforce in the United States during 1996, they accounted for 4.5 percent of the physicians and 33.2 percent of the nursing aides, orderlies, and attendants.

A minister and frequent visitor to nursing homes reflected about the problem: "Nursing homes operate like plantations: black service workers and white patients. The better nursing home administrators recognize the problem."[48]

Segregation in the Provision of Services

The civil rights movement, specifically through the passage of the Medicare legislation, set as a goal the elimination of racial segregation in the provision of health services. However, simply tearing down the Jim Crow signs, forcing random assignments to patient rooms, and requiring the racial integration of medical staffs were not sufficient in themselves to accomplish such a goal. Patterns of residential segregation, geographic separation, and economic inequalities shape where individuals receive their care.[49]

How much integration was actually achieved in health care has never been officially documented.[50] While the Medicare program forced racial integration within facilities, it also stimulated the creation of new proprietary hospital chains and the relocation of urban hospitals to the suburbs, both catering to private-pay and predominantly white markets.[51] Using Medicare program data, however, it is possible to document the current degree of hospital segregation in that program.[52] The Expanded Modified MEDPAR (Medicare Provider Analysis and Review) File for fiscal year 1993 contains records of all Medicare beneficiary discharges from short-term acute and specialty hospitals. The racial information on beneficiaries in the file is from Social Security enrollment records and subsequent enrollment surveys. Consequently, it is more uniform and complete than that provided by hospital claims data. Using these data, I constructed the most common measure of segregation, the index of dissimilarity.[53] An index of zero would show that black and white inpatients distribute themselves across facilities proportional to their numbers in the population as a whole. In such a case, each facility would have the same racial composition as exists in the total population of discharges. An index of 1 would show

TABLE 6.13. Blacks Employed in Health-Related Occupations in 1996

	N (all races, in thousands)	Percentage Black	Ratio to % Total Black Employment[a]
Managers, medicine and health	713	8.50	0.794
Natural scientists			
Chemist	149	3.70	0.346
Biological and life sciences	116	4.70	0.439
Medical sciences	73	4.80	0.449
Health-diagnosing occupations			
Physicians	667	4.50	0.421
Dentists	137	1.20	0.112
Veterinarians	54	2.90	0.271
Health assessment and treating occupations			
Registered Nurses	1,986	8.60	0.804
Pharmacists	184	6.80	0.636
Dieticians	105	29.30	2.738
Therapists			
Respiratory	64	4.50	0.421
Physical	118	3.80	0.355
Speech	97	2.20	0.206
Physician assistants	63	1.80	0.168
Technicians, sales, and administrative support			
Health technologists and technicians			
Clinical laboratory technologists and technicians	376	16.10	1.505
Dental hygienists	94	0.00	0
Radiological technicians	135	8.70	0.0813
Licensed practical nurses	395	14.00	1.308
Science technicians			
Biological	79	9.30	0.869
Chemical	78	14.50	1.355

TABLE 6.13—*Continued*

	N (all races, in thousands)	Percentage Black	Ratio to % Total Black Employment[a]
Service occupations			
Health service occupations			
Dental assistant	212	6.20	0.579
Health aides, except nursing	336	23.30	2.178
Nursing aides orderlies, and attendants	1,850	33.20	3.103
Cleaning and building service occupations			
Supervisors	166	23.90	2.234
Maids and housemen	683	29.60	2.766
Janitors and cleaners	2,205	21.10	1.972
Total	11,135	11.00	1.032

Source: Data from unpublished Household Survey Data Annual Averages, 1996, Division of Labor Force Statistics, U.S. Bureau of Labor Statistics, Washington, D.C., 1997.

Note: Index of dissimilarity for all health-related occupations = .322.

[a]Blacks represented 10.7 percent of all employed persons.

complete separation of the races. The actual value of the index represents the proportion of the two populations one would need to move to create an equal distribution of the races across all facilities.

As indicated in table 6.14, for fiscal year 1993 there were a total of 11,075,789 Medicare discharges from short-term acute and specialty care hospitals. This included 84.3 percent white, 9.8 percent black, 2.9 percent other, and 3.0 percent for whom race was unknown or missing, distributed across 5,393 providers of service. As shown in table 6.15, the index of segregation for the United States as a whole was .529 and ranged from .716 to .154. States in the Midwest and Northeast, with black populations more concentrated in urban areas, had generally higher segregation indexes than southern states. Underneath these numbers are the footprints of the great migration of black Americans that began after World War I.[54] Historically, concentrated in the rural South, the search for employment and better living conditions shifted a large portion of this population to large cities of the Northeast and Midwest. The hospital segregation indexes reflect this migration and the greater geographic separation that exists in the Northeast and Midwest.

Underlying the broader patterns of geographic separation are those of health care utilization within the more geographically concentrated medical-service areas. The same measure of segregation that was applied to the nation as a whole and to each state was applied to 126 Standard Metropolitan Statistical Areas with a black population of more than thirty thousand. Standard Metropolitan Statistical Areas have often been used as rough approximations of medical service areas. Many factors may contribute to the degree of hospital racial segregation in a metropolitan area. Five interrelated factors that were included in a model to predict the degree of hospital segregation in a service area were (1) its size, (2) the density of hospitals, (3) the degree of residential segregation, (4) the degree of racial income inequities, and (5) regional location. The larger the metropolitan area and the larger the number of hospitals per unit of population, the greater the hospital choices individuals have and the greater the potential for racial segregation to be reflected in the pattern of use of hospitals. Since geographic proximity strongly influences patterns of hospital use, it would be expected that an index of residential segregation in a metropolitan area would be strongly related to an index of hospital segregation. Differences in income or the ability to pay for care may also restrict the choices of individuals. Hence, racial differences in income levels may in turn influence the degree of hospital racial segregation. Since Jim Crow practices were historically concentrated in the South, one would expect this to be reflected in the degree of hospital racial segregation.

The results of this analysis are presented in table 6.16. A linear regression model used to predict hospital segregation in the 126 SMSAs with the largest black population had an adjusted R^2 of .52 ($p < .0001$).[55] Hospital segregation was related to the natural log of the population of the metropolitan area ($p < .001$), the relative density of hospitals ($p < .001$), and to

TABLE 6.14.   Acute and Specialty Hospital
Discharges, Medicare Patients, by Race, FY 1993

	Discharges	Percentage
White	9,338,251	84.3
Black	1,081,844	9.8
Other	322,367	2.9
Unknown	333,327	3.0
Total	11,075,789	100.0
Number of Hospitals	5,393	

Source: Data from Health Care Financing Administration, Expanded Modified MEDPAR File for fiscal year 1993, Bureau of Data Management and Strategy HCFA, Baltimore, Md.

residential segregation (p < .01). It was negatively related to related racial income inequities (p < .05) and to location in the South (p < .05).

The regression results suggest a significant transformation of the South, at least from its popular image in the pre–civil rights era. *In hospital care in the Medicare program, the South is the most racially integrated region of the country.* The sixty-four metropolitan areas in the South included in this analysis were on the average smaller than the sixty-two metropolitan areas included from other regions of the country. They had higher hospital density and more racial income inequities, but less residential segregation. Attempting to correct for these differences, however, the model showed a significant effect for location in the South. Some of this effect for the population as a whole may be mitigated by economic segregation (e.g., Medical Assistance vs. private insurance accommodations) within facilities. However, from the perspective of hospitals in a metropolitan area, reimbursement from Medicare is essentially the same for all beneficiaries. Out-of-pocket costs and physician coverage under the Medicare supplementary medical insurance, of course, may vary by income.

Mobile, Alabama, the highwater mark of the federal civil rights offensive in 1967 described in the last chapter, provides a useful benchmark for translating these numbers into more interpretable measures of accomplishments. Alabama as a whole now ranks tenth among the most racially integrated states in terms of Medicare acute hospital admissions with an index of segregation of less than half the national average. Alabama also ranks thirteenth among states with the lowest disparity between black and white age adjusted death rates.[56] In spite of a relatively high degree of residential segregation for a southern metropolitan area (.659), the segregation of Medicare admissions in Mobile is less than that of Alabama as a whole (.298 versus .335). The pattern of clustering of facilities in many southern metropolitan areas, a legacy of the pre–civil rights era now works to assure a greater degree of racial integration. Among Mobile's hospitals, the Mobile Infirmary's Medicare proportion of admissions of blacks (30 percent) corresponds closely to their representation in the Mobile service area.

On the whole, however, there remains substantial racial segregation of Medicare beneficiaries in hospitals, reflecting the geographic distribution and persistence of residential segregation of the black population. The measure understates the segregation in the medical-care system as a whole since it (1) compares a fully insured population with common benefits, (2) fails to allow for economic segregation that might take place within rather than between facilities, and (3) fails to take account of the primary and long-term care services that are less evenly distributed and for which greater racial discrepancies in patterns of use exist.

TABLE 6.15.   Racial Segregation of Medicare Hospital Discharges by State, FY 1993

| | Number of Providers | Race of Patient | | Index of Dissimilarity |
		White	Black	
Delaware	7	23,859	4,019	.154
Hawaii	22	9,004	148	.168
Puerto Rico	54	80,957	7,696	.204
South Carolina	70	97,752	33,127	.275
Mississippi	103	101,131	40,841	.275
New Mexico	44	41,336	665	.286
Louisiana	146	156,264	50,999	.288
Connecticut	35	122,126	7,033	.315
North Carolina	128	225,424	54,039	.316
Rhode Island	12	47,240	1,192	.326
Alabama	115	181,990	46,088	.335
Nevada	23	38,365	1,947	.341
Maine	40	56,905	98	.346
Alaska	22	5,403	171	.351
West Virginia	58	105,898	3,589	.362
Georgia	160	218,910	64,816	.362
Oklahoma	114	127,997	7,539	.367
New Hampshire	26	38,964	122	.368
Kentucky	104	183,922	10,932	.378
Vermont	15	20,469	52	.381
Utah	41	37,335	189	.387
Maryland	54	149,692	37,147	.389
Montana	57	36,278	75	.389
Wyoming	27	13,162	105	.393
Florida	213	612,012	50,011	.393
Virginia	99	190,836	45,699	.403
Idaho	41	31,512	56	.405
Texas	410	518,580	62,938	.410
New Jersey	91	314,838	39,053	.418
Arizona	68	120,649	2,362	.420
North Dakota	51	34,140	38	.433
South Dakota	58	37,646	75	.436
Tennessee	135	245,317	34,833	.453
Ohio	190	459,824	49,724	.458
Iowa	122	135,768	2,017	.468
Massachusetts	101	292,722	9,256	.468
District of Columbia	10	14,232	20,317	.477
Kansas	132	105,557	4,705	.480
New York	231	636,553	77,106	.485
Washington	95	148,361	3,329	.498

TABLE 6.15—*Continued*

	Number of Providers	Race of Patient		Index of Dissimilarity
		White	Black	
Arkansas	83	118,695	15,765	.503
Colorado	66	93,087	2,706	.518
California	453	723,055	62,740	.525
Indiana	118	236,474	18,673	.540
Oregon	64	99,706	1,231	.556
Minnesota	145	151,488	1,795	.570
Missouri	133	240,661	23,227	.572
Michigan	173	325,843	51,259	.575
Pennsylvania	210	643,855	57,822	.581
Nebraska	91	60,928	1,460	.607
Illinois	205	421,085	63,796	.616
Wisconsin	128	204,444	7,222	.716
Total	5,393	9,338,251	1,081,844	.529

Source: Data from Health Care Financing Administration, Expanded Modified MED-PAR File for fiscal year 1993, Bureau of Data Management and Strategy HCFA, Baltimore, Md.

The provision of hospital care under the Medicare program remains, as the racial segregation indexes show, quite separate. In the tradition of the *Brown v. Board of Education* precedent that was eventually applied to hospitals, is separate unequal? The answers are complex and ambiguous. For example, one of the few studies that have tried to answer that question reviewed medical records of 297 hospitals and 9,932 patients who were Medicare beneficiaries. They concluded that, while blacks and the poor tend to receive poorer care within a hospital, this was offset by their 1.8 times higher likelihood of receiving care at an urban teaching hospital where better overall care was provided.[57] The more basic conclusion is that, since such care *is* separate, one should not evaluate information and health policy changes as if it were not.

There are two troubling implications of the persistence of racial segregation in health care.

First, the degree of segregation suggests the potential for a systematic racial bias in reporting of health events. Uniform classification and reporting across all service providers have proved an elusive goal. The National Hospital Discharge Survey has found that hospitals in their sample not reporting race were overwhelmingly white. White hospital use rates derived from this source of data underestimates actual use.[58] Studies using hospital discharge data that have reported large racial differences in use of such procedures as coronary artery bypass grafts probably understate the differences.[59] Variations in testing and reporting practices by providers for viable live births, sexually transmitted diseases, and drug and alcohol abuse by providers may similarly exaggerate the differences in these rates. For example, a recent audit of infant deaths in the Philadelphia area found a systematic racial bias in reporting. The overwhelming preponderance of black births take place at a few teaching hospitals in the city while the overwhelming preponderance of white births take place in suburban or community hospitals. Nonviable fetuses (babies born too premature to live) are reported as live births at the major teaching hospitals while they are less likely to be reported as such at the suburban community hospitals. If one corrects for this reporting bias, about half the difference in black and white infant mortality rates in the Philadelphia metropolitan area disappears.[60]

Second, the high rates of segregation also lend support to the concern about the racially unequal impact of market reforms. The states in the

TABLE 6.16.   Regression Model for Medicare Hospital Segregation in Standard Metropolitan Areas, FY 1993

Analysis of Variance	df	Sum of Squares	Mean Square	F	P-Value
Source	5	1.246	0.2492	28.092	0.0001
Model	120	1.0645	0.0089		
Cumulative total	125	2.3105			

Root MSE = .0942 $R^2 = .5393$
Mean = .3255

Variable	df	Parameter Estimate	SE	t	P-Value
INTERCEPT	1	−0.7647	0.2098	−3.645	0.0004
LNPOP	1	0.0711	0.0129	5.49	0.0001
HOSDEN	1	0.0663	0.0108	6.127	0.0001
RESEG	1	0.2647	0.0797	3.322	0.0012
INCSEG	1	−0.3680	0.1566	−2.351	0.0204
SOUTH	1	−0.0470	0.0197	−2.366	0.0186

Source: Data from Health Care Financing Administration, Expanded Modified MEDPAR File for fiscal year 1993; 1990 United State Census Summary, Tape File 1, Bureau of Data Management and Strategy, HCFA, Baltimore, Md., and U.S. Bureau of the Census, Washington, D.C.

Note: Calculated for 126 Standard Metropolitan Statistical Areas with a black population greater than 30,000.

Midwest and Northeast that have been generally most aggressive in introducing Medicaid market reforms are also ones with higher rates of hospital segregation.[61] Urban public hospitals and teaching hospitals care for a disproportionate share of this population and may be more vulnerable to current changes proposed in the Medicare program and in state and local managed-care health care reform. The potential for racially separate and unequal impact needs to be at least a visible, measurable consequence if not a moderating influence on such changes.

Organizational Adaptation

There is, however, a largely unexplored third dimension to describing what happened and what didn't. So far we have described a flat world. We have presented evidence concerning the impact of civil rights efforts in (1) closing racial gaps in health care access and outcomes and (2) ending a segregated, racially divided health system. That third dimension has to do with how organizations behave and how the behavior of health services organizations faced with these new pressures reshaped the organization of health services in the United States. Simply stated, organizations adapt to the constraints imposed on them by their environment. Those that don't adapt don't survive. Hospitals had to adapt by complying with the Title VI requirements while at the same time being responsive to the "racial sensibilities" of their local market. I argue here that they were able to adapt to these two sometimes-contradictory constraints because of the peculiar character of those racial sensibilities and the selective imposition of Title VI requirements on the health system as a whole.

Local Market Sensibilities: Vertical Integration but Horizontal Segregation

In understanding the adaptation that did take place, it is important to note that even the most extreme expressions of those "racial sensibilities," the Jim Crow laws in the South, *never fully* segregated blacks and whites. Only those interactions that were perceived as more personal and private and that, consequently, implied more equal status, were segregated. Blacks in Greensboro, North Carolina were free to enter the downtown Woolworth and make purchases; they just couldn't sit down at the lunch counter. Similarly, in Moses Cone Memorial Hospital in Greensboro, and throughout the South, patients were segregated on hospital floors but used common areas for diagnostic and ancillary services. Those that could find humor in this would joke about the seeming contradiction.[62] As long as people were "vertical," whites had little problem mixing with blacks. However, sitting down next to them was troubling and lying down next to them was unthinkable. These acts implied an increasing degree of social equality that such "vertical integration" did not. Furthermore, segregation did not require separate facilities, only that the same space in those facilities not be occupied by blacks and whites at the same time. White private-practice physicians who did not want to go to the extra expense of maintaining separate areas for their black and white patients would simply schedule them at separate times.[63]

Board chairman Benjamin Cone of Moses Cone Memorial Hospital in Greensboro, for example, as noted in chapter 3, was quick to defend his institution against accusations of race mixing, noting,

> Actually there is no mixing of Negro and white patients in rooms. . . . Of course, they become mixed when being served in radiology, laboratory, operating room and obstetric and delivery rooms. This can't be helped, and is exactly the same situation existing all over the South in general hospitals, which do have segregated Negro wards.[64]

The Selective Imposition of Title VI Requirements on the Health Care System

As described in chapter 5, a host of constraints including political realities, practical administrative considerations, and declining support for aggressive enforcement worked against uniform enforcement of Title VI. Nursing homes never received the on-site investigations and arm twisting that the general hospitals received. Private practice physicians, whose services were reimbursed by the supplemental medical insurance program (Part B of Medicare) were exempted altogether.

Adaptation

Those familiar with organization of medical services in other developed countries struggle to explain the distinctive organization of such services in the United States. Yet taking into account local market racial sensibilities and the selective character of Title VI enforcement, the evolution of the organization of health services in the United States would seem easy to explain. In brief, the resulting organizational adaptation allowed for a measure of "vertical integration" while minimizing "horizontal integration." This was achieved by (1) restricting acute hospital admissions and lengths of stay, (2) a massive expansion of a separate nursing-home sector, (3) a shift to greater emphasis on ambulatory services by hospitals, and (4) a massive conversion of acute-hospital beds to private accommodations in markets where racial sensibilities were of particular concern.

For the past thirty years, providers, planners, regulators, and third-party payers have focused on reducing excess acute-care bed capacity and hospital lengths of stay. The average length of stay in American hospitals is now the shortest in the world. In Japan the average length of stay in a hospital is more than four times as long, and in all European countries it is at least twice as long.[65] The United States has the lowest rate of general hospital beds per one thousand population in the developed world. Yet, health care planners and policy analysts in the United States have repeatedly argued over the past thirty years that there is an *oversupply* and *overutilization* of acute-hospital beds. These reductions in hospital admissions and lengths of stay have rarely exposed patients to increased medical risk but have placed an increasing burden on patients and their families. Insurance-driven early discharges, the so-called drive-by deliveries, the one-day C-section admissions, and treatment of mastectomies as an outpatient procedure finally sparked rebellion and the recent passage of federal and some state legislation mandating minimum lengths of stay.[66] The argument for limiting inpatient use over the last three decades has been to make more efficient use of resources and eliminate unnecessary costs. Yet the logic and evidence to support such arguments is weak. In spite of the substantial reductions in inpatient use, per capita hospital costs in the United States are still higher than in any nation in the world. Much of the current effort to transfer care to the home makes little sense in managing scarce resources and staffing that could be more efficiently managed by centralizing services in a hospital inpatient setting. One health care economist recently expressed bewilderment over the "American obsession" with reducing lengths of stay and substituting home care, which he described as about "as brilliant as inventing square wheels"[67]

In addition, hospitals over the last thirty years, partly in response to payment incentives, have increasingly shifted services from inpatient to ambulatory settings. Ambulatory diagnostic services, therapies, and surgical treatments have replaced inpatient stays. Most no longer even refer to themselves as hospitals but as medical centers and health systems.

More dramatic during the first decade after the passage of Medicare and Medicaid, however, was the rapid expansion of a separate modern nursing-home sector. As knowledgeable readers will be quick to point out, the markedly shorter lengths of stay in general hospitals in the United States result from the markedly different use of beds in such hospitals. This reflects another unique feature of the U.S. health system: the almost complete segregation of long-term from acute inpatient care. In Japan and

European countries many of the hospital beds are used almost inter-changeably for acute and long-term care. Historically and, to a somewhat lesser extent, up until the passage of the Medicare legislation, U.S. hospitals provided care to long-term patients. Indeed, many of the more progressive voluntary hospitals in the United States began to implement plans in the 1950s for transforming themselves into "health campuses" that would efficiently combine education, acute care, long-term care, and assisted living for the elderly.[68] Those efforts came to an end with the passage of the Medicare legislation. In acute hospitals, as described in the last chapter, room assignments without regard to race were aggressively monitored in the acute hospitals in the implementation of the Medicare program. No similar monitoring and enforcement effort was ever mounted for nursing homes. Between 1963 and 1974 the number of persons who were residents in nursing homes grew from 25.4 to 46.2 per 1,000 elderly.[69] Between 1963 and 1973 the number of nursing-home beds in the United States grew from 510,180 to 1,107,358, exceeding the number of acute-care hospital beds in the United States.[70] Even this shift understates the magnitude of the change, since many nursing homes closed during this period, replaced by larger, more medically oriented facilities, and proprietary chains replaced owner-operated facilities. The substitution of nursing-home care for that formerly delivered in state mental hospitals and general hospitals drove some of the increasing demand for nursing-home beds.

Appropriately skeptical readers will object to the characterization of the trend toward dramatically shorter length of stays, expanded outpatient services, and a separate nursing-home sector as being driven by the motive of preserving a degree of racial separation. They would argue that the nature of hospital-based specialty practice in the United States, the way in which hospitals and nursing homes were reimbursed for services, and the subsequent payment strategies that were adopted to control costs all pressured adaptation in this direction. This is certainly true. The basic question, however, is "why were these particular approaches and strategies selected?" The argument here is *not* that racial attitudes were the sole determining cause of all these changes. No single factor can explain why the organization of health in the United States evolved in distinctively different ways than in other developed countries. Its evolution reflects the adaptation to a complex combination of pressures. The argument here is that those racial attitudes and concerns helped often subtlety and indirectly, to reinforce, magnify, and legitimize these changes in use and methods of payment.

In most cases, race was not a conscious part of the decision shaping these organizational changes. Indeed, the dramatic nature of the changes caught many physicians and other participants by surprise.

I bumped into the man that used to deliver newspapers to patients at the hospital on the street. I hadn't seen him for a long time and I asked why. He said, "Oh, I don't deliver papers to the hospital anymore, the patients are too sick." The acuity is way up and we now have "disposition problems," trying to accelerate discharge. The mentality has become "vertical"—no horizontal thinking, no integration. Nobody seems to be interested in the patient as a person. I think the patients notice this.[71]

In other words, "horizontal" *racial* integration in health care is minimized and most likely to take place only in highly medicalized settings where most patients are almost comatose.

By far the greatest irony in the post-Medicare transformation of health care, however, was that Medicare, the same program whose implementation forced the racial integration of hospitals, also enabled hospitals to adapt and massively subsidized separation. Medicare and Medicaid capital cost reimbursement was basically a cost pass-through for hospitals. Whatever costs were incurred in renovating or constructing a new hospital physical plant in terms of interest and depreciation were recovered from Medicare and Medicaid. Prior to Medicare, hospital construction had been financed through direct public subsidies, such as Hill-Burton, accrued savings from operations, or charitable contributions. Now, since the Medicare and Medicaid programs essentially guaranteed repayment, it became feasible to receive the necessary funds for construction from tax-exempt bonds and private loans. As indicated in the last chapter, hospitals such as Druid City, a trend setter in Tuscaloosa, Alabama, tried to adapt to the constraints by converting their entire hospital to private rooms to avoid biracial occupancy, and a large number of surrounding area hospitals followed suit. The constraints of old physical plants limited the ability to do this in the short term. The Medicare and most Medicaid programs, however, provided a new and attractive source of payment for covering the cost of hospital construction and conversion. Indeed, the method of payment actually provided hospitals a financial incentive to build new facilities while discouraging the integration of long-term care and hospital care.[72]

This confluence of incentives propelled a massive hospital construction and renovation boom that would insulate many patients from the room assignments made, as the Title VI regulations required, without regard to race. The lending institutions and tax-exempt bond authorities were more than willing to underwrite these projects, the bulk of whose repayment costs were essentially guaranteed by the government. The local planning agencies responsible during the 1970s for approving such projects were focused almost exclusively on controlling bed supply, not the physical arrangements of those beds. The construction of largely private room accommodations also fit the expansionist strategies of some hospitals in the face of the efforts of local planning bodies to restrain them. Built large enough, private rooms could easily be converted, if necessary, to semiprivate rooms, accommodating two patients some time in the future. In many northern urban transition neighborhoods hospitals adopted the construction of all private accommodations as a conscious strategy to stem the tide of white flight of predominantly private pay patients to suburban hospitals. In many metropolitan areas of the South, where for-profit hospital chains were acquiring and building facilities in the growing suburban areas, hospitals that integrated too quickly or did not have sufficient single-bed rooms to accommodate racial aversions faced a declining census. For example, a nurse at Providence Hospital, a Catholic hospital in Mobile, Alabama, during the time the hospital was integrated recalled the difficulties.

> We integrated the hospital before the Mobile Infirmary did, and our census went way down. One floor had been all black with all black staff. People would bring their own pillows for fear of sleeping on one that a black had. It was a difficult transition for everybody. Black patients and staff didn't like it either. They didn't feel comfortable. The Mobile Infirmary dragged its feet but finally integrated too. A lot of people would try to find excuses for moving to a private room or changing rooms if they were in with a black and would never say why. We were an older facility and didn't have as many private rooms as the Mobile Infirmary, so we were more affected.[73]

Perhaps the greatest irony was that Providence Hospital, whose greater independence from local control had enabled it to lead in racial integration, also later relocated to a growing white suburban area of Mobile. It now serves the lowest percentage of black Medicare patients in the region (13 percent), and its new facility was the first in Mobile to provide exclusively private accommodations. The other acute hospitals quickly followed suit, and now the Mobile metropolitan area offers exclusively private accommodations for all acute hospital patients. Mobile General (now University of South Alabama Medical Center) and the Mobile Infirmary geographically buffer the new Providence Hospital from the bulk of the black and low-income population in the Mobile Metropolitan area.

As the case of Mobile illustrates, once one facility in an area converted to all private rooms, the others often rushed to follow suit. There was little to stem this shift. Most patients, given a choice, would prefer private accommodations in hospitals. There is no source of information nationally or internationally that keeps track of the number of private, semiprivate, and ward accommodations in the acute hospitals, but some general observations are possible. Almost none of the large ward accommodations that were the dominant pattern in the nation's teaching hospitals up until the 1960s remain. The private and voluntary community hospitals provide a mix of private and semiprivate accommodations. Many of the more recently constructed facilities provide all private room accommodations. No other developed country has undergone such a transformation. The hospitals of other developed nations—Japan, England, France, Germany, the Scandinavian countries—continue to provide predominantly ward and semiprivate accommodations for patients. It is quite reasonable to hypothesize that the U.S. health care system may have stockpiled the majority of private-room, acute-hospital accommodations in the world.

The argument here, as with the drastically shorter length of stay in U.S. hospitals, is not that racial attitudes by themselves caused the transformation to more private accommodations when racial segregation was no longer permissible. Other things being equal, most people prefer private hospital accommodations. The argument is that racial attitudes and concerns helped, often subtly and indirectly, to reinforce, magnify, and legitimize this transformation.

Private accommodations are not in themselves a bad thing, but they come at a price. They add to the cost of operations and construction. Staffing requirements, given the greater physical dispersion of patients, are likely to be higher. Construction costs are clearly much higher. Each such room is typically constructed with a private bathroom. The cost of hospital construction is typically calculated in terms of square feet of floor space, and private accommodations require more floor space per bed. The average floor space per bed in Japanese hospitals, for example, is roughly 25 percent of that in United States hospitals.[74] Grady Hospital, the public hospital in Atlanta whose twin towers had been the symbol of "separate but equal" health care in the United States, was completed in 1958. It had mostly eight- and four-bed wards along with a few private rooms. One did not request private rooms; one was assigned those rooms based on the medical condition. This was a major improvement in amenities. The "Old" Grady hospital had almost exclusively thirty-bed wards. In 1991 a major renovation of the hospital was completed, converting rooms to all private and semiprivate accommodations. Each of these rooms included a private bathroom. The construction costs of the "New" Grady hospital in 1958 was 25 million. Its renovation in 1991 cost approximately 325 million.[75]

Duke Medical Center used to have open wards. Long Ward, for black male patients, and Osler Ward, for black female patients, have now been converted to physicians' offices. The new hospital facilities are all private rooms.

One black physician who lived through the period of integration in North Carolina reflected on the ironies.

> In the South, in order to avoid having to put people in rooms together irrespective of race, part of the rebuilding of hospitals was to build all private rooms. "Wise" men have made "wise" choices! It's costs us a tremendous amount of money for "someone's" emotional well-being. What one comes to find out in the end is that black and white people are not really bothered about each other. Life is such a simple thing. All those terrible prognostications about what would happen with integration never happened. Yet we have all those private hospital rooms![76]

In Durham the two hospitals, historically all-white Watts Hospital and all-black Lincoln Hospital, merged. A single county hospital, Durham Regional, was built to replace the two facilities. Heated discussion about whether there should be any semiprivate accommodations surrounded the planning of the new facility. A black physician who had participated in these discussions reflected on the experience and the decision to include these accommodations in the new facility.

> It was one the best sociologic things that happened. It brought black people in contact with white people who never had any contact with them before.
>
> I saw an older man who got into difficulty with cancer of the colon. He was referred to me, and I took care of him at Durham Regional. He was in a semiprivate room with an old white fellow who had severe arterial sclerosis and had lost both of his legs. They were both baseball hounds. They watched it every day in their room on TV. By the time he'd left the hospital they had exchanged addresses and telephone numbers. He told me later that they visited each other, got to be friends, and went to baseball games together.
>
> There was another patient I had, a younger woman who was in a room with an older white lady in her seventies who was very feeble. Once the younger woman was able to get out of bed, she was busy helping the older woman. The day the younger woman was discharged, the older woman took her home with her to wait for her husband to get off of work and pick her up that evening.

I can think of many small acts of kindness that happened that you wouldn't have expected. I don't remember any incident. Yet we argued in the planning for weeks about whether it should have any semiprivate rooms because of the race problem. It took care of itself.[77]

In many cases, of course, it was not permitted to take care of itself. As the pressures to shorten length of stay increase, as the pressure to do diagnostic and surgical procedures on an ambulatory basis increases, as hospital occupancy drops and competition for a shrinking market share increases, even semiprivate rooms have become de facto private ones. People now recover and die in ever more splendid isolation.

Research and Teaching: The Persistence of the Old Accommodation

Teaching programs were expected to be the area most directly affected by the improved access afforded blacks and the poor. Such programs had always been an awkward marriage of convenience. Local municipalities, public hospitals, and clinics traditionally had contracted with medical schools through affiliation agreements and other arrangements to care for the medically indigent. Such arrangements have offered better quality services to the poor at a cost well under market value. Yet, those providing care in such settings do not have the same relationship to their patients as does a physician in private practice. Teaching and research needs to compete with patient care. The scheduling of clinics, the nature of their services, and their location are all shaped by these competing needs. In general, the outpatient services provide little in the way of amenities and convenience for patients. In contrast, the inpatient care tends to be very good. Disagreements about the quality of such care often involve confusion over which of these different sites one is talking about. The passage of the Civil Rights Act and Medicare and Medicaid legislation threatened this long-standing marriage of convenience. What would happen to teaching programs if there were no medically indigent and patients were free to seek care from any provider? Many in academic medicine voiced alarm.[78]

Yet teaching programs remained surprisingly insulated from the changes in access afforded blacks and the poor. Physicians in the United States continued to learn, as they have traditionally learned, from the urban poor, who happen to be mostly blacks and Hispanics, and then set up practices mostly for better-heeled patients who are predominantly white. An implicit understanding between state Medicaid programs, private-practice physicians, and the teaching centers accommodated the interests of all three parties. Medicaid physician payments rates proved to be below those charged private patients, and state budget pressures forced eligibility cutbacks. Private-physician participation in the Medicaid program was limited. In addition to the low rates, private physicians chose not to participate because of the difficulties they experienced with red tape and payment delays. The net effect of the Medicaid program and demographic shifts resulting in the loss of private paying patients in most inner city areas was an exodus of private physicians. While Medicare payments were more attractive to private physicians, Medicare beneficiaries in inner city neighborhoods had few private-practice alternatives.

Race, in some disconcerting ways, appears to continue to play a role in these divisions between teaching and nonteaching hospital patients. One of the few published studies reported that the likelihood of having an inguinal hernia repair or a cholecystectomy performed by a resident rather than a more experienced surgeon was 2.5 times higher for a black patient than for a white counterpart in 1962; a decade later, in 1972, it was 4.3 times higher.[79] These racial differences most pronounced for private and self-paying patients as well as for emergency cases but not significantly different for Medicaid patients.

Physicians in internship and residency programs must deal with the disparate arrangements that exist for the management of private and indigent patients in teaching hospitals. These divided arrangements often roughly correspond to divisions by race and often make little sense in terms of patient care or training. For example, residents in anesthesiology, sharing their time between a medical school's private hospital and the county hospital for the indigent, faced the problem described below.

> Staff anesthesiologists do the majority of work at University [the medical school's hospital for private patients] so the scheduler originally thought what a good place to send our beginners to observe. Wrong theory. Surgeons complained they did not want beginners taking care of THEIR private patients. This was rectified in July when we had enough residents. Then, the residents in anesthesia complained. Why were they doing work virtually independently at County (the county hospital for indigent patients) and then coming to University to assist and watch the staff? In other words, the teaching was backwards.[80]

The troubling separation between learning and practice in a divided two-class system has essentially remained unbroken.

Conclusions

Profound changes in the organization of health services took place in the wake of Title VI enforcement in the Medicare program. The structure of health care and the patterns of use of services were dramatically altered. The black hospitals died. Access to services improved for blacks and for the poor. Yet, troubling discrepancies remain. There is disparate use of the fruits of the medical revolution. While for most outcomes there has been marked improvement for both blacks and whites, the disparities in mortality rates have not closed. Much care continues to be provided in largely racially separate settings. At least in terms of crude statistics, the most segregated health care is now provided in the Northeast and Midwest. By far the least segregated area is the South. Racial segregation in health care, if it ever was just a regional issue, confined to the South, is certainly no longer so. The racial divisions in terms of where individuals receive care raise concerns both about the racial neutrality of health policy changes and potential bias in the reporting of health events by race.

The story, however, is not over, and the journey remains incomplete. Three questions concerning the organizational adaptation of the health care system to the conflicting constraints of Title VI and local market sensitivities need to be answered. First, what really happened to the nursing-home sector, which was effectively insulated from Title VI enforcement? Second, what happened to private medical practice, which was exempted altogether? Finally, how do all of these changes shape the persistence of racial disparities and what should be done about them? The next three chapters will address these questions, rethinking what needs to be done to heal a health care system that continues, to a large extent, to be racially divided.

CHAPTER 7

Race and Long-Term Care

Harland Randolph was recruited to the Office of Equal Health Opportunity to head the long-term care program at the end of 1966. He established an elaborate set of procedures, and we all worked very hard, from eight o'clock in the morning to eight or nine o'clock in the evening. We had hoped to develop some kind of formula from the forms, to follow up on the nursing homes, as we had done with the hospitals. Nevertheless, President Johnson decided during the first part of 1967 that he was not going to require anything. All he was going to do is require a good-faith effort. The nursing homes had to advertise in the papers saying that they were nondiscriminatory. The advertising was put in the classified ads. They couldn't use very small print, but nothing in large bold print was required. I didn't like that, but I understood why, because nursing homes are different from hospitals. . . . It is as much a social kind of environment as a medical one. There were also nursing-home associations and politicians from the South who ran a lot of committees then, who said if you don't do that, you're going to lose votes. I don't know that if I had been in President Johnson's shoes then that I would have done differently. Nevertheless, I was disappointed.

The real problem was that we didn't understand the admission process in nursing homes, and it was all done so quickly. We needed to know more precisely the mechanisms of admission and how it really works. It is much more complicated than in hospitals.

It was very difficult to define what compliance with Title VI was in nursing homes. If you need a hospital, you want to go into a hospital; if you need a nursing home, you don't necessarily want to go. It's not necessarily a good thing to have equivalence. The very character of it in the sixties was that it was not a good place to be, and it still isn't. Once you get in you are dealing with a social problem. You've got people in their seventies and eighties and nineties, who have had, all their life, certain feelings, and some of those feelings are very strong. How do you change those feelings? That, of course, is what President

Johnson was dealing with, too. Anyway, that program was not a success in my judgment, because we didn't change much.[1]

The Office of Equal Health Opportunity was approaching the end of its useful life as the nursing-home portion of the Medicare program came on line in January 1967. A combination of political events and the distinctive characteristics of nursing homes themselves had left them insulated from the initial federal efforts to enforce Title VI. That insulation produced a subtle chain reaction of events that contributed to the current crises in the Medicare and Medicaid programs and also to the broader pressures for health care reform. This chapter tells the nursing-home part of the story. In doing so, it will suggest ways of seeing the forces shaping this chain reaction of events that reconfigured the organization of health services in the United States. Within the "box" that encompasses the interplay of forces, which shape the organization of health services at the national level, is another one that captures the state and local dynamics. In contrast to the hospital story, nursing-home financing and regulation is predominantly a state function, and the dynamics take place largely inside the state and local box. For illustrative purposes, the chapter will focus mostly on the Pennsylvania and, more specifically, the Philadelphia story. It is representative of the patterns that have evolved in other states and metropolitan areas. As will be described later in this chapter, nothing in the supply of nursing homes, the nature of their regulation and payment, or in community racial tensions would suggest that Pennsylvania, or Philadelphia, is an extreme case, much different than that of other states and metropolitan areas. Yet just as in most other states and metropolitan areas of the United States, race continues to matter for persons growing old.

In order to get the full story of the relationship between nursing homes and race in the United States, one needs to dig through three levels of analysis. The first level describes the forces that gave rise to the evolution of a separate long-term care sector in the United States, unique among developed countries. Racial divisions contributed to producing that separate long-term care sector, but it is also a useful story to recount since it helps reinforce the idea of how the larger environment shapes the evolution of health care organizations. This idea will be an important theme through the remainder of this book. The second level describes the guerilla war that ensued from the creation of this divided system. Those divisions pitted state agencies against federal ones and general hospitals against nursing homes. Race played an indirect role in many of these struggles. The third level focuses in detail on Philadelphia and Pennsylvania and describes efforts through litigation and reform to bring to an end the war and the resulting racial disparities in health care.

Level 1: The Organizational Evolution of Long-Term Care

Imagine the organizations providing long-term care as individual organisms living in an environment, just as biological organisms do. Their size, shape, function, and diversity reflect the adaptations they have made to their environment.[2] The features of that environment include patterns of financing and regulation as well as the underlying social values about race, the poor, and the frail elderly, which shape those patterns of financing and regulation. When the environment changes, so do the organizations that populate it. Certain "species" of organizations become extinct and new ones emerge, better adapted to the changes. As illustrated in the last chapter, the passage of Title VI of the 1964 Civil Rights Act and the implementation of the Medicare and Medicaid program altered the environment for hospitals. Black hospitals closed or merged; public hospitals in many large cities either closed or became increasingly marginalized. Similar shifts in the population of organizations providing long-term care services have taken place throughout the twentieth century.

Nursing homes and acute hospitals in the United States began the twentieth century as essentially indistinguishable organizations. Both voluntary and public hospitals provided mostly long-term care to indigent residents. Over time, long-term and acute care was provided increasingly by separate institutions. This shift reflected scientific advances in medicine and surgery as well as changing social attitudes about race, the poor, and the frail elderly. Nursing homes in the United States, as a "species" of organizations distinct from hospitals, evolved in response to the forces of three distinct periods in their development.

Controlling Blacks and the Poor: The Era of the Prison and
the Poor Farm (1865–1935)

Embracing the British Elizabethan Poor Law tradition, the United States in the nineteenth century defined indigence as a problem of maintaining public order and as the responsibility of local government. County workhouses and farms were established to control vagrancy. These were, for the most part, not designed to assist the unfortunate but to demean and punish those who did not work. The lowest pay and the most difficult working conditions would thus be elevated by the contrast.

The South developed repressive local arrangements to tie black sharecroppers and farmworkers to the land. Cotton production in the black belt of the South after the Civil War was dependent on preserving the supply of cheap black labor. Black codes passed by most southern states included vagrancy provisions providing that "idle" blacks could be arrested and hired out at public auction for as long as a year. In Mississippi, a freedman had to have written proof of lawful employment (a labor agreement with a plantation owner) or be subject to arrest. Florida went further in defining vagrancy to include a laborer with such an agreement who disobeyed orders or was "impudent." Other statutes empowered courts to remove children from parents declared unwilling to provide for them and bind them over to their former owners in an apprenticeship system.[3] The county prison farms and convict labor system grew out of the post–Civil War arrangements. County and municipal nursing homes also evolved from these historical roots. This legacy, still fresh in the memories of many black families, chilled local civil rights groups' interest in the issue of access to nursing homes after the passage of the Medicare and Medicaid legislation. It was too closely associated with the methods used to control blacks in the post-Reconstruction era in the South.

Those too old, disabled, or sick to work, however, presented local communities with an increasingly difficult problem. The prisons and poor farms were predicated on the assumption that such operations could pay for themselves and thus not burden local communities. The prevailing system also blamed the victims of misfortunes. One didn't want one's own relatives, friends, and neighbors who, through no fault of their own, needed help, to be subjected to this treatment. This solution to this problem required the application of moral judgment, separating the "deserving" from the "undeserving." The private charitable institutions concentrated on caring for the "deserving poor," suitable candidates for private charity. Race, ethnicity, and religious preferences played a role in assigning such moral labels. Those with drug and alcohol problems, sexually transmitted diseases, and criminal records were unlikely to be defined as deserving of private charity. The county or public hospitals, poorhouses, and poor farms provided the indoor relief for those who were deemed ineligible for the private charitable facilities. Various ethnic groups in the nineteenth century established charitable hospitals and homes to care for their "own kind" who were deserving of charity. Blacks were excluded from many of these voluntary facilities and struggled with limited resources in establishing places of their own. Often lacking the wealth of other local ethnic groups, the only option for blacks in many communities were the county homes.

However, in the twentieth century, most of these voluntary charitable institutions began to be slowly transformed into workshops for their medical staffs. Even Johns Hopkins Hospital, the prototype of the tertiary-care teaching hospital, was originally planned with one hundred convalescent beds. This plan was then abandoned.[4] Other hospitals were slower to shed their original mission of caring for longer-stay residents. Up until

1960, for example, Einstein Hospital in Philadelphia continued to operate a nursing home and, in keeping with the poor farm tradition, a vegetable farm on its grounds, supplying food for the residents.[5]

The predominantly rural character and continued growth of the nation left this locally financed public and charitable system of "indoor relief" unchanged from colonial times until 1930. Public attitudes concerning the individual's responsibility for his or her own financial well-being were reinforced by an expanding demand for labor. Indolence needed to be discouraged and controlled. Direct subsidies were felt to be too costly to administer, and many feared they would encourage indolence. By 1920, roughly 1 percent of the elderly population in the United States was housed either in county or municipal facilities or in institutions operated by private charities initiated by immigrant self-help organizations or by religious groups.[6] A larger proportion of the elderly was housed in state psychiatric hospitals. From the perspective of local welfare administrators, the shift to the state psychiatric hospitals had the effect of shifting most of the financial burden from the local municipalities to the state. (A similarly motivated migration of elderly psychiatric patients back to local nursing and boarding homes took place after the passage of Medicare and Medicaid, when state officials discovered that they could shift much of the financial burden they had assumed from local municipalities on to the federal government.) In addition, many long-term care patients continued to be cared for by general hospitals.[7] Few general hospitals had made the full transition into workshops for physicians in 1930. Many local community hospitals were just beginning to be influenced by the American College of Surgeons' hospital standardization program.

Providing Security in Old Age: The Era of the Private Boarding Home (1935–65)

The Great Depression beginning in 1929 forced the collapse of the welfare system based on local responsibility and the resulting patchwork of private charitable institutions and county or municipal facilities. By 1935 as many as twenty million people were forced to rely on public assistance. In the 1920s, a combination of the political pressure exerted by pension advocates, a scathing report on poor farms produced by the Department of Labor, and a national muckraking expose supported by a dozen fraternal orders had imposed an indelible stigma on county homes in the mind of the public and politicians. The magnitude of the relief problem during the depression overshadowed the problems of the fewer than two hundred thousand persons over sixty-five living in local charitable and county institutions. Initially, the proposed Social Security Act of 1935 disallowed aid to persons who were "inmates of public or other charitable institutions."[8] Quick to defend the financial interests of their members, the voluntary-hospital associations objected. The final bill excluded payment only to inmates of public institutions. So-called outdoor relief, or providing direct payments to recipients rather than committing them to institutions, had gained broad acceptance in the height of the Great Depression, when the stigma and practicality of "indoor" relief no longer made sense. Legislators also wanted to promote a clear distinction between old-age assistance as honorable and deserved public aid in contrast to the old-fashioned poor relief. In the process, the Social Security Act of 1935 redefined the nature of the relationship between citizens and the federal government. For blacks, the Social Security system meant a significant shift toward greater equality. Many locally financed and administered welfare programs had not provided equal treatment for blacks.

Completely without plan or intention, however, the Social Security Act stimulated the growth of private boarding homes and their gradual evolution into the proprietary nursing-home sector. Local welfare administrators, denied a federal subsidy to support inmates of county and municipal facilities, now shifted them to private boarding homes, where Old Age Assistance payments could reduce the local financial burden. While, in theory, they could have shifted residents to private charitable institutions as well, such a course of action was often not feasible. Private charitable institutions were (1) largely concentrated in the northeastern part of the United States, (2) generally not interested in growing and expanding beyond the religious and ethnic communities they had historically served, and (3) typically more costly. The combination of this new source of funding, the exclusion of the use of public institutions, and the lack of private charitable alternatives produced the dramatic growth of the proprietary boarding-home sector. Since elderly persons now had "outdoor" relief in the form of Old Age Assistance and Social Security, only those who were physically unable to live independently ended up in the private boarding homes. As a consequence, the residents in the private boarding homes became increasingly older, frailer, and sicker. In response, these boarding homes were transformed into nursing facilities. By 1963 an estimated 502,242 residents lived in 16,370 nursing and personal-care facilities in the United States. Eighty-two percent of the homes and 61 percent of the beds were proprietary.[9] Yet, nursing and personal care for the aged and chronically ill continued to be provided in the nursing-home units and chronic-disease wards of general hospitals as well as in freestanding geriatric and chronic-disease hospitals. In 1963, 728 such institutions and units of general hospitals were identified with a total population of 77,076 residents. Government-operated facilities accounted for

68 percent of these residents. Black access to nursing homes and personal-care facilities was more restricted than their access to the chronic-disease hospitals. The rate of use of personal-care and nursing homes by adult nonwhites was only 35 percent that of whites but was roughly equivalent for the use of publicly operated geriatric and chronic-disease hospitals.[10]

In the 1950s many general hospitals revisited the idea of integrating long-term care into the medical mainstream. A "Continuing Care Department" established at Thayer Hospital in rural Maine in 1950 attracted widespread attention. Many studies were conducted documenting the need for an integrated approach to the care of those with chronic illnesses. In 1956 the Commission on Chronic Illnesses, an organization created by the American Hospital Association, the American Medical Association, the American Public Health Association, and the American Public Welfare Association, convened a national conference. The recommendations of that conference included the following:

> The most desirable approach to providing hospital care to long-term patients is through extension, organization, and coordination of the facilities and services of general hospitals. . . . On the basis of its studies and analysis of the problems, the Commission believes that development of these (nursing home) institutions as elements of general hospitals is one of the best ways of raising standards, and recommends this arrangement.[11]

Some hospitals, such as the Jewish Hospital of St. Louis, a five-hundred-bed teaching hospital, set up chronic-disease units and documented significant improvements in a formerly neglected population, reducing lengths of stay and death rates. The conclusions from this well-documented success were as follows:

> Long-term care services properly belong in the professional and administrative purview of the general hospital. Chronically ill patients require access to the same medical, nursing and technical staffs, and to the same facilities and equipment, as do short-term "acute" patients. . . . Because of superior resources of personnel, equipment, and physical plant, the services rendered to chronic-disease patients tend to be more comprehensive and of higher quality when incorporated in the organic envelope of the general hospital than when provided by an independent chronic disease institution.[12]

These recommendations and conclusions were not only ignored; massive development soon proceeded in exactly the opposite direction.

Adapting to Medicare and Title VI: The Era of the "Modern"
Nursing Home (1965–95)

The passage of the Medicare and Medicaid legislation in 1965 produced a massive increase in federal funding of health care and, as described in the previous chapters, compelled hospitals to comply with Title VI of the 1964 Civil Rights Act. The percent of national health expenditures accounted for by the federal government jumped from 10.9 percent in 1960 to 24.3 percent in 1970.[13]

All the elements of a continuum of services (acute-hospital care, con-valescent-hospital care, home care, and institutional long-term care) were included, but no mechanisms existed for their integration into a single sys-tem. The Medicare legislation had initially provided benefits for extended-care facilities, usually units of acute-care hospitals to which patients might be transferred during the postacute convalescent period. High Medicare hospital costs produced a drastic curtailment of eligibility for this benefit in 1969, and, as a result, the federal Medicare program ceased to play any significant role in the provision of long-term care. Nevertheless, federal dollars flowing through state Medicaid programs to nursing homes grew dramatically. National expenditures for nursing-home care jumped from $800 million to $4.2 billion during the 1960s, the bulk of this increase com-ing from state Medicaid funds. Expenditures for nursing-home care during this decade grew at an average annual rate of 17.4 percent, faster than any other health expenditure.

Nursing-home bed capacity in the United States more than doubled between 1963 and 1973, expanding to 1,174,900 and exceeding the bed capacity in acute-care hospitals.[14] This growth signaled a major watershed in patterns of use of inpatient care in the United States. The number of long-term hospital beds dropped from a high of about 1,019,000 beds in 1960 to 207,000 in 1995.[15] Some of these declines were absorbed into nurs-ing homes. In addition, nursing-home stays were also increasingly substi-tuted for more extended stays in hospitals.

The massive growth in nursing-home beds alone understates the watershed that took place in long-term care. At the beginning of the 1960s, many of the proprietary nursing homes were conversions of private homes. The average size of proprietary homes in 1963 was 25.9 beds. Mrs. Murphy might have been a nurse by training, but it was still the image of Mrs. Murphy's Boarding Home that prevailed. At least half of the nurs-ing-home beds that existed in the 1960s closed and were replaced with new facilities. New nursing homes constructed between 1965 and 1975 included approximately one million beds. The character of what was then described as the nursing-home "industry" had changed dramatically. Proprietary chains, some becoming national in scope, operated an increasing share of these beds. The greater standardization and predictability imposed by federal regulation of payment and care created the potential for real economies of scale that had not been possible before through locally administered programs. There was also a dramatic shift in the character of the care provided in these homes. The homes became more medicalized, treating sicker patients. Nursing homes that had previously served as part of the welfare system became, increasingly, an extension of the hospital and medical system. Many of the older "ma and pa" operations were closed in the process. In New York state, for example, 291 of the 339 homes closed between 1967 and 1974 had fewer than fifty beds, and 251 of these smaller homes were proprietary. Most of these smaller, owner-operated homes could not meet the stricter building-code standards now imposed on all medical facilities. An operator of one of these smaller homes that closed wrote the following protest letter to the editor of a local paper.

> What are you doing New Year's Eve? Would you and all the residents of Monroe County like to cancel your previous plans and join the non-conforming nursing homes in Monroe County? There won't be any liquor, balloons, or an orchestra, but there will be dancing. The dancer will be the geriatric patient, who is literally being pushed out on the street by New York State.
>
> You see we aren't built right. We aren't fire-resistant—but check out with the fire departments as to how often they have answered a fire call to one of us. Our hallways aren't eight feet wide but more love and compassion travel down our narrow pathways than any 8–10 foot one. Ours expand with all the tender loving care one could desire and need, not by a carpenter's tool![16]

The small, non-code-compliant, owner-operated homes in New York, in spite of protests, closed as they did elsewhere, replaced by larger, more medically oriented and more institutional facilities. Even the nursing-home operators themselves were ambivalent about the changes taking place.

> A group of nursing-home operators at a conference were asked to describe their own facilities. Some described brand new facilities with elaborate recreational and physical therapy programs and over 300 beds. One facility was a thirty-bed operation run by a religious order. The home had a garden, some chickens, and a stream for fishing. The Sisters spoke with great affection and interest about each of their res-

idents. At the end of the session the participants were asked to vote for the homes in which they would prefer to be a patient. The thirty-bed home of the Sisters was the unanimous choice![17]

The patient in the acute-hospital bed began to look more like the patient in intensive care before 1965, and the resident in the nursing home began to look more like the patient in the acute-hospital bed, pre-1965. In the first decade after the passage of Medicare, a new, more impersonal set of institutions had emerged. Organizationally separated from acute hospitals and from the welfare system, these institutions exceeded the general hospital in bed capacity. Nationally in fiscal year 1995 the Medicaid program paid more than $27 billion to nursing homes, more than it expended for inpatient care in acute hospitals.[18] Public funds accounted for more than 58 percent of all nursing-home revenue in 1995.[19]

No one could make much sense out of the long-term care system that was emerging. In 1975 the Senate Special Committee on Aging published a report, *Doctors in Nursing Homes: The Shunned Responsibility,* bemoaning the medical neglect. For every one thousand nursing-home beds there were 250 costly transfers to hospitals, a rate five times that which takes place in Great Britain's more integrated system.[20] Health policy analyst Anne Somers lamented the search for solutions in 1982: "Although many of the current remedial proposals recognize the importance of long-term care they appear to be prepared to settle for a second-class program, separate in both organization and financing from the mainstream of acute care." A position paper from the American College of Physicians Health and Public Policy Subcommittee on Aging surveyed the barren landscape in 1984.

At present, there is not a comprehensive system of long-tern care for the elderly in the United States. A confusing, fragmented, and expensive system exists that contains both gaps and duplication of services. Consequently, many elderly do not receive the services they need, while others receive services inappropriately. . . . Reimbursement procedures, both public and private, tacitly recognize the existence of two separate systems of health care: one for acute care and another for long-term care. Such a division is unrealistic and results often in inadequate responses to the medical needs of the elderly.[21]

No one, in terms of public policy, had consciously planned for this to happen. It was in direct opposition to what most clinicians, managers, and policy analysts would have envisioned as an optimal way to organize services for the frail elderly and chronically ill. It was certainly not a "market driven" result of consumer preferences. Stand-alone nursing homes still retained the stigma of the poor farm. People might be willing to go to a "step down unit of a general hospital," but no one wanted to go to a nursing home. Why did it happen?

Level 2: The Guerilla War in a Divided System

Race played a role in the growth of the nursing-home sector and its increasing separation from acute-hospital care. The combined effect of Medicare, Medicaid, and Title VI was to pit the nursing-home owners against the hospitals, state governments against the federal government, rich against the poor, and blacks against whites. Many pressures in addition to race, of course, contributed to the growth and increasing separation of long-term care. The aging, urbanization, and increasing geographic mobility of the United States population played a role in expanding demand, as did the influx of federal funding through the Medicaid and Medicare programs. The interests of hospital medical staffs powerfully influenced the direction of development of acute hospitals. Specific strategies adopted through reimbursement and regulation to control the growth of public expenditures in the Medicare and Medicaid programs played a part in shaping the population of organizations providing such services. Diverse pressures, resonating with and amplifying each other, produced an environment more conducive to certain species of organizations at the expense of others. I will focus here, however, on the role of race. Race has had a ripple effect, producing a growing instability in the complex network of provider and payer accommodations emerging out of the Medicare and Medicaid programs and Title VI.

The Insulation of Nursing Homes from Title VI Enforcement

The Medicare program's implementation treated hospitals and nursing homes differently. The Department of Health Education and Welfare mounted a major effort to bring hospitals into compliance with Title VI before the beginning of the program on July 1, 1966 (chap. 4). Nursing-home participation lagged six months behind and resulted in a half-hearted pro forma paper compliance effort that everyone understood was cosmetic. These actions both acknowledged and amplified the differences between the environments to which hospitals and nursing homes had to adapt. Title VI added to the pressures forcing greater separation of acute and long-term care.

A combination of characteristics insulated nursing homes from the Title VI enforcement pressures faced by hospitals. These are summarized

TABLE 7.1. The Stake of Key Resources in Hospitals versus Nursing Homes

Key Resources	Hospitals	Nursing Homes
General community (patients)	Medicare payment for care of all persons over 65	Medicaid payment for the care of the indigent
Medical staff (referrals)	Active involvement: a major source of practice income	Limited involvement: a minor source of practice income
Third-party payers (reimbursement)	Medicare full-cost payments; few self-paying patients	Medicaid less than full-cost payments; many self-paying patients
Regulators (approvals to operate)	Federal accountability; enforcement budget-neutral	State accountability; substantial fiscal implications for state government
Advocacy groups (influence over other key resources)	Strong interest of constituency groups; symbolic importance	Little interest of constituency groups; persistence of stigma of nursing-home care

Source: Adapted from David Smith, "The Racial Integration of Hospitals and Nursing Homes," *Milbank Quarterly* 68, no. 4 (1990): 576.

in table 7.1. Both nursing homes and hospitals had to attract the same five key resources. These resources were (1) patients, (2) medical staff who provided the referrals and care for the patients in the facilities, (3) adequate revenue—from patients, third-party payers, private endowments, or government subsidies—to cover the cost of facility stays, (4) approval from state regulators who established the conditions for licensure and operation, and (5) the support or at least the acquiescence of civil rights and consumer advocacy groups who could potentially influence the flow of all of the first four resources. Yet, hospitals and nursing homes faced starkly different constraints in assuring the flow of these five resources.

Title VI compliance for hospitals was a rational business decision. Hospitals didn't need to worry as much about the flight of white professional staff or the loss of white patients. The other institutions would face the same identical requirements. The hospitals would also receive generous cost-based reimbursement from Medicare and Medicaid for many of their new black patients and thus faced little financial risk. For the white, racially separate hospitals, integration offered the opportunity for almost risk-free expansion of their market. For the racially segregated hospitals, it offered risk-free elimination of costly duplication of services. In addition, local civil rights advocacy groups were an aggressive, visible presence. Those groups included hospital employees and local physicians and dentists in their membership. Little would escape detection and subsequent Title VI complaints.

Title VI compliance for nursing homes made less sense as a rational business decision. Title VI had far less potential financial leverage over the nursing homes. Only indigent patients in the community would lose access if a facility was decertified. For most physicians, Medicare and Medicaid payments for the care of nursing-home patients constituted at best a marginal contribution to their incomes. Indeed, the inconvenience and the relatively low payments accorded nursing-home visits has been a long-standing source of dissatisfaction among physicians. Hospitals also provided physicians the opportunity to participate in teaching programs and in continuing education, providing important nonremunerative rewards that nursing homes did not provide. The two public payments programs lacked the overwhelming financial leverage over nursing homes that they possessed over hospitals. Medicare's limited benefits for long-term care produced little income for nursing homes. Nursing homes preferred almost all other forms of payment to the stringent reimbursement of most state Medicaid programs.

Most nursing homes were unenthusiastic about admitting minorities, and first-day-eligible Medicaid patients and most state governments were equally unenthusiastic about forcing the issue of equal access. Medicaid costs for nursing-home care represented the largest and most rapidly growing cost in most state Medicaid programs, itself usually the most rapidly growing component of state budgets. Nationally, nursing-home expenditures account for 26 percent of all Medicaid expenditures. Control of such costs quickly became a major focus of state governments.[22] Greater access for black patients, either by expanding the supply of nursing-home beds in poorer minority neighborhoods or by exerting greater control or surveillance over the admission processes of homes, would increase costs. In most cases, the lack of access would simply cause these patients to be backed up in acute hospitals, shifting the expenses for their care from the state Medicaid program to the federal Medicare program, and thereby easing pressures on the state Medicaid budget. Nursing homes themselves were dependent on private-pay, predominantly white patients, and in many communities they faced serious risks of white flight. They were sensitive to the racial attitudes of their customers.

This reluctance of nursing-home operators to insist on strict Title VI enforcement of access and room assignment could have been overcome by the efforts of local civil rights groups. These groups played a pivotal role in assuring the integrity of Title VI compliance efforts in hospitals. It was, however, not a pressing concern to their constituencies, who tended to be younger black professionals. Discrimination in employment, housing, education, and in the criminal-justice system were pressing concerns. Preserving the "right" of access to nursing homes, which for many black families was still too closely associated with the Jim Crow era methods of controlling blacks through the county prison and poor farm system, could hardly be expected to generate much civil rights fervor. Unlike the issue of access to hospitals, which had produced a strong coalition between the National Medical Association and the NAACP, no vital economic interest was at stake for these practitioners. Nursing-home medical-staff privileges offered neither the promise of professional development nor the potential for income that hospital privileges provided. In short, access to nursing homes never became a grassroots civil rights issue.

As a result, concerns about nursing-home minority access and discrimination were relegated to periodic reports that collected dust. In reviewing federal Title VI enforcement efforts in 1970, the Civil Rights Commission observed that "since most extended care facilities and nursing homes also have never been subject to field review, their current status with respect to Title VI can only be a matter of conjecture." A year later, the commission observed that compliance surveys had highlighted extended-care facilities as an area of concern.

An analysis of the individual reports demonstrated that a substantial number of facilities continued to serve patients of exclusively one race, despite the fact that they had signed assurances of open admission policies. . . . On the whole, there is very little detailed information available concerning the distribution of most minority group citizens, and little data available which can be used to assess compliance by HEW recipients with civil rights legislation and regulations.[23]

A decade later, the more academically credentialed Institute of Medicine of the National Academy of Sciences focused on the issue of access to long-term care in their own review of civil-rights-related issues in health care. The committee's conclusions underwent careful internal reviews over the wording.[24]

The evidence . . . including published studies, anecdotal observations, and testimony presented to the committee . . . is consistent with the hypothesis that blacks are discriminated against in nursing home admissions. Nevertheless, little direct, systematic documentation of such discrimination exists. Most of the evidence that leads the committee to conclude that racial discrimination may play a role in nursing home admissions pertains to inadequacies of competing explanations for the low rates of nursing home use among blacks. . . . On the basis of this evidence, the committee concluded that there is a strong likelihood that racial discrimination is an important factor in the admission of blacks to nursing homes, though how widespread a factor is not clear.[25]

In its review, the Institute of Medicine (IOM) Committee systematically eliminated most of the alternative explanations for the differences in black and white use of nursing homes. They were not attributable to superior health status, since black elderly health status was generally poorer and blacks had more chronic and disabling conditions. Black elderly tend to be more likely than white elderly to be located in mental and chronic-disease hospitals, thus undercutting arguments about extended family supports. Differences in rates of black use also appear to vary markedly from city to city, further undercutting the notion of cultural differences. A survey that was reviewed by the committee also suggested that the lack of personal assistance at home showed little difference between blacks and whites. The committee was frustrated by the lack of data and by the complex interplay created by Medicaid access to nursing homes and variations in the supply of nursing-home beds reflecting the racial composition of different areas. The issues that the IOM study identified, like previous reports, were left to collect dust.

Long-Term Care and Hospital Services Drift Further Apart

In the meantime, race influenced the increasing division between long-term and acute care, while rarely surfacing as a conscious, explicit part of such decisions. If hospitals had evolved, as many had advocated in the 1950s and earlier, as integrated networks of services providing a continuum of care, their long-term care components would have shared after the passage of Medicare the same Title VI requirements as the rest of the network.[26] No part of a hospital, whether it directly involved Medicare patients or not, was immune from Title VI review, and the potential sanctions in terms of withdrawal of all federal funds would apply to the entire institution. Discrimination, whether it surfaced in a training program for technicians or in admissions to a hospital-operated nursing-home wing, could trigger sanctions affecting the entire organization. An integrated delivery system that encompassed both acute and long-term care would have forced an integrated approach to Title VI enforcement. However, the implementation of the Medicare and Medicaid programs propelled an increasing organizational separation of long-term from acute care. The most common explanations for this shift were (1) the Medicare and Medicaid policies adopted to control the cost increases of these two payment programs and (2) the economic self-interests of hospital medical staffs that diverted resources to more costly medical technology. Resonating with these influences, however, sometimes consciously and sometimes unconsciously, were the issues of race and Title VI compliance.

In the 1970s, the nursing-home sector became a part of the civil rights legal struggle over the relocation of hospitals from inner-city areas. Many metropolitan regional health planning agencies were singling out the "shortage" of nursing-home beds and the "surplus" of acute-hospital beds in their planning regions as major issues that needed to be addressed. A primary focus of cost reduction concerns of these bodies was to constrain the growth or reduce the overall supply of acute-hospital beds. In Philadelphia, as in other communities, there was an almost 1:1 correspondence between the "shortage" of nursing-home beds and the "surplus" of hospital beds. The physical relocation of frail elderly patients from one facility to another exposes them to a risk comparable to that of undergoing major surgical procedures.[27] The stress and disruption associated with these relocations, or "transfer traumas," argue strongly for organizing a broad continuum of services under the same roof, rather than bouncing patients back and forth between acute and long-term facilities. The obvious solution would have been to convert the surplus of acute beds to fill the shortage of long-term care beds in Philadelphia. The obvious in Philadelphia, as in most other medical service areas in the United States, was avoided.

Many have been frustrated by the perverse lack of integration of acute and long-term care and the resistance to blending of acute and long-term care beds. One recent administrator of the Health Care Financing Administration, which operates the Medicare and Medicaid program, argued for the logic of reintegrating long-term care into the acute hospitals.[28] Others have looked admiringly at the ability to integrate services for the elderly into a continuum of services on a hospital campus as has been developed in England.[29] Indeed, as noted in the last chapter, almost none of the complete organizational separation of acute and long-term care that exists in the United States exists in any other developed country. The only organizational integration that has taken place in the United States is through the development of multi-institutional systems. Until very recently, however, the few systems that have owned *both* acute hospitals and nursing homes have operated them as *separate* product lines, with little patient flow between the two.

Predictably, the organizational separation of acute and long-term care produced increased friction. The division of responsibilities for the elderly between the state Medicaid programs and the federal Medicare program added to this friction. The Medicare program paid for almost all of the costs of hospital care for elderly persons. State Medicaid programs paid for the majority of the nursing-home care of elderly persons. State budgets could be reduced by shifting more of the cost of caring for the "dually eligible" (indigent elderly eligible for both Medicare and Medicaid) onto hospitals, thus forcing the federal Medicare program to absorb more of the costs. Federal costs could be reduced by shifting persons out of hospitals and into nursing homes. As the state Medicaid and the federal Medicare program both struggled to control their own costs, the hospitals and nursing homes struggled to respond. A chaotic guerilla war ensued with each party seeking temporary alliances and launching assaults and counterassaults.

The State Medicaid Programs' and the Nursing Homes' Cease-Fire

Nursing-home care provided by the Medicaid program absorbed an increasing share of state budgets, and states struggled to control these costs. By 1995 Medicaid costs for long-term care in the United States had grown to $40 billion, representing 26 percent of all national Medicaid expenditures. The cost of nursing-home care to the Pennsylvania Medicaid program had grown to $2.6 billion, or 37 percent of all of its costs. States such as Pennsylvania were faced with slowing economic growth, competition to keep and lure large employers by reducing their tax obligations, and a more general tax revolt among the electorate. As a result, states struggled to contain the growth of their budgets. The seemingly unlimited potential for the expansion of Medicaid nursing-home expenditures has represented and continues to represent a major threat to such control. Nursing homes, on the other hand, are dependent on state Medicaid payments. Almost 60 percent of nursing-home revenues nationally come from public sources, predominantly Medicaid. There are no other third-party payers. Private insurance accounts for only 3 percent of nursing-home expenditures.[30] The remainder comes from out-of-pocket payments by patients and their family members. Few facilities, however, can afford to concentrate on just the out-of-pocket payers. Long nursing-home stays can quickly deplete the assets of most families. As a result, the nursing-home industry in most states were locked in a protracted battle with state government. The economic viability of one party to this conflict seemed possible only with the bankruptcy of the other. Both parties struggled for accommodation. In most states, a fragile accommodation was worked out to protect the financial self-interests of both parties. It is centered on two basic principles.

1. *The state will control the number of persons who will use Medicaid nursing-home benefits.* Without some way of capping the number of persons using nursing-home benefits, the state Medicaid agency would have no control over the cost of the Medicaid program. Such caps could be achieved by (1) restricting the number of nursing-home beds, (2) reducing payment to the homes and thereby reducing the willingness of homes to admit Medicaid patients, (3) restricting eligibility for nursing-home benefits under the Medicaid program, or (4) by a combination of the first three strategies. Capping bed supply in many states was the most politically acceptable approach. This both served the interest of the state Medicaid program and protected the investments of nursing-home owners. High occupancy levels were essentially guaranteed. Facilities could be selective about which patients they admitted and avoid ones whose only source of payment was Medicaid. The arrangements, of course, varied from state to state. In states without strong laws imposing restrictions on expansion of nursing homes, it was possible to control Medicaid patient use of nursing homes by reducing their rates of payment and thus reducing the willingness of nursing homes to accept Medical Assistance patients.

2. *The nursing homes will control admissions.* In contrast to hospitals, for whom laws greatly limit their discretion, nursing homes in most states

have preserved the absolute right to control who gets admitted to their facilities. In this way they have been able to control (1) the payer mix and (2) the case mix within the facility. Private-pay rates are in some cases as much as twice the Medicaid rates, which are often below the cost of providing services. Not surprisingly, nursing homes prefer private-pay patients. In addition, since payments have been typically set at a fixed per diem rate, patients who will be less costly to care for, the "easy care" patients, are preferred. (New "case mix" payment systems have altered the attractiveness of the "easy care" patients but not the importance of controlling admissions.) Behind the admission process in most nursing homes lies a set of risk calculations not unlike those that govern the marketing and enrollment strategies of managed-care plans.

Through this accommodation, at least in the short run, the interests of the nursing-home operators and the state coincided. From the nursing-home operator's perspective, their franchise would be protected from competition, and they could shape their admissions practices to maximize their revenues and minimize their costs. From the state's perspective, the so-called first-day-eligible Medicaid and heavy-care patients would be backlogged in the hospitals; their costs would be absorbed for the most part by the federal Medicare program, and not the state Medicaid program. Even if these patients were discharged to the care of their families, the Medicare program would cover their care on an ambulatory basis or for home care.

What made this a particularly elegant accommodation, however, was its broader public appeal. Not only did this arrangement exert at least some fiscal control over nursing home and state Medicaid budgets; it also converted a program designed to care for the poor into one that provided a catastrophic long-term care insurance policy for the middle class. Income for nursing homes comes from two sources: the pockets of patients and their families or the state Medicaid program. These two sources account for more than 90 percent of nursing-home revenues. A person unfortunate enough to need nursing-home care but with some income and other assets could become eligible for Medicaid nursing-home payments by (1) spending down his or her assets, (2) converting these assets to a category, such as a home, exempt from Medicaid income eligibility calculations, or (3) transferring them to his or her children. Self-help books, financial-planning seminars, adult education courses, and newsmagazine articles designed to assist individuals in making such arrangements are a growth industry.[31] Nursing homes, however, often impose their own admission requirements that require the ability of an applicant to pay private-pay rates for an extended period of time. One study in Pennsylvania estimated that the average spend-down period in nursing homes before eligibility for Medicaid was thirty-six months, and considerably longer for not-for-profit homes.[32] Thus, for homes either unable or reluctant to discharge patients no longer able to pay the private rates, the Medical Assistance program provided a catastrophic insurance policy for the homes as well as for their private patients.

Critics, of course, argued that these arrangements (1) restricted access to nursing homes for the poor or first-day-eligible Medicaid recipients and (2) limited the total amount of Medicaid funds going to the indigent for which the program was intended. Many of the elderly first-day-eligible Medicaid recipients needing nursing care were, in fact, backed up in hospitals.

The Guerilla War Escalates

The accommodation between nursing homes and state Medicaid programs that restricted access to first-day-eligible Medicaid nursing-home patients "solved" the problems of the nursing-home industry and of state governments at the expense of the federal Medicare program. The federal government, the state Medicaid programs, the hospitals, and the nursing homes all worked to shift the costs from themselves onto the other parties. Restrictions in the access of Medicaid patients to nursing homes increased use by the medically indigent elderly of hospitals and drove up the cost increases in the Medicare program, particularly in inner-city minority neighborhoods. The number of hospital days per thousand elderly in many of these areas was more than twice that of higher-income neighborhoods.[33] A series of defensive measures and countermeasures resulted. For example, in 1983, after a protracted and ineffective effort to control hospital costs through utilization review, federal legislation devised an effective strategy to prevent state Medicaid program cost shifting. Hospitals under Medicare would no longer be reimbursed based on their cost but would be paid set rates for care. The Medicare prospective payments system paid a flat rate per admission for diagnostically related groups (DRGs). This destroyed the remaining loophole that had provided Medicare payment for indigent nursing-home-eligible patients who had been backed up in hospitals.

The implementation of DRG-based hospital reimbursement probably helped to dampen cost increases in the Medicare program. It did not, of course, eliminate the underlying problem. Urban hospitals, including many influential teaching institutions, served a large proportion of indigent patients. These hospitals experienced longer lengths of stay and higher costs per admission that were, in part, a reflection of the difficulties they faced in placing patients in nursing homes. The hospitals with large indigent care populations lobbied Congress hard and, as a result, a system of "disproportionate share adjustments" was devised. These payments tried to compensate for the larger volume of free care and for the nursing-home access problems faced by hospitals serving a disproportionate share of indigent patients. In 1996, these adjustments cost the Medicare program 4.4 billion dollars, or more than 10 percent of what the Medicaid program was spending for nursing-home care.[34] The state Medicaid programs were similarly pressured through legislation and lawsuits into providing similar disproportionate-share payments to many urban inner-city hospitals.

State Medicaid programs, in the wake of pressures to provide disproportionate-share payments to hospitals, began to get very creative about financing these programs. Medicaid programs "match" state dollars with federal ones. Faced with state budget restrictions, state Medicaid programs invented a "tax" on providers that was used to inflate the state matching contribution for federal Medicaid dollars. The state program would temporarily "borrow" the money from the hospitals, and these funds would be used to draw down a larger federal match. This classic pyramid scheme helped to provide roughly 19 billion dollars in disproportionate-share payments to providers in fiscal year 1995.[35] These manipulations, of course, increased the costs incurred by the federal part of the Medicaid program, which stimulated federal efforts to close this loophole. Increasingly blocked from being able to shift costs onto the federal government, state Medicaid programs have turned to shifting those costs onto health plans, providers, and beneficiaries through managed-care contracting.

The chaotic guerrilla war between the state and federal governments, health plans, hospitals, and nursing homes grew in intensity. Black elderly Medicaid beneficiaries were a disproportionate share of the casualties in these battles. The third and final phase in this war is yet to be fully written.

Level 3: The Philadelphia Story of Race, Long-Term Care, and the Endgame

The dynamics within the state of Pennsylvania and in the metropolitan service area of Philadelphia mirror those in most other states and larger metropolitan areas. While this section focuses on Philadelphia, it is representative of the stories played out in most urban communities across the nation and suggests some ways that the cumulative contradictions described in the first two levels of analysis may be resolved.

Black Access to Nursing-Home Care in Philadelphia,
1940–70

Access to nursing homes for blacks in Philadelphia is an old problem. Its basic dimensions were well described in a 1946 article published in the *Social Security Bulletin.*

> Nonprofit institutions care for only a fraction of the aged population because of the scarcity of such institutions and their restrictions on admissions. Some of these homes operate on a contractual basis that automatically excludes recipients of public assistance. Many are limited with respect to church affiliation or race. Few will accept non-ambulatory persons or persons with progressive ailments. Staff limitations in the Department of Welfare have greatly curtailed the possibilities of constructive work with the commercial homes in maintaining standards and improving services. The Department is also handicapped in supervision of nursing homes by its recognition of the shortage of homes in the face of increasing need for sheltered care, and is therefore reluctant to eliminate any existing resources by too rigid insistence on high standards.
>
> The consequence of these circumstances, coupled with the fact that proprietors are operating the homes as a business and that receipt of monthly payment to the homes is usually $40 or less, is that the caliber of the care leaves much to be desired. . . . The exclusion of alcoholic, mental, and cancer cases is almost universal. The need for nursing home care for indigent Negroes is practically unmet. Only three homes (out of 52) now accommodate Negro recipients on assistance, although Negroes constitute one-fourth of the old-age assistance caseload in the city.[36]

The problem has remained essentially unchanged. Philadelphia's Home for the Indigent had changed its name to Riverview in 1953, perhaps in an effort not to continue to stigmatize its residents. Unfortunately, the stark accommodations shared grounds with the city's House of Correction, located in the northeastern section of the city along the Delaware River. Riverview had opened in 1914. Until 1937, aiding the indigent in Pennsylvania had been solely the responsibility of county and municipal government. In 1937, the state was made responsible through public assistance for providing for the noninstitutionalized indigent. The city's public facility assumed responsibility for caring for those who could not care for themselves independently and could not find accommodations in private

or not-for-profit facilities. Blacks were among those cared for in these aus-
tere accommodations, which included 850 nursing-home and custodial-
care beds. As previously noted, the Old Age Assistance provisions of the
1935 Social Security Act prohibited the use of these funds to support people in public institutions. This had stimulated the growth of private boarding homes/nursing homes in Philadelphia, as it had in other parts of the
country. In Philadelphia it had also stimulated the addition of some nonprofit nursing homes by fraternal orders and church groups. By 1968
Philadelphia had accumulated a total of fifty-three proprietary and fifty-
five nonprofit nursing homes, in addition to the original city facility. There
were a total of 9,357 beds: 34 percent proprietary, 56 percent not for profit,
and the remaining 10 percent in the county home, Riverview.[37] The rate of
use of nursing homes was estimated at 2.0 per 100 white persons over the
age of 65 and 1.0 per 100 nonwhites over age 65, in line with rates found in
national surveys. (Current rates of nursing-home use are more than two
times these rates, in part reflecting the shift of long-term care patients from
general hospitals into nursing homes.)

Social workers in the public-assistance office of the Department of
Welfare reported in 1967 that it was difficult to find vacancies in nursing
homes that would accept patients at the public-assistance rates, and at the
end of October there were seventy-five names on a central waiting list.[38] A
sequence of events over the next thirty years would, in spite of periodic
protests and legal actions, leave the problem, at best, unaltered.

First Shots Fired: Boarding-Home Exposés and the
Medicaid Consumer Advisory Subcommittee

In the 1970s the problem worsened. Department of Welfare workers found
it increasingly difficult to place public-assistance patients in nursing
homes. Under pressure, they found themselves bending the criteria and
placing persons with medical problems in boarding homes. Hospital discharge planners, faced with backlogged public-assistance patients and
increasing utilization review pressures, began to bend under the same
stresses. The boarding homes, now referred to as personal-care or assisted-
living facilities, did not come under the mandated inspection programs of
the health department and were only loosely supervised by the Department of Welfare. A 1966 state law that had required licensure and inspections of these facilities had never been implemented. An estimated fifteen
thousand persons were being housed in some fifteen hundred unregulated
boarding homes in Philadelphia.[39] Pressures to reduce occupancy in state
mental hospitals had added greatly to the expanding demand for placements in these homes. Acute hospitals unable to gain access to the

restricted supply of nursing homes for their indigent patients also began to look at boarding homes as destinations for their patients. These pressures, and the resulting living conditions afforded residents, as one report observed, had produced the development of "an enormous and frightening capacity to endure human suffering."[40]

A fire killing seven residents in a facility in the Germantown section of the city, reports of the beating of residents resulting in death, the theft of residents' funds, starvation of residents, and, in some cases, the use of residents as chattel to be traded from one home to another finally precipitated state action.[41] A disproportionate share of the cases dealt with blacks that had been relocated to boarding homes because of a lack of access to nursing homes. In April 1980 the Pennsylvania Department of Welfare began to license and inspect personal-care boarding homes. Still the problems persisted.

Meanwhile, in 1979, Louis Brookings, director of the Philadelphia Welfare Rights Organization, filed a complaint with the Office for Civil Rights alleging that the admission policies and procedures of Philadelphia area nursing homes discriminated against minorities in violation of Title VI of the Civil Rights Act of 1964 and that the Pennsylvania Department of Health had failed in its responsibilities to enforce Title VI and its implementing regulations. The Office for Civil Rights' subsequent investigation found that many of the homes in the Philadelphia area required application fees and that many patients were required to pay the private rate for 18 months. The Baptist Home admitted 91 percent of private-pay applicants and required an application fee of all members, although about half of the nursing home's residents were being paid for by Medicaid. The home, located in a racially mixed neighborhood, housed 321 patients, all of whom were white. Subsequent to the Office for Civil Rights investigation, the Department of Health revised its methods of reviewing Title VI compliance for nursing homes. Yet a decade later, in 1989, the access barriers and racial composition of the homes remained essentially unaltered.

Discussions over the black nursing home access problem took place between welfare rights activist and nursing home industry representatives in the 1980s. Federal statute requires each state Medicaid program to have an advisory committee including providers and consumers to provide advice and information to the state Medicaid agency. Pennsylvania's Medical Assistance Advisory Committee included an extensive structure of subcommittees, one for each major provider group and one for consumers. Louise Brookings chaired the consumer advisory committee. A subcommittee of Medicaid recipients, lacking any staff or technical support, hardly posed a threat to the Pennsylvania Department of Welfare or to its providers. Brookings, however, was angered by the boarding-home scandals. Access to nursing homes, where many of the patients would have been more appropriately placed, would have averted some of the worst abuses. Too often, the victims were blacks. Ann Torregrossa, an attorney with the Delaware County Legal Assistance group who was involved in the Pennsylvania Health Law project, joined Brookings's consumer sub-committee in 1982 to provide legal advice. The group soon focused on the issue of access to nursing homes, and a joint task force was formed between the consumer and long-term care subcommittees. According to one participant, these protracted negotiations could be distilled into three cryptic lines of dialogue.

> *Providers.* The issue is reimbursement. Until the rates for Medical Assistance become more comparable with private-pay rates, the problem of access will persist.
> *Consumer Reps.* If we support higher reimbursement, will you support access requirements?
> *Providers.* No![42]

Conditions Worsen: The Medicaid Capital Cost Moratorium for Nursing Homes and Medicare Prospective Payment System for Hospitals

Two events exacerbated the problem of access to nursing homes in the Philadelphia area for indigent blacks and strengthened the hand of the nursing-home operators. First, in an effort to constrain the rapidly grow-ing Medicaid budget, the Department of Welfare declared a freeze on reimbursement of cost of new construction in 1982. In effect, this further exacerbated racial disparities in access. No new homes could be built in areas with a large concentration of Medicaid patients. It was financially feasible to construct homes only in areas likely to attract a large propor-tion of private-pay patients. Second, in the same year at the federal level the Tax Equity and Fiscal Responsibility Act of 1982 began a wave of changes in Medicare and Medicaid payments to hospitals that would effectively eliminate the ability of acute hospitals to absorb the blacks that needed nursing-home care but could not be placed. Up until then, hospi-tals had absorbed the excess demand for long-term care, shifting the cost from the state Medicaid obligations to cover the cost of nursing-home care for the elderly indigent to the federal Medicare program responsible for covering the cost of the bulk of their hospital care. These changes culmi-nated in the July 1, 1984, introduction of a DRG Prospective Payment System in both the federal Medicare program and the state Medicaid pro-gram in Pennsylvania. Hospitals would be paid a flat rate per admission for a particular diagnostically related group based on the average cost of treatment. The length of the patient's stay in the hospital, which is strongly related to the cost of the care provided, would no longer have any bearing on how much the hospital would be paid for that patient's care. Average length of stay in Philadelphia hospitals had remained stable for more than a decade. In a responsive to these new financial incentives that surprised most observers, average length of stay in Philadelphia area hospitals now dropped by more than a day within a year.[43] For nursing-home eligible but medically indigent hospital patients it was a classic catch-22 that said (1) you can no longer be cared for in the hospitals because long-term care will be reimbursed only in a nursing home, and (2) there are no nursing homes that will accept you.

The freeze on capital-cost payments for new nursing homes and the prospective payment system for hospitals gave nursing homes new leverage over the hospitals. They could be much more selective in picking and choosing residents. Many Philadelphia hospitals soon found that, in order to get any placements of first-day-eligible Medicaid patients, they had to "guarantee eligibility." State determination of a patient's Medicaid eligibility for nursing-home payment could take weeks. If, for some reason, the state Medicaid program determined that a patient was not eligible for reimbursement, the hospital had to provide assurances that it would pay for the patient's nursing-home stay. Hospital discharge planners begged for nursing-home slots for patients. They were pressured by hospital administrations to find places for patients now hemorrhaging hospital financial projections. The homes were increasingly picky. The discharge planners learned the rating systems used by different homes. They knew when it was pointless to contact a home about the placement of a particular patient. Nursing-home ratings systems were based on four criteria: (1) payer status (private pay vs. first day eligible), (2) level of care required (light vs. heavy), (3) duration of stay (short vs. long), and (4) race (white vs. black).[44] Some, it seemed, would accept only white, private-pay, light-care patients, and at the other extreme, only a few were willing to accept first-day-eligible, Medicaid, heavy-care, black patients. These differences between facilities roughly reflected the proportion of private paying patients they accommodated. Nursing homes were also concerned about the estimated duration of stay of both Medicaid and private-pay patients. A young private-pay patient, permanently and totally disabled but without a life-threatening condition, could be expected to convert to Medicaid at some point and become a long-term drain on the financial health of the home. A projected short-stay Medicaid patient could be admitted to fill an empty bed but not jeopardize the opportunity to acquire a "hot one," a long-term, private-pay, light-care patient.

Hospitals, however, needed the nursing homes not just as a place to discharge patients who required long-term care. The hospital's income was now driven by admissions. Philadelphia area hospitals faced declining occupancy rates and had plenty of excess capacity. More than one in every four Medicaid nursing-home patients is admitted to a hospital each year. Since Medicaid-eligible nursing-home patients are least likely to have a private physician managing their care, the nursing home and its medical director have considerable influence over where to hospitalize patients. A metropolitan nursing-home chain with several thousand Medicaid beds had considerable economic clout. What hospital nursing-home residents were steered to could make a greater than five-million-dollar difference in hospital revenues.

Most nursing homes in the Philadelphia area survive as businesses on the basis of their ability to attract private-pay patients. A decline below a certain proportion of private-pay patients spells financial disaster. White flight of private-pay customers was a concern of some operators. As operators would say in unguarded moments of candor, "I'm not a racist, but if the private-pay customer doesn't want mama next to a black lady in a home, then I'm not going to let the black lady in. They will get what they want." Some hospitals, through the efforts of their discharge planners, became complicit in the selective placement of nursing-home patients. As one critic observed:

> No one wanted to rock the boat. There was a fear of being blacklisted by the nursing homes that they had become dependent upon. There was no leadership. There was an openness and blatancy about such practices.
>
> In some sense, the whole industry operated above the law. Federal statutes prohibit extra payments by individuals and families as a condition of acceptance of a Medicaid patient. That prohibition also extends to duration-of-stay requirements as private-pay patients. Yet, in the Area Agency on Aging *Directory of Nursing Homes,* these requirements were included in the information. Here was a public agency, responsible for acting as an advocate of seniors, publicly acknowledging and providing legitimacy to practices that are against the law.[45]

Stalled Negotiations with the Welfare Department

Efforts to address the problem began to focus directly on discussions between lawyers for the Pennsylvania Health Law project and Department of Welfare Official. The negotiations dragged on inconclusively.

We focused on negotiating directly with the Department of Welfare, but the department refused to do anything. We tried to empower the department. It is very unusual in Pennsylvania for a regulatory agency to take on anything as powerful as the long-term care industry without there being some stink somewhere about it. So we helped a reporter, Gill Gaul, do a series of articles about the black nursing-home access issue for the *Philadelphia Inquirer*.

The Medicaid program was paying for 70 percent of the patients in Pennsylvania nursing homes; you would think that this would give you some leverage. In reality there was no rate setting for private-pay patients, and the homes had unfettered control over admissions.[46]

The *Inquirer* articles presented gross disparities in the racial composition of the homes and the ritualistic paper-processing of Title VI certifications of the homes. Yet, the traditional civil rights watchdogs for the Philadelphia black community remained silent.[47] There were no protests by the local chapter of the NAACP or other local advocacy groups. There were, as there had been thirty years before with hospitals, black business interests in nursing homes that were comfortable with the status quo. Probably more significant, however, was the stigmatized legacy of nursing homes. As mentioned in the first part of this chapter, they were not an attractive focus for civil rights advocacy. Focusing on improved opportunities for education, employment, and housing would seem to do more to close the racial gaps in income and quality of life than getting people into a place they didn't want to go to in the first place. Yet, equal opportunities for education and employment for individuals are constrained by the other needs of their families.

If we don't have the traditional African American groups pressuring things, it borders on the hopeless. Maybe there are so many more critical issues for these groups than worrying about the end-of-life-issues. Yet, the intergenerational effects we see in our legal-assistance office are often cataclysmic. There was a mother who cleaned house for a living, off the book, as was the tradition at the time, and had no savings. The daughter had to quit her job to care for her at home, losing the opportunity to qualify for a pension that would have prevented repeating the experience of her mother. There was a young man age sixteen who had to quit high school to care for his grandmother. The family needed the mother's income to support the household. The intergenerational ramifications are huge.[48]

The Numbers

The numbers told an important part of the story, invisible to most of the participants. These are summarized in tables 7.2 through 7.5.[49]

Table 7.2 shows that, using the index of dissimilarity as the measure of segregation, nursing homes in Pennsylvania are highly segregated by race. In part, this is a reflection of the geographic concentration of the black elderly population in Philadelphia. Since black elderly are concentrated in Philadelphia, Philadelphia area nursing homes have a higher concentration of black residents than the rest of the state. Based on surveys of nursing homes that are participating providers in the state's Medicaid program, the overall index of segregation in Pennsylvania nursing homes is .68. In other words, 68 percent of the black and white residents in nursing homes would need to be moved in order to create an equal distribution by race across all facilities. In terms of ownership, the public homes in Pennsylvania are the least segregated (.55); the proprietary homes are slightly more segregated (.62); and the not-for-profit homes are the most racially segregated (.85). These differences perhaps reflect the different historical role each type of ownership has played in the development of health care and race relations in the United States. (Prior to the civil rights era, public hospitals were the most integrated and not-for-profit or voluntary hospitals were the most segregated.) Geographic separation, however, *does not account* for all of the segregation of nursing homes. In Philadelphia, the segregation of nursing homes is .63, almost as high as the figure for the state as a whole. In contrast, the racial segregation in Philadelphia hospitals is .33, half the rate found in nursing homes.

As shown in table 7.3, based on estimates from the 1990 census, the count of Pennsylvania elderly located in group quarters shows that black elderly use of nursing homes is approximately 73 percent that of the white elderly. This understates the discrepancies, since it is generally acknowledged that black elderly, with their higher rate of chronic conditions and lack of alternative assisted-living arrangements, have a substantially higher need for nursing-home care.[50] Racial discrepancies in access are often attributed to differences in income, not race. However, if one controls for this by looking only at the black and white elderly who are eligible for public assistance, black elderly on public assistance are only .55 times as likely as white elderly to be located in homes for the elderly. In other words, race is a better predictor of use than income.

The Pennsylvania Health Department's own analysis of need for nursing-home beds in 1989 showed that half the total estimated shortage of beds in the state were located in Philadelphia. Other counties had substantial surpluses. Philadelphia had an estimated shortage of 4,304 nursing-home beds.[51] The city includes 62 percent of Pennsylvania's over-sixty-five black population and less than 10 percent of Pennsylvania's white over-sixty-five population. Taking the number of beds per hundred population in each of Pennsylvania's sixty-seven counties and weighting them with the proportion of black and white elderly in each produces strikingly different ratios of nursing-home bed. As indicated in table 7.4, there are on the average 4.55 beds available within the county per 100 white elderly in Pennsylvania and 3.06 beds per 100 black elderly. The odds that a black

TABLE 7.2.   Index of Dissimilarity for Nursing Homes in Pennsylvania, 1989

Pennsylvania	
Voluntary	.85
Proprietary	.62
Public	.55
All nursing homes	.68
Philadelphia[a]	
Hospitals[a]	.33
Nursing homes[a]	.63

Source: Updated from David Smith, "Racial Integration of Health Facilities," *Journal of Health Policy, Politics, and Law* 18, no. 4 (1993): 851–69.
[a]Listed separately for purposes of comparison.

TABLE 7.3.   Use of Nursing Homes by the Elderly, by Race and Receipt of Public Assistance

	White	Black	Total	B/W Ratio
All Elderly				
In home	95,816	4,638	100,454	
Not in home	1,609,889	109,142	1,719,031	
Total	1,705,705	113,780	1,819,485	
Rate in home per 100	5.62	4.08	5.52	0.73
Elderly with Public-Assistance Income				
In home	6,459	787	7,246	
Not in home	68,253	15,883	84,136	
Total	74,712	16,670	91,382	
Rate in home per 100	8.65	4.72	7.93	0.55

Source: Updated from David Smith, "Racial Integration of Health Facilities," *Journal of Health Policy, Politics, and Law* 18, no. 4 (1993): 851–69.

elderly person will have a bed available in the county where they reside was .67 of that of a white elderly person. While Philadelphia had a deficit of 4,304 beds, the four surrounding suburban counties had a projected surplus of 3,110 beds. Thus, before even beginning to negotiate the admission process that has been molded by the preferences of nursing homes to favor private-pay, easy-care, and other patient characteristics, the deck is stacked. Nursing homes in shortage areas can be more selective and those

TABLE 7.4.   Nursing-Home Beds and Estimated Bed Needs

	White	Nonwhite	Total	B/W Ratio
Projected 1992 population aged 65+	1,747,002	180,637	1,927,639	
Beds per 100 elderly	4.55	3.06	4.34	0.67
Projected bed deficit per 100 elderly[a]	−0.17	−1.66	−0.38	9.76

Source: Updated from David Smith, "Racial Integration of Health Facilities," Journal of Health Policy, Politics, and Law 18, no. 4 (1993): 851–69.

[a]Within county of residence.

TABLE 7.5.   Distribution of Residents in Pennsylvania Nursing Homes Subjected to State Health Department Licensure Action, by Race and Receipt of Medical Assistance

	White	Nonwhite	Total	NW/W Ratio
Action	12,528	2,131	14,659	
No action	63,001	4,670	67,671	
Total	75,529	6,801	82,330	
Probability of action	0.17	0.31	0.18	1.89

	Non-MA Patient	MA Patient	Total	MA/Non-MA Ratio
Action	4,651	10,008	14,659	
No action	26,497	38,833	65,330	
Total	31,148	48,841	79,989	
Probability of action	0.15	0.20	0.18	1.37

Source: Updated from David Smith, "Racial Integration of Health Facilities," Journal of Health Policy, Politics, and Law 18, no. 4 (1993): 851–69.

in areas of excess less so. A first-day Medicaid-eligible patient will face shorter delays and greater choice of facilities if that person resides in a suburban county.

Unequal treatment does not appear to end once a nonwhite person is admitted to a nursing home. As indicated in table 7.5, nonwhite person is 1.89 times more likely to be admitted to a facility that has been subjected to adverse state health department licensure action. Such adverse licensure actions take place when inspections identify what are judged to be serious deficiencies in patient care or in the physical plant. These actions result in a temporary provisional licensure and sometimes in a ban on new admissions or readmissions. In a few cases it results in the revocation of the license and the transfer of patients to other facilities. Race again is a better predictor than Medicaid status of location in such a home. Medicaid patients are only 1.37 times as likely as non-Medicaid patients to be located in such facilities.

In short, nursing homes were highly segregated in Pennsylvania. Race was a better predictor of access than income. Race was also a better predictor than Medical Assistance status of a patient's chances of being located in a substandard facility. The federal Medicaid program was passed at the height of the civil rights tide in the 1960s. It was envisioned as part of a way to assure health access as a right to all persons. The largest expenditures in the program were now for nursing homes. Those expenditures provided a catastrophic insurance policy for nursing-home operators and middle-class, mostly white, nursing-home patients. They conferred far fewer benefits on the poor and minorities. All of this had happened mostly through impersonal, usually unconscious, institutional forces. There were few fingerprints and no smoking gun. In the words of the person whose story began the discussion of health care prior to the civil rights era in chapter 1, "It was the way it was."

Taylor v. White Class Action Litigation

On August 15, 1990, a class action suit was filed in the United States District Court for the Eastern District of Pennsylvania by the Pennsylvania Health Law Project against the Secretary of Welfare, the Secretary of the Budget, and the Secretary of Health of the Commonwealth of Pennsylvania.[52] The plaintiffs all faced the same predicament. One, a sixty-year-old black woman, had been living at home with three elderly sisters in Philadelphia until her latest episode of illness. She suffered from hypertension, diabetes mellitus, morbid obesity, and the catastrophic effects of a severe cerebrovascular accident. Until her illness she was employed as a floral designer and was an active church volunteer all of her adult life. At the time of the lawsuit she was unable to speak, understand verbal messages, or cooperate in her care. During hospitalization for her stroke, she had developed bed-sores. She weighed 250 pounds and could not be cared for adequately by her three elderly sisters at home. She was placed in a nursing home only after several months and after being refused admission to homes that were nearer her sisters and better able to care for her condition.

Another plaintiff was a thirty-two-year-old black man who was a patient at the Jefferson Hospital Spinal Cord Center. He had attended college, studying to enter the ministry in the footsteps of his grandfather and uncle. Attempted suicide had left him paralyzed from the waist down. His acute phase of care was over, but his hospital social worker was unable to get him admitted to a nursing home because of his age, handicap, race, and status as a Medicaid patient. The third plaintiff was a forty-seven-year-old black male Medicaid patient who remained at Presbyterian-University Hospital because the hospital had been unable to find a nursing home to accept him. Admitted for pneumonia five months earlier, his course of treatment was complicated by frequent seizures and encephalopathy that produced severe mental impairment. He was confused, unable to understand the nature of his current circumstances, and required restraints to control his actions. He was unable to manage either his daily living needs or more complex needs for medical care, but no longer required hospitalization. Remaining in the hospital rather than being more appropriately placed in a nursing home, he was at greater risk of contracting infections. The final plaintiff was Louise Brookings.

The suit challenged the legality of *(a)* allowing nursing homes which received federal funds to have admission practices and policies which subjected the plaintiffs to discrimination because of their age, race, color, and handicap, and *(b)* the state moratorium on reimbursement for depreciation and interest, which had the effect of defeating or substantially impairing the objectives of the Medicaid program to provide access to, and improvement of the quality of care for, indigent individuals. The suit invoked the Medicaid legislation's requirements and regulations for state design to assure the accomplishment of those objectives. It also invoked Title VI of the 1964 civil rights bill prohibiting the use of federal funds that discriminate on the basis of race. Not leaving any stone unturned, it also invoked subsequent federal legislation that borrowed the language of Title VI and applied it to barring the use of federal funds that discriminate on the basis of age or disability.

The Lawsuit from Hell

Only a small tip of the structural and institutional forces allied against addressing these issues had been visible, and now their massiveness became evident. The judge, who had a reputation for juggling many cases and managing an unusually heavy caseload, ceded an advantage to the state as defendant. As one of the lawyers bring the suit observed:

> This is a very frustrating judge to practice in front of because he's always trying to get his docket cleared. So what he did with this case, without motion of any party, he dismissed from the active docket and instructed the parties to work out a settlement. It's great for the defendant, but as a plaintiff you've lost any pressure you can bring to force a settlement.[53]

In the meantime, the voluntary and proprietary nursing-home associations intervened on the side of the state. The nursing-home industry was reeling from a federal district court decision in a class action suit against the Tennessee commissioner of health.[54] The state had previously permitted "spot certification" of Medicaid beds. In other words, a home could limit its Medicaid certification to a floor or even an individual bed. This had permitted the homes to provide care to private-pay patients who spent down to become eligible for Medicaid without opening the home to any Medicaid admissions or, in some cases, segregating first-day-eligible Medicaid patients from those who had spent down from private pay. The federal district court had concluded that these arrangements violated certain federal Medicaid requirements regarding assurances of access to Medicaid beneficiaries and Title VI of the Civil Rights Act. Under court instructions to come up with a remedial plan, the state had negotiated a plan with the plaintiffs that required (1) Medicaid certification of all beds in the facility, (2) admissions on a first-come, first-served basis without regard to payer status, (3) prohibition of involuntary transfer or discharge based on source of payment, and (4) arrangements to beef up civil rights compliance and enforcement. The court had accepted this plan without change.

In preparation for trial, both sides began to depose witnesses. These depositions became crowded affairs. The new partner defendants didn't trust each other. Separate legal council represented the state, the proprietary nursing-home association, and the voluntary nursing-home association. All had to be present. A lawyer from the NAACP Legal Defense Fund joined the three legal assistance attorneys on the other side. In one such session, ten lawyers, along with statistical consultants for both sides, crowded into the cramped space of the legal assistance office in Chester. The Philadelphia area hospitals were reluctant to be drawn into the dispute. Only two, Jefferson and Hospital of the University of Pennsylvania, the two largest, wealthiest, and most influential institutions in the city, agreed to allow discharge planners on their staffs to be deposed.

The defense was well financed by the state associations and attracted the support and interest of the national associations. A session of the National Health Law Association conference in Las Vegas was devoted to a presentation by the attorneys handling the defense, who warned that the conditions in Pennsylvania that led to the suit were present elsewhere and that a wave of similar suits in other states could be expected.

The Demise of a Draft Settlement

As the protracted negotiations dragged on, a draft settlement began to take shape in June 1994. In exchange for the plaintiffs' withdrawal and dismissal of the matter, the state would agree to support some expansion of nursing home beds in Philadelphia and more effectively monitor admission practices. The agreement was contingent on the receipt of about $100 million made available by "provider tax" funds used to increase the state Medicaid match and thus increase federal Medicaid funds available.

Negotiating all the details acceptable to the Pennsylvania Health Law project, state, and nursing-home association attorneys were finally worked out in the fall 1994 and remained for the governor's final approval. However, in the last days of his administration, Governor Casey, not wishing to "tie the hands of the new governor," declined. The Ridge administration, with welfare reform at the top of their political agenda, refused to sign the agreement.

While some preliminary steps were taken in anticipation of the agreement by the Department of Welfare in addressing access and civil rights compliance issues, negotiations began again at square one. Adding to the difficulties, the Department of Welfare and other parties to the *Taylor* case negotiations were now embroiled in working through the details of implementing a mandatory Medical Assistance managed-care program for the Philadelphia five-county metropolitan area. In November 1993 the Department of Welfare received approval from the Health Care Financing Administration for its "HealthChoices" program. The delayed but long anticipated implementation of this mandatory Medicaid managed-care program for the region began in November 1996. The HealthChoices program requires Medicaid beneficiaries in the five-county Philadelphia metropolitan area to enroll in an HMO plan. The plans receive a fixed payment per enrollee per month from the Pennsylvania Department of Welfare. The attraction to the program for the Department of Welfare is that it controls the cost of the Medicaid program, since those costs will be fixed by the rate it negotiates with the HMOs for assuming the responsibility for the care of its Medicaid enrollees.

HMOs contracting with the HealthChoices program are responsible for the payment of the first thirty days of nursing care for a member who is admitted to a nursing home. After this period, the Medicaid program assumes responsibility for paying the costs of the individual's nursing-home use. The Department of Welfare is concerned about the incentive HMOs have to shift the costs of the chronic care of their members back to the Department of Welfare and is interested in extending the HMO's period of responsibility for the cost of nursing-home care to reduce this incentive. Persons who were dually eligible for Medicare and Medicaid benefits must join one of the HealthChoices HMOs. That is, the HMO is obligated to pay these costs as a part of their capitated payment. Persons who become eligible for Medical Assistance while residing in a nursing home (e.g. the "spend-downs" as opposed to the "first day eligibles") are not enrolled in HealthChoices.

These arrangements raise other troubling questions. With which homes will the HMOs develop arrangements for the care of their members? Will they provide a reasonably full range of choices, or will those choices be restricted to a few of the less desirable homes with which they are able to negotiate low payments? What will be the effect on nursing-home segregation of the poor and, by nature of the distribution of income and wealth, segregation by race into separate and unequal systems of care?

In its request for proposals from HMOs, DPW acknowledged the problem and placed importance on "mainstreaming" Medicaid recipients.

> The HMO must ensure that their networks of providers do not intentionally segregate HealthChoices members in any way from other persons receiving services. . . .To assure mainstreaming of HealthChoices members, the HMO shall investigate complaints and take affirmative action so that members are provided covered services without regard to race, color, creed, sex, religion, age, national ancestry, marital status, sexual orientation, language, MA status, health disease or pre-existing condition, anticipated need for health care or mental handicap.[55]

The list of protected groups has expanded since the 1960s, but the devil is still in the details.

One of the more troubling details of the plan is the ability of the Medical Assistance program to magically make the estimated shortage of nursing-home beds in Philadelphia disappear without adding a single additional nursing-home bed. Regulations by the Department of Public Welfare were implemented on September 30, 1997 to replace Certificate of Need regulations that had sunset on December 18, 1996. The CON regulations controlled expansion of acute-hospital beds and capital equipment as well as the number of nursing-homes beds. The new regulations focus only on MA nursing-home beds, freezing the existing stock of MA beds in Pennsylvania. DPW intends to do this by exercising its discretion to reject new nursing-home applications to become MA providers and to terminate contracts with existing nursing-home providers which expand their bed capacity. It intends to make exceptions to this general policy only on a case-by-case basis. The policy objective is to shift care away from nursing homes to presumably less costly home care and to personal care homes. Attempting to put the most favorable spin on this plan, DPW explained their intent in the following way:

> This policy of exercising our discretion regarding MA nursing care provider participation is a key element in the Administration's goal to broaden the use of home and community based services for citizens who might otherwise be forced into high-cost, less preferable institutional settings. . . .The Department views home and community-based services to have several important benefits. Among other things, many older Pennsylvanians and Pennsylvanians with disabilities prefer home and community-based services to institutional services. Given a choice, we believe that many people would choose to remain in their own homes and communities rather than reside in a nursing facility. Moreover, in many, if not most instances, we have found that home and community-based services are less expensive than institutional services.[56]

In effect, the guidelines for considering exceptions appear to encourage growing racial disparities in access to long-term care. First, the Department of Public Welfare plans to abandon any intention of looking at the broader community needs for nursing-home beds, as the Department of Health had done under the CON regulations. There will be no attempt to restrain the construction or expansion of private nursing-homes beds for operators not seeking to serve MA patients. Expansion of such beds will inevitably take place in more affluent and predominantly white areas, most of which, according to the State Health Department, already have a substantial surplus of nursing-home beds. This excess capacity will siphon off some of the private-pay patients from currently MA-enrolled homes in these overbedded areas, freeing up additional slots for MA patients. These same communities also tend to have better-developed networks of home care services. In contrast, Philadelphia is unlikely to have any expansion in beds and has the majority of the estimated nursing-home bed shortage in the state and an inadequate supply of home care services for the indigent. The guidelines stipulate that, even in such areas of shortage, if the average occupancy in the service area is less than 95 percent occupancy, the need for MA beds will be considered met. Philadelphia has the largest share of first-day-eligible Medical Assistance patients. The admission of these patients to nursing homes must pass increasingly formidable hurdles erected by the managed-care health plans concerned with minimizing their costs. The impact of these restraints is likely to be sufficient to reduce average occupancy in nursing homes well below the 95 percent threshold. The "shortage" of beds thus evaporates. The racial disparities in use of nursing-home care are likely to widen.[57] Negotiations related to the Taylor suit settlement continue under these changed circumstances.

The Era of Postcapitation Long-Term Care in Philadelphia

> *It's not hard to be a brilliant entrepreneur in health care—Just find something really stupid and do the opposite.*
>
> *—Anonymous*

Thus, as the parties to the *Taylor* suit struggled to resolve their differences, the terrain shifted. Just as in the earlier evolutionary shifts of organizations providing long-term care services, powerful forces were again at work drastically changing the long-term care environment and reshaping the population of organizations able to survive and adapt to those changes. The strained accommodation between acute and long-term care and its two major sources of payment, the federal Medicare and the State Medicaid programs, had produced a growing vacuum.

The search for ways to fill that vacuum began in the early 1980s with a few hospitals acquiring nursing homes. There was no thought of integration; it was just a new form of cost shifting. The former administrator of Presbyterian Hospital reflected on the experience: "We purchased some predominantly private-pay homes that we thought were underperforming in the suburbs. We thought of it purely as a way of making money, of taking the profits from the suburbs and supporting our inner-city hospital, and it worked."[58]

The first-day-eligible Medicaid nursing-home patients had new value, since they rarely had ties to a private attending physician who would decide where they should be admitted if they needed hospital care. The nursing-home medical director, by default, would become their attending physician. Presbyterian Hospital's administrator described their business strategy during this period.

> We began to see it as a way to capture hospital inpatients, but you had to be sensitive to doing the right thing. You could say, "When you need to admit to a hospital, we'd like you to think about us first."

It all follows what we have described as the 90–60–30 principle. If the nursing home was adjacent to the hospital, you'd get about 90 percent; if it was somewhere in the primary services area you might get 60 percent; outside the primary service area you might get 30 percent of these dually eligible patients. The focus was on capturing the hospital admission, not an integrated delivery system. Each hospital admission generated about ten times as much as what you could save from early nursing-home discharges. People talk about the continuum of care, but the real way to make money is to fill the hospital bed, not empty it. In fact, if you're able to fill an empty bed, you can afford to keep the other patients. If Willie Sutton were in the hospital business he would have concentrated on primary-care physicians and nursing homes who admit, and not worry about outplacement. So my friends who talk about this in the game talk about it as dual issues, outplacement and inflow. Economically, forget the outplacement, it's the inpatient admissions that really count to the hospital. A Medicare inpatient admission is between ten thousand and twelve thousand dollars a hit in terms of cash flow. Just putting in a medical director, however, didn't seem to take full advantage of the opportunity to capture inpatient hospital market share, and Presbyterian began to experiment with the idea of a "Quality of Life Campus" surrounding the nursing homes, adding services to the residents and exploring the possibilities for adding assisted living. We had the idea of building a prototype of such a campus next to the hospital.[59]

In 1995, however, the tail began to think about wagging the dog. One consequence of the increasing competition and declining hospital occupancy, driven by the efforts to block the cost shifting from long-term to acute-hospital care, was a growing consolidation of hospital services in Philadelphia. Presbyterian Hospital was acquired by the University of Pennsylvania Health System. That left the Presbyterian Foundation with its evolving network of nursing homes and a greatly expanded endowment. The endowment began to support the infrastructure that was missing, the "quality of life campus," the inner-city equivalent to what exists in suburban continuing-care communities for the affluent. Investment in job training, business development, and supportive cluster housing was also required so that local individuals could provide services to the population (food, beauticians, etc.). What began to emerge was a plan for a capitated delivery system for the elderly, similar to On Lok, a program established in San Francisco's Chinese community that began almost twenty years ago.

I learned this from the On Lok model: you pay attention to quality assurance and data collection. You contract out the hospital and nursing-home pieces. The only thing that's missing is the housing part. What we want to do is get in the food chain. The PACE demonstration [Program for All-inclusive Care of the Elderly; a Medicare/Medicaid demonstration in Philadelphia with an at-risk contract for managing the care of nursing-home-eligible patients] now gets an all-inclusive, per member per month rate of $4,500. It's $1 billion per year for the 65,000 dually eligible elderly population in the Philadelphia metropolitan area. That's how much money is going into the system now. One billion dollars. The PACE program will get $4,500 per member per month to do this. The trends from these kinds of demonstrations are encouraging: less nursing home, less hospital care, more outpatient, but the problem is scale. How do you go from a population of 350 persons to 65,000? That's the only thing that worries me. We learned the 80:20 principle. Twenty percent of the people are using 80 percent of the resources. Medicare remains the golden goose for insurance companies, for enrollment of the aging yuppies. Eighty percent just need proper monitoring.

All that money is going to go to one person; the hospital thinkers are inside the wall. It's great, though; the best and the brightest minds aren't even looking at it. You think there's money in poor people; there is. All you have to do is interdict and stop the hospital admissions. Right now, there is every incentive to maximize hospital admissions. I'm guessing we could cut 20 to 40 percent of the cost out of the system. The hospital and the nursing home are dead. Whoever captures those 65,000 persons wins. We're out there setting up our network, and no one else is even hunting.[60]

The environment is changing, and the population of organizations that will inhabit the emerging one will change. That much is clear. Many states are now working to get federal waivers or to develop demonstration programs combining Medicare and Medicaid for the dually eligible, ending the cost-shifting battles between the two programs.[61] The impact on ending the racial differences in access to inpatient hospital and nursing-home care are unclear but not encouraging. More care is likely to be provided in office practices and in the home. Yet such settings, unlike nursing homes and hospitals, are exempted from federal Title VI enforcement efforts. That final part of the story will be addressed in the next chapter. It is the part that describes not just how much race matters to those growing old but, more importantly, how much it matters to those being born.

CHAPTER 8

Race and Prenatal Care

Introduction

> Not only does the Constitution stand in the way of the claimed immunity but there are powerful countervailing equities in favor of the plaintiffs. . . . Racial discrimination in medical facilities is at least partly responsible for the fact that in North Carolina the rate of Negro infant mortality is twice the rate for whites and maternal deaths are five times greater. (Federal Court of Appeals for the Fourth Circuit, *Simkins v. Moses H. Cone Memorial Hospital,* November 1, 1963)[1]

In 1995, thirty-two years after the *Simkins* decision and thirty-one years after the passage of the Civil Rights Act of 1964, the black infant mortality rate in the United States, despite overall declines, stood at a level 2.4 times the white rate. The largest black-white differences in infant mortality in 1995 were not in the South but in the Northeast and Midwest. In Pennsylvania, black infant mortality rates were almost three times those of whites.[2] If discrimination had indeed played a role in accounting for the differences in black and white infant mortality in North Carolina in 1963, as concluded by the court in *Simkins,* perhaps in more complex and subtle ways it continues to play a role today. If not, why had the gap between black and white infant mortality widened over the three intervening decades? These differences can't simply be dismissed as the result of differences in income and poverty levels, since most of the differences persist even when controlling for income and poverty.[3]

Most studies have concluded that good prenatal care plays an essential role in improving birth outcomes and longer-term life chances.[4] Many argued in the 1980s that eliminating economic barriers to prenatal care could help reduce racial disparities in the use of such care and consequently, in birth outcomes. Pressures from a broad coalition of organizations with roots in the earlier civil rights struggles succeeded in expanding health care insurance coverage to provide essentially universal coverage of prenatal care. These efforts laid the groundwork for expanding coverage to all children under eighteen. The gap between the proportions of white and black women receiving prenatal care in the first three months of their pregnancy has narrowed. Yet the gap in birth outcomes remains. Differences in rates of infant mortality, prematurity, and low birth weight not only persist, but also contribute to the relatively poor health performance of the United States as a whole. The United States ranks twenty-fifth among developed countries in infant mortality. It ranks first in per capita health care expenditures, spending more than twice that of most of the better-performing nations.[5] The persistence of racial disparities in infant mortality is a warning signal, indicating underlying problems that reach beyond financial barriers in preventing blacks from receiving adequate care. This chapter will explore how the role of race and the organization of medical practice might contribute to these problems.

At the core of how prenatal care is organized, just as all health care, are the encounters between the physician, nurse midwife, or other care providers, and the patient. The relationship that evolves from such encounters serves as the basic building block for organizing the health system. Hospitals and nursing homes exist to provide some of the infrastructure to support this relationship. In the pre–civil rights era, the quality of that provider-patient relationship, if not the technical quality of care, provided was often inferior for blacks. Blacks and whites used different providers, often sat in separate waiting rooms, were referred to different places for more specialized services, and were admitted to different hospitals and nursing homes. Not only were the location, content, and qualitative character of the care different, the expectations that providers and patients brought to these encounters were different.

Yet, in spite of the central importance of such provider-patient encounters, they were excluded from any civil rights review. While civil rights groups and the Civil Rights Commission protested this exclusion, private office practices receiving payment from Medicare for the medical rather than the hospital portion of the program, as well as those participating in Medicaid, were exempted from Title VI compliance. State Medicaid programs never addressed the issue. There were plenty of practical administrative and political reasons for exempting private practices from reviews. There were too many providers and too few civil rights staff members to consider undertaking an effort of such magnitude. There was no obvious set of easily enforceable standards, nor were there data that could have been used for developing such standards. Given the widespread opposition of organized medicine to the Medicare and Medicaid legislation, the enforcement of Title VI in private physician practices would have almost certainly failed and, in the process, crippled these two fledgling programs. In addition, most physicians and most of the American public believed that the relationship between a patient and physician was a voluntary, private, and personal relationship into which neither the government nor any other third party had any business intruding. No one involved in the implementation or operation of the Medicare or Medicaid program had any interest in jousting with such windmills.

As a result, the issue of discrimination in private medical practices was never publicly addressed. There were no reviews of office practices, no testing by local civil rights groups, no legal cases, no requirements in the submission of forms describing the racial composition of the practice—not even the pro forma signed assurances that were required of participating nursing homes. State Medicaid programs could have, in theory, made an issue of Title VI compliance with private practitioners. The states, however, were not in a position to take the lead. If the staffing and level of expertise necessary to conduct compliance reviews were limited in the federal government, they were nonexistent in state government.

Unlike Medicare, the states have continued to have trouble getting private physicians to participate in the Medicaid program. According to many private-practice physicians, the rates of payment and administrative red tape made participation in the Medicaid program unattractive. Some, like many of the nursing homes, would use the Medicaid program as a catastrophic insurance plan for their own patients. They would continue to care for their own, long-standing private patients who had "spent down" through illness or employment problems when they became eligible for Medicaid. Few private practices, however, were open to accept new or first-day-eligible Medicaid patients. Even fewer private practice obstetricians, facing substantially higher malpractice insurance coverage costs than those of primary care physicians, were willing to accept Medicaid patients.

As a result of federal and state reluctance to use the 1964 Civil Rights Act and the Medicare and Medicaid program to impose requirements on private physicians, the racial differences in the relationships between ambulatory care providers and patients remained essentially unchanged. Indeed, no overt acts of discrimination were needed to assure the perpetuation of largely segregated care and, perhaps, the perpetuation of disparate outcomes. Many blacks, particularly the medically indigent, continued to rely on the care provided by hospital emergency departments, public clinics, and the clinics of teaching hospitals. Such care was often fragmented and lacked continuity. Attempting to respond to these problems, the Office of Equal Opportunity funded the establishment of neighborhood health centers, a part of President Lyndon Johnson's War on Poverty program. Located in low-income inner-city neighborhoods and impoverished rural communities, the health centers were initially envisioned as part of a larger strategy of community and economic development. They received the bulk of their funding directly through federal grants, circumventing state and local government control. It proved a politically popular program and expanded in the 1970s. The neighborhood health centers provided a concrete, tangible accomplishment for communities, one that a local congressional representative could take credit for. More systematic reform of the Medicaid program or through universal health insurance coverage was a far more costly and illusive goal.

A tenuous accommodation evolved between ambulatory-care providers and the state Medicaid programs, similar to the accommodation worked out with the nursing-home providers described in the last chapter. This accommodation balanced the vital interests of teaching programs, the state Medicaid program, the neighborhood health centers, and private-practice physicians. Teaching programs were able to sustain an acceptable volume of "clinical material" to maintain the accreditation of their medical school and residency programs. The state Medicaid programs saved money by reimbursing for outpatient services below their actual costs. The neighborhood health centers continued to receive a direct stream of federal funding separate from the state Medicaid programs, providing needed services but undercutting more costly Medicaid reform. As a result, private-practice physicians were buffered from pressures to assume greater responsibility for the socioeconomic and racial integration of their practices by using the Medicaid program just as the predominantly private-pay nursing homes did.

This accommodation, however, began to break down in the 1990s, as the growth of managed care began to drastically reshape the relationship between private-practice physicians and their patients. The chairman of a Philadelphia area teaching hospital obstetrical department observed the beginning of these changes in prenatal care with concern in 1992.

> We just don't have the physical space to provide the prenatal care. We're working as we did in the fifties and sixties, with the Philadelphia General Hospital–type approach, with long benches and long waits. GA [an elective Medicaid managed-care plan] is very competitive with other third-party private insurance carriers. My concern is, as the chairman of a department in a teaching hospital, it's going to cut into my volume of patients, as a teaching basis for my residents and medical students. The Medicaid patient can present herself to a private practitioner's office, doesn't have to wait on long benches, and doesn't have to partake of all the activities which we provide them. I

think its going to be reflected in an increase in the morbidity. Even though our patients have long waits, we provide them with nutritional care, food supplements, with a lot of support, which they probably don't see as patients, but which reflects itself in statistics. When they go to a private doctor's office, they are going to be more comfortable in terms of the social amenities. Sooner or later there is going to be a for-profit group of obstetricians that are going to come in here and set up practices to provide obstetrical care for Medicaid patients. Our private physicians do not accept Medicaid patients. However, when they are allowed to avail themselves of GA and other third-party carriers that provide competitive payment to private physicians, then, of course, it would be discrimination if they didn't take these patients in their office. My concern is that I'm going to lose the teaching patient here, which means we'll lose our ability to train residents and medical students, unless we can upgrade the physical facilities I have to provide those services. I'm losing about 10 percent of our Medicaid patients to managed care right now. There are plenty of private obstetricians and there is a lot of competition for patients.[6]

The environment faced by ambulatory care providers changed precipitously. State Medicaid programs began to control their budgets by providing flat payments per enrollee to managed-care health plans. The plans, in turn, were responsible for providing whatever services were needed and bearing the costs. Most state Medicaid programs were in the process of converting to mandatory managed-care arrangements by 1997. As Medicaid, Medicare, and private employer health plan coverage through managed-care plans increased, few private practices could afford to avoid accepting such patients. The differences in both payment and red tape between the private plans and Medicaid narrowed. Hospitals, concerned about protecting market share and faced with increasing competition, began to buy up physician practices. The character of the relationship between the physician and patient had been redefined.

This chapter pieces together the story of race, prenatal care, and the relationship between its providers and patients. The racial nuances are explored by contrasting the experiences of two cities, Charleston and Philadelphia. Addressing racial disparities in birth outcomes, each city chose to redefine the relationship between providers and patients in starkly different ways. The stream of the health care civil rights struggle had reached flood stages in the 1960s before being blocked. Now those waters flowed through other channels, merging with an expanding women's movement and focusing on maternity care and the health of children. Through the battles in Charleston, Philadelphia, and many other communities across the nation, the health care civil rights struggle continues. It is first, however, necessary to provide some background on other forces shaping differences in the relationship black as opposed to white patients experience in receiving medical care.

Background: Race and the Patient-Provider Relationship

The relationship that a pregnant black woman typically experiences with her health care providers differs from that of her white counterpart. She uses different providers, and, as a result, the way in which her care is managed is different. White pregnant Medical Assistance patients are more likely to receive care in private practices. These differences result mostly from patterns of racial residential segregation and where physicians choose to locate their practices.

The Location of Private Medical Practices

Physicians starting up practice focus on location. For patients, a major determinant in choosing where to go for care is distance. Few patients will choose a primary-care provider outside relatively narrow geographic boundaries. Primary-care physicians and dentists have historically tended to space their offices almost equidistant from each other. Specialty practices, however, tend to be more geographically concentrated. This reflects both their greater dependence on physician referrals, rather than choices by the lay public, and their greater reliance on the more centralized services provided by hospitals to support their practice. Obstetricians fall somewhere between the primary-care and specialty-care pattern of practice location.

Like any small business, physicians locate their practice or join ones in places they can make a living. Unlike nursing homes, whose construction tends to be controlled by state laws that regulate supply, physicians face few constraints regarding the location of their practices. However, just as in the case of nursing homes, a large proportion of their income has historically been dependent on the out-of-pocket payments of their patients. As a result, physician-to-population ratios are directly related to the income levels of different areas. The more a particular specialty practice is dependent on out-of-pocket rather than insurance payments, the greater its concentration in higher-income areas. For example, in Lower Merion Township, a community in the affluent Main Line suburban area outside Philadelphia, the physician-to-population ratio is double that of the United States as a whole. However, in terms of specialty practices,

Lower Merion Township has 3.5 times as many pediatricians, 4.2 times as many obstetrician-gynecologists, 6.3 times as many plastic surgeons, and 18.6 times as many psychiatrists per 100,000 population as in the United States as a whole.[7]

Private-practice physicians followed the flight to the suburbs that accelerated at the end of the 1960s, just as de jure forms of racial segregation of medical care crumbled. This forced hospitals in many urban areas to either follow their physicians, relocating to the suburbs, or lose out to newly formed or expanded suburban hospitals. The urban hospitals were financially dependent on the admissions of these physicians, particularly because of the more attractive forms of private insurance payment associated such practices. The civil rights legal battles in the 1970s in Wilmington, Delaware; Gary, Indiana; Bexar County, Texas, New York City, and other communities were all involved with the efforts of hospitals to prevent the loss of their medical staffs by relocating with them (see chapter 5).

Separate and Unequal Care

Residential racial segregation persists in most metropolitan areas of the United States. This segregation in turn shapes the use of obstetrical care. The racial disparities in private health insurance coverage further separate white and black obstetrical patients. For example, 15,754 babies born in the five-county metropolitan area of Philadelphia in 1994 were identified in hospital discharge records as black.[8] Nine urban teaching hospitals out of a total of forty-two acute hospitals in the region providing obstetrical care accounted for 74 percent of these black births. These same nine urban teaching hospitals, however, accounted for only 8 percent of the 32,011 white births in the region. The majority of births in each of these nine hospitals were black, and the percentage of black births was as high as 85 percent. Applying the index of dissimilarity, the measure of segregation used in the last two chapters for Medicare hospital admissions and nursing-homes census, the degree of racial segregation of hospital obstetrical care in the region was .63. In contrast, the segregation of elderly Medicare discharges is somewhat lower (.47) and the overall residential segregation in the region is higher (.76) in the Philadelphia metropolitan area.[9] However, this estimate of the degree of racial segregation of obstetrical care in the Philadelphia area of .63 understates the actual degree of segregation. Some hospitals provide separate accommodations for private and Medical Assistance patients, and the obstetrical practices, using the same hospital, differ substantially in the racial composition of their practices.

Blacks and whites don't just tend to use separate practices; they use

distinctively different ones. In 1993, for example, adjusting for age differences the two populations, blacks visited physician offices only .66 as
many times as whites. In contrast, black use of hospital emergency departments was 1.69 times that of whites, while the use of hospital outpatient
departments was fully 2.04 times that of whites.[10] Teaching-hospital clinics, urban hospital emergency departments, and public-health clinics have
filled the vacuum produced by the absence of private practices in poorer,
inner city areas. In such clinic settings, the relationship between a patient
and the provider of services that usually exists in a private practice is often
absent. Care tends to be more fragmented and episodic. There is little of
the continuity and ongoing relationship between patient and provider that
exists in private practice, and often there is less attention to routine examinations and preventive care.

In the Philadelphia metropolitan area, the bulk of black children are
born in a few of the city's larger teaching hospitals. These are major teaching institutions that set the standards in prenatal and neonatal care. One
could make an argument that such children receive superior care. In narrow terms of technical standards of care this is certainly true. Most of
these institutions also provide outreach, counseling, and supportive services that are typically absent in a busy private suburban obstetrical practice. Yet, they are also separate and different from the providers and institutions experienced by the average white. The relationship between the
provider and the patient is more transient and less central to the activities
of the provider. Such differences may contribute to the differences in black
and white birth outcomes. Metropolitan areas with a lower degree of residential segregation and thus, by implication, a lower degree of segregation
in the provision of maternity services tend to have narrower disparities in
black and white infant mortality rates.[11]

Private Practices Adapt

Private medical practices, just as hospitals and nursing homes, have struggled to adapt to the residential segregation of the communities they serve
and the disparities in payment they received from private and Medical
Assistance patients. Obstetricians, just like other physicians in private
practice on the periphery of inner-city neighborhoods, have been fearful of
opening their practice to Medical Assistance patients, who are also more
likely to be black. One Philadelphia doctor who had opened his private
practice to Medical Assistance patients voiced concern about the "chicken
bone syndrome." He claimed he had little problem with accepting lower
payments and with treating Medical Assistance patients. He was afraid,

however, that the chicken bones left in the waiting room might result in a loss of some of his private patients.[12] Physicians in the more middle-class neighborhoods of Philadelphia and the bordering suburbs shared similar concerns about being overwhelmed with Medical Assistance patients, as an in-depth discussion with ten such primary-care physicians revealed. The willingness to accept new Medical Assistance patients into their practice varied inversely with the concentration of Medical Assistance patients in their practice area.[13] Areas with higher concentrations of Medical Assistance patients also tended to be areas with a higher concentration of blacks. Thus, access to private-practice care by black patients on Medical Assistance was disproportionately affected. Here is how it works, according to these physicians.

> If they're patients we've had any contact with or are down on their luck, have switched to Medical Assistance after losing employment, we always accept them. . . . Patients we've had no contact with before are generally referred elsewhere. If our practice were one hundred percent Medical Assistance, our doors would be closed. We could not provide service. It would be beyond our expenses. That's the bottom line.[14]

> There are two sorts of "underground" issues that I see. One is that there are a lot of institutions and doctors that don't accept Medical Assistance. If there's a growing trend toward more people needing Medical Assistance, there's always the possibility of your being overwhelmed. There has to be a more global system so that everybody is sharing responsibility, so that it makes it more readily available.[15]

> If the problem gets big enough, if the numbers get big enough, then people start walling themselves off because it just doesn't pay.[16]

There were also, according to these physicians, more qualitative reasons for avoiding taking on too many Medical Assistance patients. The patients were seen as taking more time to care for, often failing to fit comfortably in the style of practice that the physician was accustomed to, and more likely to sue.

> You definitely spend more time with them. They tend to be more limited in their understanding of things. It takes longer to teach them, and you get more phone calls. Our nurses have to go over things, and then the patients will go home and have more questions and they'll call again.

Some Medical Assistance patients are more apt to be unhappy with their care and more apt to sue you. Especially those you get through the emergency room.

The malpractice costs don't bear it out, but it seems so to me too.[17]

You don't have the same bond with them as you have with some of your other patients you've seen for years. A lot of these people are transient: you see them for a short period of time, then they disappear and go see someone else. So you don't have the same interpersonal relationship with them. They're more apt to be unhappy. The patient-doctor relationship is a two way street. You just don't get the rapport.[18]

These same physicians also reported performing an informal balancing act in referring Medical Assistance patients to specialists, similar to that used by hospital discharge planners in dealing with nursing homes in the last chapter.

You wouldn't send a surgeon a Medical Assistance patient if you didn't also send him Medicare or Blue Cross-Blue Shield patients. If you have one surgeon you use only for Medical Assistance people, he's not going to like you.[19]

The Patients Adapt

The episodic patterns of care and reliance on emergency departments and hospital clinics seen among black patients are often attributed to the characteristics of the patients rather than to the manner in which care is organized. More educated and motivated patients, some argue, would make more intelligent use of the medical-care system. Yet, in depth discussions with black mothers of small children in an inner-city neighborhood of Philadelphia reveal wary, but sophisticated, consumers.[20] One mother, familiar with the long waits at the health center and knowing that a weekday afternoon was likely to be a slow time at the hospital's emergency department, had called a friend working as an aide at the hospital to check this. Discovering that her hunch was correct, she had gone to the emergency department. As a result, she avoided a long wait at a local clinic and was seen immediately. These same discussants were contemptuous of those who got lost in the cracks. They viewed them as lazy. "You got to be able to work the system."

Most of these mothers, however, were wary of the intentions of the large Philadelphia teaching institutions. When showed a picture of a van that a medical-school hospital was considering purchasing to provide better access to services in their neighborhood, one asked, "What I'd like to know is, if I use this to get care, what happens when the grant funding runs out?" At the teaching-hospital clinics where some of the mothers received care, they did not trust the residents or "student doctors" they saw. They were sensitive to feeling like guinea pigs and as part of "experiments." While not mentioned by name, the "Tuskegee" sense of distrust was palpable.

The mothers were not happy with the local city health centers either. The city had historically provided care to the medically indigent population of Philadelphia through these centers. "You have to wait several hours and sometimes all day. It's run down now, and the services are not what they used to be. The people are overworked, and they feed back that attitude to you." Lack of childcare, inadequate transportation, and "being afraid of being told you're a bad person" were major factors that these individuals felt prevented women from getting early and complete prenatal care.

In short, separate care is perceived as unequal. Some of the mothers, perhaps those more adept at "working the system," had sought maternity care outside the immediate service area, at hospitals in the adjoining suburbs and more affluent neighborhoods of the city. These facilities catered to predominantly private-practice patients. The services they received had more of the look and feel of a private office practice.

Beyond differences in the nature of the practices where they received care, the environment these patients returned to was different from the one most white Medicaid patients returned to. Beyond those who could "work the system" were younger and more isolated women who were overwhelmed.[21] A program was developed by one of the teaching hospitals employed registered nurses as care coordinators to seek out such high-risk women and get them into prenatal care. The care coordinators themselves were sometimes overwhelmed. "Sometimes, when I go into these cramped, decaying places, it is so dark. I'd say, 'Let's open the blinds and let in some light.' They are sealed in, and there is such a sense of hopelessness." The program had originally intended to provide more convenient and familiar neighborhood locations. It was soon discovered that patients were bypassing these locations to get to the more distant clinic on the medical-school campus. The stated reason was the greater sense of security that the medical-school surroundings provided. For all the foreign character of a large medical center, they felt safer there than in their own neighborhoods. The fear was justified. One of the nurse-care coordinators visiting a patient in a high-rise housing project was chased five floors down a dark stairwell by a man with a knife. Rescued by the driver and supervisor waiting on the street below, the supervisor suggested that she take the rest of the day off. The nurse said, "No, I'm going back in, my patient is in there."

Practices and Patients Struggle to Adapt to Managed Care

For the physicians, the conversion of the Medical Assistance program to managed care offered some relief from billing hassles, but transformed their relationships with their patients in unwelcome ways.

> All the primary-care physicians are frustrated because they are being put into impossible situations by managed care. Good medicine is crumbling down because of this. We are having labor pains of the new era of health reform. This is a doctor-bashing era. So patient attitudes have changed. They are demanding, impatient and they yell at doctors. How did they change from decent citizens to being hostile to doctors? You reach out to them, but after a while you get disgusted. People are picking physicians for new reasons, because they are on a "list." It becomes adversarial from the start.
>
> Capitation gives a doctor a disincentive to treat social problems. For example, Attention Deficit Disorders take one to one and one-half hours to explore and make decisions with the parents. Now you can charge them a fee for that time. With managed care in a capitated system, you don't get anything. The loyalty to physicians has been lost.[22]

Implications for Racially Disparate Outcomes

In short, without the need for a single conscious act of discrimination, the manner in which services are organized would seem to guarantee disparate racial outcomes. The implications suggested here are similar to those for nursing homes described in the last chapter and supported by many of the statistical results presented in chapter 6. The residential and geographic segregation of the black population and its greater relative dependence on Medical Assistance produces a cumulative series of barriers. White Medical Assistance recipients are more diffused through the region and thus more easily absorbed into private physician practices. The white Medical Assistance patient faces a less impersonal setting, a more stable relationship with the provider, and greater ease of access to specialty referrals. Even when forced to rely on the teaching hospitals and public clinics for care, the white Medical Assistance patient is less likely to bring along the legacy of distrust that a black Medical Assistance patient brings. The black patient is more likely to carry into the relationship the assumption that in such a divided system they are receiving second-class care and that they will be used primarily as teaching material. The physician and other providers bring to such encounters the expectation that the patient will be more hostile and more likely to be noncompliant. There will be less of an affinity with the patient and a more detached approach to the encounter. The provider will be less aggressive in recommending more complex, specialized care to the patient and in serving as the patient's advocate for this care with other providers and with the Medical Assistance program.

In addition, managed care places an added burden on an already strained relationship. Providers may go out of their way to serve as an advocate for a patient if they have has a strong relationship with or affinity for that patient or if they are being paid to perform this role. They are less likely to do so if neither of these conditions is met. Given the diversity of organizational arrangements and incentives in managed-care plans, it is difficult to come to any broad generalizations about their impact on racial differences in referral rates and health outcomes. Nevertheless, an early study of an HMO in Detroit for United Auto Workers employees and their families found that specialty care referral rates for blacks were significantly lower than for whites, and a more recent study in California notes troubling disparities in outcomes by race in managed care as opposed to fee-for-service insurance programs.[23]

Substance abuse during pregnancy, more likely to be detected in a public clinics, which do routine screening, became a focus of increasing concern toward the end of the 1980s. The failure of patients to take individual responsibility became a recurring theme among many providers. Health care providers and their prenatal care patients across the country were drawn into a political firestorm as the crack epidemic grabbed headlines in the early 1990s. In Charleston, South Carolina, a new partnership was forged, redefining the relationship between providers and their patients.

Charleston's Interagency Policy

The first shots of the Civil War were fired in Charleston, and the last struggle to integrate acute-care hospitals in the United State ended here. Roper Hospital, owned by the state medical society, had sought to avoid integration by refusing to participate in the Medicare program. In 1969, the hospital lost in a suit brought by the Justice Department and was forced to integrate.[24]

In October 1989, Charleston declared war on a group of indigent black obstetrical patients. The Medical University of South Carolina

(MUSC), after consultation with the local solicitor for the state's Ninth Judicial Circuit, began to institute what became known as the Interagency Policy on Management of Substance Abuse During Pregnancy.[25] This policy was designed to "ensure appropriate management of patients abusing illegal drugs during pregnancy." It applied only to patients attending the MUSC obstetrics clinic, which were predominantly black and indigent. It did not apply to private obstetric patients at MUSC or other facilities in the area, which were predominantly white. The less controversial part of this policy eventually required patient education. This included watching a video on the harmful effects of substance abuse during pregnancy at the time of their initial visit. The more controversial part of the policy was the presentation to them of a written statement warning that the protection of unborn children from the harmful effects of illegal drugs could involve the Charleston police, the courts, and protective services. The MUSC staff intended to back up this threat. Patients who met certain subjective criteria were required to undergo urine screening for illegal drugs. Perhaps mindful of the legal implications of such subjective profiling, the criteria were eventually made more objective and included inadequate prenatal care and a variety of poor medical outcomes that could possibly be related to drug abuse. If the patient tested positive, she was warned, "If you fail to attend substance abuse treatment or prenatal care you *will* be arrested by the Charleston City Police and prosecuted by the Office of Solicitor."[26] Arrest warrants were indeed issued to some that failed to keep appointments for substance abuse therapy or prenatal care. In addition, some who tested positive for a second time were taken into police custody. Those patients who delivered a child and tested positive for illegal drugs were arrested immediately after their release from the hospital. Their newborn children were taken into protective custody by the Department of Social Services.

The MUSC staff had adopted a policy that involved a breach of patient confidentially, medical coercion, and participation in punitive incarceration. It would be, however, too simplistic to dismiss these efforts as racist. At the very least, the key staff were not indifferent to the fate of the infants, as one observer recounted about the nurse in charge of the program.

> She may have totally pulled the wool over my eyes, but my impression was that she was compassionate, really distraught about the babies. The first time I went to meet with her, I was in her office for about seventeen minutes and the phone rang twice. One call was that a baby had died and tears came to her eyes. She was just talking on the phone. That baby that had died had tested positive for cocaine. She

then asked for an autopsy of the organs, because she thought there was a lot more drug involvement than just coke. From the physical symptoms that the baby had that there was something else going on there and we owed it to the infant to find out what it was. The second call was for another infant that had come in and they had tested and it did have drugs. She said that we better notify the Department of Social Services. She then explained to me that the woman had other small children in the home and she thought social services should go in and take a look. I think they were genuinely caring, compassionate, and concerned. They were trying to do something. Maybe it wasn't the smartest and best thing to do and maybe they didn't do it the right way but they totally convinced me that they were trying to deal with what the thought was the problem of babies dying.[27]

Nevertheless, not all the alternatives to such Draconian measures had been exhausted. There were other steps that could have been taken in providing transportation, child care, or residential treatment in lieu of incarceration. There were, in fact, no residential treatment centers in South Carolina for pregnant, drug-abusing women. Clinical encounters are intended to be personal, private, based on trust, voluntary, and therapeutic, while criminal-justice encounters tend to be impersonal, public, based on rules, coercive, and retributive. Now they became linked in the same system. MUSC staff became arresting officers. They were delegated a great degree of authority by the criminal-justice system in determining who should be arrested. According to the sworn statements of the women involved in these arrests, these were not auspicious beginnings for their new infants.

Women subject to arrest were, in some instances, denied the opportunity to change out of their hospital gowns or to make a phone call to family members to make arrangements for care of their babies. Some women were arrested while still bleeding, weak, and in pain from just giving birth. Some women were put in handcuffs that were attached to a 3-inch wide leather belt that was placed around their stomachs. Some were also put in leg shackles when they were taken into custody. A blanket or sheet would be placed over the woman and she would be wheeled out of the hospital to a waiting police car. One woman, ——, was arrested while in the hospital and kept shackled to her bed until she was taken to jail. . . . Some of these women were never referred for treatment even after arrest. MUSC neonatology division nurses complained to the NICU medical director that "women would be discharged and that they would be handcuffed and shackled and then they would be wrapped in a sheet so that people couldn't see them and then kind of shuffled out of the hospital." . . . Ms. ——, who was still pregnant, remained in jail until the time of delivery. Each week, Ms. —— was transported to MUSC for prenatal care from the jail in handcuffs and leg shackles. With one exception she was kept in hand-cuffs and shackles throughout her doctor's visit. Almost three weeks after Ms. —— was first arrested, she went into labor. She was again transported in handcuffs and leg shackles to MUSC; she went through labor and gave birth while handcuffed to her bed. A uni-formed security guard waited outside her door.[28]

What had begun with what most involved felt may have been the best of intentions in coaxing individuals into treatment to protect their unborn children now became the center of a national maelstrom of political pos-turing and deeper, more anguished ethical debate. It produced a three-mil-lion-dollar civil suit against the parties involved on behalf of ten of the mothers, an investigation by the Office for Civil Rights, and a review by the National Institute of Health in regard to MUSC's procedures for pro-tecting human subjects. American Civil Liberties Union (ACLU) attor-neys had brought suit on behalf of the mothers claiming, among other constitutional violations, a violation of equal-protection provisions of the Fourteenth Amendment. They argued that Charleston's interagency pol-icy applied only to MUSC patients and only to non-private-clinic patients, not to other hospitals or to MUSC's private-pay clients, who were pre-dominantly white. They also argued that the policy had targeted only cocaine use and that drug-testing criteria included the failure to obtain prenatal care. Both of these behaviors had been shown to be more preva-lent among blacks. While the ACLU suit failed, the Office for Civil Rights investigation resulted in a settlement agreement in September 1994.[29] MUSC agreed to cease any activities related to the arrest of patients. A review completed the same month by the National Institutes of Health Office for Protection from Research Risks concluded that certain activities involved in the interagency policy constituted research involving human subjects, and required that corrective action be taken. Local response to the federal intervention was reflected in the November 1994 elections when the solicitor of the Ninth Judicial Circuit, who had initiated the policy, was swept to a landslide victory as state attorney general and to national con-servative political prominence.

The subsequent debate over the interagency policy was confusing because there was a lack of evidence, other than anecdotal arguments, of its impact. Proponents of the policy claimed that the number of positive urine drug studies dropped from about twenty-four per month to five or six per month after the implementation of the policy.[30] Such conclusions were (1) based on tests done selectively and not on the entire clinic population, (2) limited to the institution in which the policy was implemented and well publicized (logic would suggest that drug-using women would seek to avoid that hospital), and (3) lacked population comparisons or comparisons from other institutions for which such policies were not adopted. These subtleties did not deter the newly elected attorney general of South Carolina, the program's architect, from claiming success and going on a national public policy offensive.

The MUSC participants in the interagency policy were less effusive. A preliminary analysis submitted as an abstract to the National Perinatal Association's 1993 poster session documented a significant increase from 0 percent to 22 percent in the number of women testing positive for cocaine who had received no prenatal care prior to the delivery of their baby, and the number of women testing positive for any drug who had received no prenatal care jumped significantly as well from 3 percent to 14 percent.[31] Since early prenatal care is widely acknowledged as key to preventing adverse outcomes, particularly for drug-using women, these were troubling statistics. In May 1994, however, as the "swarm of federal officials" descended on Charleston, and as the difficulties in coming to definitive conclusions about a policy that had never been purposely designed as a research evaluation became evident, the MUSC participants wrote an addendum to the abstract, concluding that the "data cannot be definitively interpreted."[32] A paper coauthored by the institution's own medical ethicist also arrived at different conclusions on the interagency policy.

> The lesson of the Charleston experience, therefore, is not so much that medicine ought to avoid involvement in difficult social problems, but that it should exercise great care in conceptualizing the problem and in tailoring intervention appropriately. Clinical approaches that individualize complex social problems are unlikely to succeed by themselves and may involve health clinicians and administrators in external agendas that compromise the clinical encounter. If medicine is to play a constructive and responsible role in addressing problems such as cocaine use among pregnant women, it must pursue strategies that take the social and economic context into account. Medical professionals need not be social reformers, but they must involve others from the community, such as community leaders, substance abuse counselors, social workers, clergy, the affected community itself and law enforcement officials, so that the larger social and economic context will be addressed along with the individual pathology. Policies designed in consultation with various community groups and through

a process of internal review that ensures that divergent perspectives will be fully aired and considered will help promote accountability and discourage alienation from the health care establishment. Policies subjected to a "test of publicity" are far less likely to breach prevailing moral and legal standards, and may avoid costly after-the-fact scrutiny from the media, courts and research sponsors.[33]

As the Philadelphia experience was simultaneously demonstrating, that was easier to advocate than to implement.

Philadelphia's Healthy Start Initiative

Philadelphia's experience in addressing the disparities in birth outcomes tried to take the larger social and economic context into account by involving from the outset a diverse array of community participants.[34] Most of the organizations locally and nationally pushing to address the disparities between black and white birth outcomes were new ones, but linked in many ways to the century-long civil rights struggle. A small network of health professionals, community leaders, and activists in Philadelphia worked to develop a more concerted and organized approach to addressing the disparities in birth outcomes. Their efforts eventually culminated in Philadelphia's Healthy Start initiative.

Healthy Start is the most recent major federal initiative focused on reducing infant mortality. Philadelphia became one of fifteen targeted sites for this effort. More than $540 million had been invested nationally in this five year effort by the end of fiscal year 1997 and $33 million in Philadelphia alone.[35] What follows is the perspective of the diverse participants involved in getting the project set up in Philadelphia.

The Social and Economic Context

Infant mortality rates are a commonly used crude proxy for comparing the quality of life in different population groups. After consistent declines for decades, these rates leveled off for the black population of Philadelphia in the 1980s. The differences between black and white infant mortality rates and rates of adequate prenatal care widened. The infant mortality rate for blacks in Philadelphia in 1890 was roughly 500 per 1,000 births and for whites, 250 per 1,000. By 1993, those rates had declined to 18.7 for blacks and 5.5 for whites. In 1890, black infants in Philadelphia were twice as likely as white infants were to die before their first birthday. In 1993, black infants were 3.4 times as likely as white infants were to die before their first birthday. However, infant mortality, reduced to a rare abstract statistical event, was "not on the radar screen" of issues for local community-based organizations and community members. Adequate housing, employment, and safety from crime remained the major concerns of these neighborhoods, as they had been a century before.

The distinctive role of the wealthy, leading-family elite of Philadelphia also serves as an important backdrop to the Philadelphia Healthy Start story. As University of Pennsylvania sociology professor E. Digby Baltzell observed, Philadelphia's upper class continues to be influenced by the egalitarian individualism of its Quaker founders.[36] In contrast to the Puritan hierarchical social structure of Boston, Philadelphia's upper class has never had a socially valued position in the broader society. As a result, it has typically disengaged from public life and concentrated on accumulating private wealth, thus insulating itself from the consequences. Philadelphians, in contrast to Bostonians, are remarkably absent from any national lists of outstanding public citizens. Whatever public leadership has existed has been largely provided by self-made men, like Benjamin Franklin or Stephen Girard. While William Penn's statue sits atop City Hall, he never held any elected public office. Many of Philadelphia's institutions and hospitals, perhaps in part reflecting the inclination of the proper Philadelphia family members on their boards, have done the same. The health care institutions serving West Philadelphia have collectively amassed almost $2 billion in endowment. They have begun to use these funds in acquiring medical practices to respond to increased managed-care competition and curtailed Medicare and Medical Assistance payments and increased competition.

In the meantime, Philadelphia's performance in maternal and infant care has been less than mediocre. It has consistently ranked dead last of all Pennsylvania counties in infant mortality and related statistics. On a composite indicator of maternal and infant care in Pennsylvania cities, Philadelphia was narrowly edged out by Chester, a concentrated pocket of poverty.[37] Pennsylvania has consistently been one of the three states with the largest difference of white versus African American infant mortality rates for decades. The concentration of the black population in its two major cities, Philadelphia and Pittsburgh, each with striking differences in birth outcomes between its white and black populations, accounts for this.

The Evolution of the Civil Rights Movement

The successes of the civil rights movement had historically come from focusing on those concrete, visible symbols of inequities whose elimination could mobilize broader public support. The early targets were electoral politics, and then segregated schools, buses, lunch counters, and, finally, hospitals. Infant mortality now became a target symbol. The political environment had changed, and new organizations, loosely connected to the older civil rights movement, emerged to take advantage of those changes.

The population of civil rights organizations had changed rapidly after World War II. The middle-class-based, political-action-oriented NAACP was eclipsed by the NAACP Legal Defense Fund, as it began to demonstrate the ability to get results in the more responsive federal courts of the 1950s. Internal Revenue Service pressure to revoke the Defense Fund's tax exempt status forced full separation of the two organizations in 1957, and this produced increasing friction over fund-raising and the respective leadership roles of the two organizations. The Southern Christian Leadership Conference, the Student Nonviolent Coordinating Committee, and other loosely organized direct action groups, however, soon eclipsed both these older organizations. Yet, by the 1970, these direct action organizations were in disarray, fragmented by internal divisions over leadership and direction and weakened by the inability to focus on targets that could attract broad-based political support.

Part of the void began to be filled by organizations emerging out of the women's movement. The black civil rights and the women's movements had historically resonated with each other, and they would now do so again. The early leaders of the women's movement had emerged out of the pre–Civil War abolitionist movement, and the woman's suffrage movement emerged out of the post-Civil War passage of the Fifteenth Amendment extending suffrage to black men. Similarly, the black freedom movement of the 1960s, paired with the almost inadvertent inclusion of sex as part of the antidiscriminatory employment provisions in Title VII of the Civil Rights Act of 1964, stimulated a new surge of activity. The National Organization for Women (NOW), consciously modeled after the NAACP, was formed in 1966 and focused on equal employment opportunities. Similar to the black freedom movement, more radical coalitions formed shortly after this.

The Children's Defense Fund, founded in 1973, represented a distinctive synthesis of these forces, seeking broader political support for social programs in a more conservative political environment—one that saw increased constraints on public dollars. Its founder, Marian Wright Edelman, had been one of the NAACP Legal Defense Fund's first interns and had directed the Legal Defense Fund's office that opened above a pool hall in Jackson, Mississippi, in 1964. She was the first black woman admitted to the bar in Mississippi and one of only four black lawyers practicing in the state. The office handled the more than 120 cases generated from the Mississippi Freedom Summer.[38] Edelman served as council to the Poor

People's March in 1968. The Children's Defense Fund then became a part of a remarkably effective coalition that expanded coverage to children and the prenatal care of mothers under the Medicaid program. The marriage of the civil rights and the women's movement forces, the skillful use of the "preventive investment" argument to assuage newly ascendant fiscal conservatives, and the increasing recognition of the resonance of such issues with the broader women's vote (which no politician could afford to ignore) created a potent force for change.

This force helped transform infant mortality rates—vivid, easily accessible numbers with an emotional impact—into something with a political momentum all its own. There is a certain tyranny in measurement. What is measured becomes important even in the absence of well-organized political pressure. At a national policy level, as the per capita cost of health care grew, increasingly unfavorable comparisons began to be made. Both health care costs and infant mortality rates were much lower in other developed nations than in the United States.

Thus, maternal and infant care began to appear on the national political radar screen in the 1980s. The Omnibus Budget Reconciliation Act of 1981 substantially reduced Medicaid eligibility for poor families. This, combined with the effects of the 1981–82 recession, produced a decline in women who received adequate prenatal care. By the mid-1980s it was estimated that the percentage of women of childbearing age who lacked any insurance coverage for prenatal care had grown to 26 percent.[39] By 1986, the low-birth-weight rate for blacks was 12.5 percent, in contrast to 5.6 percent for whites, the largest racial gap since such comparisons were first made in 1969.[40] A variety of studies pointed to the importance of access to adequate prenatal care in reducing adverse birth outcomes.[41]

Early political efforts focused on expanding Medical Assistance coverage. First there was the Deficit Reduction Act of 1984, which expanded Medicaid eligibility beyond the Aid to Families with Dependent Children (AFDC) eligibility requirements for pregnant women. More importantly, the Omnibus Budget Reconciliation Acts of 1986 and 1987 uncoupled Medicaid income-eligibility criteria from those of the Aid to Families with Dependent Children program, permitting states to expand thresholds up to and above the poverty level. In addition, the Consolidated Omnibus Budget Reconciliation Act of 1985 (COBRA) had permitted state Medical Assistance programs to expand the content of services provided to pregnant women. When the budget reconciliation bill in 1987 extended optional Medicaid eligibility for pregnant women to 185 percent of the poverty level, coverage was quickly expanded in many states to include additional pregnant women and children. In 1988, the Medicare Catastrophic Coverage Act required states to provide Medicaid coverage for pregnant women and infants below the poverty level, and in 1991 federal Medicaid amendments expanded this requirement to cover pregnant women with incomes of up to 133 percent of poverty level. By 1989, twenty-four states had started programs of enhanced care in their Medicaid programs, including care coordination, risk assessment, nutritional and psychosocial counseling, health education, home visiting, and transportation. By 1992 twenty-five states had initiated the optional 185 percent-of-poverty level Medicaid eligibility requirements for pregnant women.

In Pennsylvania, the Medical Assistance program expanded eligibility to 133 percent of poverty in 1989. It also provided presumed eligibility to pregnant women applying for Medical Assistance, guaranteeing payment to prenatal care providers. In 1992, the Healthy Beginnings Plus program began providing Medical Assistance payment for expanded support services for pregnant women at qualifying sites.

In effect, in Pennsylvania, as in the rest of the country, pregnant women not only now had something close to universal insurance coverage, but the services that could be provided to those eligible for Medical Assistance had been greatly expanded. It was, however, a two-edged sword. The substantial expansion in Medical Assistance coverage for pregnant women and infants was accompanied by a profound shift in the rationale that was used to support it.[42] The expansions were justified not so much because the recipients deserved coverage as victims of events beyond their control (the traditional "deserving poor" argument), nor because it was a right of citizenship (the civil rights era Medicare argument), but because coverage made economic sense. Expanded coverage for prenatal care, it was argued, would reduce overall Medicaid costs by reducing low birth weight and the associated costs of medical complications related to such an outcome. However dubious these claims, they helped sell the expansion in coverage. Yet, while the expanded coverage did increase the proportion of births covered by Medical Assistance, it resulted in almost no decline in the number of Medical Assistance clients receiving late or no prenatal care.[43] The economic argument said that this was costing taxpayers money.

The Philadelphia Offensive

The local Philadelphia efforts to address the problem mirrored national efforts. The Maternity Care Coalition (MCC), an informal group of community activists and care providers that had originated a decade earlier (at about the same time the Children's Defense Fund became part of the national scene), became increasingly influential. MCC helped orchestrate a city council hearing for Council Member Angel Ortiz in the spring of

1989. The hearings were harshly critical of the Philadelphia Health Department. They concluded that the Health Department lacked creativity, policy, and programs for addressing the city's unacceptably high infant mortality rate, a core public-health responsibility.

The hearings represented an important watershed. For the first time, infant mortality became a local political issue. Predictably, the city picked the most "media-genic" idea, and MCC got the contract for the "Mom Mobile." The Mom Mobile van project patrolled high-risk neighborhoods, providing information and assisting residents in accessing prenatal care. MCC had long advocated more systemic approaches. It had also begun a transformation from an informal advocacy group into a provider of services. It was a transformation that the Healthy Start program would later duplicate on a larger scale for many community groups.

Almost simultaneously with the hearings, a spring 1989 report sponsored by the Pew Charitable Trusts described a "crisis of caring" in Philadelphia. It identified infant mortality as one of several key interconnected problems and outlined a broad consensus strategy for addressing the problem. The report gave the issue new legitimacy.

The city health commissioner recruited the chairperson of the Maternity Care Coalition to join the city's Office of Maternal and Child Health (MCH) as director. He signed on a young pediatrician from the Children's Hospital of Philadelphia as an assistant commissioner. Under this new leadership, MCH shifted from a primarily passive recipient of state funds to an initiator of projects. The city was designated as a local Title V agency for maternity services and, eventually, for child health services as well. Title V was part of the Reagan block grant programs to the state. The city allocation had been routinely distributed to hospitals for the care of indigent maternity patients and for support of programs for this population. The redesignation of the city as a local Title V agency provided an opportunity to propose and design programs and then secure approval from the state health department, rather than simply participate in state-initiated activities. The federally stimulated expansion of eligibility for pregnant women under the state's Medical Assistance program provided the opportunity to rethink the use of local Title V funding and to expand the efforts of MCH. As the new director of MCH observed, "We concluded that, because of the change in Medicaid eligibility, the hospitals did not need the Title V funds for those purposes. There was some friction, but it was diffuse. Overall it was not a big deal to the hospitals, since it accounted for such a small fraction of their income. In contrast, our MCH budget was $4.5 million per year and Title V accounted for most of that."

While the activities of MCH began to grow, the Health Department in which it was embedded continued to face cutbacks. The city was struggling with a shrinking tax base and growing obligations to an increasingly indigent population. In the last decade, the department has experienced a reduction of the equivalent of eight hundred full-time employees.[44] MCH, four levels down in the Health Department's organization chart, faced the inevitable problems that such cutbacks produce in any large organization.

The odds that the Philadelphia Health Department would create an innovative new partnership in maternal and infant care were stacked against it. The department faced (1) a federal administration seemingly indifferent, if not hostile, to providing funds to address the problems of the urban poor; (2) local health care institutions that had, for the most part, opted out of any leadership role in addressing the problems (they were preoccupied developing marketing strategies and expanding satellites in suburban areas to attract private-pay patients); (3) a city administration preoccupied with avoiding bankruptcy; (4) a Health Department struggling to assure basic services; and (5) a black community hostile toward and distrustful of all of the above and itself preoccupied with the more immediate problems of securing adequate housing, employment, and safety for their families in neighborhoods with growing drug and crime problems. Yet, through a series of federal and city Health Department decisions made between 1990 and 1993, combined with the efforts of an informal local coalition, an unlikely partnership focused on maternal and infant care began to emerge.

The Federal Decisions: What to Do, How to Fund It, and Whom to Fund

In the federal executive branch, the Bush White House in 1989 had convened a task force of maternal and infant care experts to review possible policy options. A confidential draft report had recommended spending an additional $500 million a year to reduce the infant mortality rate in the United States.[45] It reminded President Bush of his campaign promise in 1988 to "invest in our children," which appeared to have been put on hold. The task force urged him to raise the issue of infant mortality to the top of the pubic policy agenda because "this country cannot afford its current infant mortality rate in economic or human terms."

The Bush White House Task Force on Maternal and Infant Care floated many ideas. The least costly and least ambitious one became the kernel of the Healthy Start initiative. It would be a selective and narrowly focused program. The White House wanted to get as much political mileage out of it as possible.[46] Media plans concerning the program included joint handling of the announcements with the White House and a kickoff of the initiative with a visit by President Bush to one or more perinatal service delivery sites.

The original plan was to pay for this narrowly focused initiative through community health center funds and Maternal and Child Health Block Grants (Title V). Predictably, this smoke-and-mirrors design—presenting the program as a new initiative while raiding existing program funds—drew a storm of protest from Philadelphia and elsewhere.[47] Congress eventually appropriated $25 million in new money, explicitly prohibiting the use of Maternal and Child Health Block Grant and community health center funds from being used for this purpose.

The Bush administration decided to bypass the states. The Title V MCH block grants to the states, the invention of the Reagan era, had left a bad taste even with the Bush administration. "There was no accountability and you couldn't determine the value added by the funds the MCH director observed." It is perhaps a conclusion that is instructive given the current Republican legislative efforts to reinvent block grant state funding on a more ambitious scale. As with the Neighborhood Health Centers, this approach combined the attraction of getting the biggest political bang for the buck without incurring the far greater costs that would be incurred by further expanding and reforming the Medicaid program.

In spite of the lobbying efforts of the maternal and child care interest groups to expand the number of projects and create less competition for scarce new dollars, the final federal Request for Proposal (RFP) issued April 17, 1991, had four specific requirements:

1. The grants would be for five years: one year for planning, and four years of operation.
2. The project area must be limited in size, including more than fifty infant deaths per year but no more than two hundred.
3. The overall infant mortality in the project area must be greater than 15.9 per one thousand live births.
4. Only ten projects would be funded, and only one project grant would be awarded in any one state. Federal officials tentatively identified nineteen cities as eligible for grant funds.[48]

Philadelphia's Decisions: Whose Grant, Which Neighborhoods, and What Should Be Done?

"The first thing we had to recognize was that we were competing for a grant. It was a grant that peculiar and arbitrary decisions about the rules of the game had been set by Feds. I can remember questioning them about this at the briefing in Philadelphia in May 1991 at the Sheraton in Center

City and not getting any answers," one of those involved in writing the grant noted. The rules forced some painful decisions in preparing Philadelphia's proposal.

The Health Department wanted to be the applicant. No one else was in a better position and the Director of Maternal and Child Health felt the Health Department should take the leadership role. The RFP specified that there would be only one application per city and that the mayor was to serve as gatekeeper, endorsing only one application. MCH, at the request of the mayor, had completed a well-reasoned action plan for reducing preventable infant mortality in the city in November 1990. This would serve as the basic outline for the city's response to the Healthy Start RFP. A lot of groups could have strongly objected to the Health Department being the grant applicant. The Delaware Valley Hospital Council, the Maternity Care Coalition, a consortium of community organizations could have claimed this role, but they didn't. Other communities seeking Healthy Start grant applicants appear to have tried to avoid such rivalries by proposing the creation of a new, not-for-profit Healthy Start Corporation. Some who had previously worked with the city and were veterans of the difficulties of extracting payments for contracted services saw serious risks for small community-based organizations that might become financially dependent on providing Healthy Start services.

Federal requirements restricted the size of the Healthy Start service area that could be proposed. For Philadelphia, that required triage. Two areas of the city, North and West Philadelphia, cried out for help and clearly met all of the requirements. A citywide group had been pulled together as a steering committee but declined the offer of MCH to make a choice between these two areas. The MCH director and the health commissioner, poring over the statistics, struggled with the decision. According to the MCH director, the final choice hinged largely on the differences in the patterns of prenatal care use in the two communities. North Philadelphia women traveled to many more outpatient sites for prenatal care. Each of these outpatient sites, in turn, saw only a small proportion of the patients from what might have been designated as the North Philadelphia Healthy Start area. They were unlikely to be willing to set up separate programs and services for this population. Even if they were, such a project area would make the project complex and unmanageable. Later in the project, some attributed the choice to the strength of the community people, the five participating medical centers, and the advantages of the greater residential geographic concentration that West Philadelphia provided. The friction the selection of the West Philadelphia site might have produced was muted by assurances that any additional new funds for maternal and infant care would be allocated to North Philadelphia. The steering committee then shifted their focus to West Philadelphia and invited West Philadelphia community groups to participate. The steering committee's core workgroup began to meet weekly.

This workgroup now stared at the irony of their situation. The highest infant mortality rate in Philadelphia lay in a narrow corridor due west of what everyone judged to be premier clinical services for OB-GYN and neonatal care. The clinical services were not the problem: in terms of technical quality and geographic availability, the Healthy Start neighborhoods were enviably well situated. In addition, managed care, now widely being embraced as the panacea for assuring access and continuity of services, had been made mandatory for the ninety-five thousand Medical Assistance beneficiaries in West and South Philadelphia in 1986 through the Health Pass program. A comparison of matched managed-care and regular Medical Assistance obstetrical patients at the Hospital of the University of Pennsylvania revealed equally bad prenatal-care outcomes.[49] A GAO audit of the program would later reach similar conclusions.[50] The problem, whatever it was, lay in the organization of these services and the large chasm between the attitudes, perceptions, and assumptions of community members and providers. "There was nothing in terms of medical technologies that could be enhanced. We didn't know why the babies were dying," observed a neonatolgist. A nurse midwife also struggled for an explanation. "The reason for the higher infant mortality rate in the black population is a large part of what we don't know. It could even be the nutrition of the grandmother affecting the mother that affects the baby. We do know that stress in a pregnant woman's life is a major predictor of pregnancy outcomes. Treating pregnancy like a sickness compounds the problems. The closer the providers and the services are to people, the better, but some have already learned not to trust the system." The group chose to focus on the simple basics, the community development side of the equation. "We know what works in terms of prenatal care, but it's never been adequately funded. Let's do it. It's stupid to stretch and try to think of something new and innovative." Most believed this would weaken the position of Philadelphia in the grant sweepstake's competition. "I knew we had to do more and come in technically better than the other applicants. We were not glitzy and not focused on centralized case management, which was very trendy. Ours would be a messy and highly decentralized approach," one of the nurses involved in planning the project recalled.

The basic questions, however, were never completely put to rest and would resurface again as the process later became infused with real dollars. Whose grant is it? What should be its political message? Some felt family planning and choice should be a more important part of the program's message. Who would control it? Initially it was seen as George Bush's idea in an election year and there was a lot of concern about the kind of strings that would be attached. All of the participants brought some of their own agendas and political baggage to the table.

Making the Awards

The completed application met the July 15, 1991, deadline. The mayor signed off, there was some last minute confusion over the governor's office failure to include a signed form, and the waiting began. The proposals were reviewed over the summer of 1991.

Everybody involved knew that the summer of 1991 included the campaign between Richard Thornburg and Harris Wofford for Senator Heinz's vacant seat. Wofford, who had been involved in the early stages of the movement as an advisor to Martin Luther King Jr., had a brief and frustrating stint as civil rights advisor to President John Kennedy. He had resigned prior to the formulation of Kennedy's civil rights bill, which Johnson would later sign. Wofford had unexpectedly pulled ahead in the polls and appeared to be scoring points on the need for health care reform and improved access. The awards would be announced about a month before the November election. If either Philadelphia or Pittsburgh was awarded a Healthy Start program, it could give a boost to Thornburg and, possibly, head off a major political embarrassment for the Bush Administration.

Pittsburgh was not on the initial list of ten project sites. The assumption of several of those who were interviewed was that a call was made. In the mind's eye of one informant it was a direct line call to George Bush from the prominent Republican fund raiser in Pittsburgh that said, "George, I want one of those programs for Pittsburgh." In any event, the agency seemed to break its own jealously defended guidelines. The number of sites awarded was expanded from ten to fifteen and Pennsylvania was the only state awarded two sites.

In September, Philadelphia application was funded. It was as if the city had won the World Series of maternal and child health. On October 17, 1991, the mayor held a celebration in the Mayor's Reception Hall.

The Planning Year

By June 1992, MCH had to (1) pull together a project staff, (2) reconstitute the consortium, and (3) develop a plan. Much of the planning took place before the staff was on board. Beginning in October, the larger planning group was reconstituted. One proposal for governance favored by the MCH director would have created a smaller consortium and provided it a greater degree of control. It was rejected by the group in favor of a more decentralized model, with more committees and teams and a larger central decision-making structure. Amazingly, things worked quite smoothly. Staff was hired and in place by February 1992, breaking city government records. Ten workgroups were constituted, and a steering committee was elected. One major problem was external, no clear budget.

The early efforts culminated in a two-day orientation session at Miseracodia Hospital for the new staff and coalition members, held in February 1992. The session was not without its rough edges. Nevertheless, the Healthy Start project was eventually able to focus on five goals that had been outlined as part of the application for the planning grant. MCH staff saw them as central to reducing infant mortality and improving maternal and infant health. As presented in the project plan submitted at the end of June 1992, these were to "(1) increase the capacity of communities to improve maternal and infant health among consumers, (2) raise public awareness about the incidence of and factors contributing to infant mortality and strategies of prevention, (3) establish effective support services for health for childbearing families; (4) establish effective linkages between and among community-based and clinic-based services, and (5) build public policy that promotes maternal and infant health."[51] The workgroups had focused on fleshing out the activities under each of these broad objectives. The steering committee attempted to create logical groupings of the often-overlapping activities. They also made recommendations about the resource allocations. Since no one knew what the actual amount would be, these allocations were made based on percentages and on two hypothetical dollar estimates of what the grant award would be. (The lower hypothetical estimate was close to the $4.4 million awarded for the Philadelphia project in its first year of operations.) A variety of activities were proposed under each of these broad objectives, envisioned as decentralized and community based. The Health Department had long contracted with local hospitals and agencies for many services and would follow a similar pattern in the Healthy Start Project. Each of the ten workgroups produced their priorities, and the steering committee attempted to honor the wishes of the workgroups in their recommendations. The final 174-page Request for Proposal put together by the City of Philadelphia Health Department was an impressive distillation of the ideas developed by these groups. The twenty-eight project areas identified in the Health Department's RFP included a wish list of every service for pregnant women dreamed of by providers and community leaders. It included requests for proposals for outreach, transportation, "health corners" to improve access, incentives for extended service hours and for making care settings more attractive, interpreters, assistance for housing and transitional living, a lending closet, child care, career preparation and placement, health education, and peer teen counseling programs. It also included requests for proposals to create community initiatives for consumer assessment of health care sites and for consumer advocacy for Medical Assistance reform. The RFP was a blueprint for major structural change in the way services were provided and in the relationship between those services, their consumers, and the communities. The initial RFP was announced in April 1992 with a June 4 deadline for the submission of proposals.

Most people felt good about the process in the planning stage. A complex and potentially divisive process under a tight schedule had been handled well. But the sudden new volume of work dealing with the Health Department's RFP and the contracting process overwhelmed some MCH staff. The June 4 RFP deadline brought in a flood of more than 250 applications, and the summer of 1992 was spent reviewing the applications. They were all distilled into an elaborate set of charts for the new health commissioner's final approval.

 MCH wanted to ensure that small community-based organizations participated, and because of the desire of the Health Department to open the process up, many agencies that received contracts had no previous funding history. Providers complained about the complexity of procedures and delays in receiving funds in the early stages, but procedures were simplified as the program developed more experience.

Implementation Pains

The Health Department, expecting less and not being sure what the real numbers would be, had submitted a budget of $10 million for their plan in June. They received $4.4 million in September. Now the stakes became real, and, as one participant remarked, "Most of the tension concerned who had power over the money." The Health Department, as recipient of the grant, had a fiduciary responsibility, but the community-based organizations felt they should have a say. The chairperson of the Healthy Start Consortium tried to keep these discussions on an even keel. As a respected community representative, she saw jobs for community members as an important part of her interest in the project and in assuring its credibility. About fifty people from the community would eventually be employed on the three outreach teams and other activities related to the Healthy Start project. Race added fuel to these tensions. There had been a concerted conscious effort to hire black staff. Three community development people were hired and have stayed with the program. Nevertheless, there was an outcry when a white project manager was appointed. As the project evolved, it began to experience a perhaps almost inevitable turnover of both staff and volunteer leadership. Many early volunteer leaders disengaged, and new ones emerged. For the volunteer leadership the time commitments were sometimes overwhelming.

The Health Department, the Healthy Start Consortium, and those that received contracts to provide services faced deeply conflicting goals. Many wanted to use the program to build a grass roots movement similar to those of the civil rights era. They saw such empowerment as the only way to have a real impact on birth statistics. A patchwork of community organizations received contracts to provide outreach, education, and help for expectant mothers and newborn infants, but these lacked a cohesive unifying vision. At the same time, a city government agency was managing a federal grant with all of the top down requirements that such arrangements impose.

The Work That Remains

Nobody felt that the national objective of reducing infant mortality by 50 percent in the Healthy Start services areas was an achievable goal. A more systematic accounting of the possible impact of various Healthy Start interventions on infant mortality supports this assessment.[52] Three major challenges must be met to assure a lasting legacy for Healthy Start.

First, the development process needs to be sustained. Philadelphia's Healthy Start created by design new lines of communication that had not existed and, perhaps, the beginnings of a more supportive, user-friendly infrastructure. People and organizations that had never talked or worked together were now doing so. Everyone involved in Healthy Start saw what they learned from process as an important personal benefit. The project forced people to learn how to work in new, organizationally diverse, and undefined situations.

Strikingly, it was not just the professionals and the researchers that seemed to learn the most, but the people in the community-based organizations. One community organizer spoke with gleeful amusement about her discovery of the osteopath and MD rivalry in West Philadelphia. The image of a monolithic, all-powerful medical fraternity was shattered forever—they weren't even as unified as the African American community groups!"

Second, there needs to be a way to sustain the success stories of the process. Most of those involved could identify, out of the diverse array of projects, ones of which they were particularly proud. They guessed that, whatever more objective evaluation was conducted, they would prove worth preserving. Some felt the lay home visitor program should be incorporated into the basic Medicaid benefits package: "They work with mothers until the baby is a year old. One of them who is responsible for seventeen teen clients reported to me that all are back in school, and three are in college. That's a wonderful record." Other candidates for the Healthy Start success stories included low cost programs addressing basic needs: "The Lending Closet . . . gives people a lot of very concrete things and it costs almost nothing." "The archdiocese nutrition program really works." A physician, reflecting on all the difficulties, had a different spin on empowerment as a key to what should be preserved. "What we really need to do is save the programs that empower providers. Sometimes we feel so frustrated and powerless in giving people what they really need: food, baby supplies, housing. TAG [tenants' action group] has a poster with an emergency phone number for people who need help. It's posted in the nursery at HUP. How did it get there? The nurses stuck it on the wall. It was powerful to them. It gave them a sense that they could do something. Those are the things that make providers burn out a little slower."

Finally, there needs to be a way to add the key elements that seemed to be missing. Many felt there were pieces left out in the early group decision making. Several felt more attention should have been placed on the development of a clearly articulated reproducible model that could be replicated in North Philadelphia and other areas. Some felt there had not been enough attention placed on changing the provider attitudes and insensitivities. Others felt more should have been done to develop stronger links with the schools. The service gap most frequently mentioned was the relative lack of emphasis on pregnancy prevention. The funding and organization of these services represented a more pervasive problem in the delivery system and in values within society not unique to Philadelphia's Healthy Start. The major gap that concerned the early participants in the Healthy Start initiative, however, was the failure to sustain and expand upon the early involvement of the major providers of services and the HMOs.

Lessons of Philadelphia's Healthy Start

Philadelphia Healthy Start is part of a larger story of efforts to address unacceptably high infant mortality rates that are a legacy of deep racial divisions. It is a story that takes place in a period of major transitions, posing many risks for vulnerable populations. It also takes place in a period that poses many opportunities for redefining the relationships between public health agencies, health care providers, and the communities that they serve. The key to taking advantage of these opportunities lies in creating (1) a persuasive vision and (2) practical mechanisms for realizing that vision.

A Persuasive Vision

At a conceptual level, projects such as Healthy Start need to articulate clearly and convincingly what they are doing in a way that can build a broad consensus. Specifically, the program must address three key issues raised by the Monday morning quarterbacks and those who view themselves as spectators in what has been a bruising contact sport.

1. *Risk:* Achieving the goals of Healthy Start means doing things differently and taking risks. Some efforts will succeed, but probably more will fail. Efforts to address infant mortality need to design for such eventualities. That means defining when to pull the plug on projects. It should be defined in such a way that terminating a particular project is not construed as failure for the program or for those involved in that project. It is evidence of their strength.

2. *Ownership:* What does empowerment mean in the context of a federally funded project?[53] Who is accountable to whom and for what? How does one mediate between the legitimate but often conflicting demands of community groups and funding sources? While the rhetoric surrounding the project embraced empowerment, the realities reflected the need for centralized control and accountability in the use of federal funds by both the Health Resources and Services Administration of the Department of Health and Human Services and by the Philadelphia Health Department.

3. *Impact:* Efforts to assure adequate prenatal care that are made in isolation from a larger and more difficult social and economic transformation may have limited impact. Are the efforts an attempt to compensate or are they part of a larger strategy? Do you focus on the outer Chinese box or the inner one? Focusing on the inner box is a more manageable task, but also a potentially ineffectual one.

Effectively Addressing the Operational Imperatives

It is, of course, far easier to create a persuasive common vision than it is to put it into operation. Healthy Start faces three critical, hardly unique obstacles in accomplishing this.

1. *Sustaining funding:* Most projects of this kind have struggled with temporary demonstration funding. It takes a tremendous amount of effort

and time, as the Philadelphia experience with Healthy Start shows, to get such programs started. They too often experience a short, wasteful life cycle that results in either dissolution, after a costly period of development, or worthless dilution of their efforts.[54] The conventional wisdom is that there should be a way to sustain funding for services that have a real impact on outcomes in a capitated environment. Certainly such efforts are far more difficult to support in a fee-for-service environment. Some ongoing support could be crafted by taking advantage of the current "feeding frenzy" among Medical Assistance HMOs.

2. *Sustaining a vision through organizational evolution:* There is a limit to what can be accomplished through loosely connected consortia. The participating organizations all respond to their own institutional imperatives, culture, and operating procedures. Initiatives such as Healthy Start and any common vision it might create are unlikely to be more than a small part of these operational realities. The key to such longer-term survival and, perhaps, the ultimate test of the success of the Philadelphia Healthy Start project will be its ability to evolve and change as an organization. It must shift from a coalition influencing the allocation of a federal grant program to one influencing the rapidly changing medical-care system in Philadelphia. The RFP, contracting, and evaluation processes expended a tremendous amount of energy in the Healthy Start program.

Such a contracting process has the advantage of flexibility and adaptability. It is currently an attractive approach in developing managed-care networks.[55] The process can create "virtual" organizations and systems overnight. They are, however, inherently unstable, temporary solutions. If health plans and providers become a part of the sustained support of the Healthy Start vision, they may choose to either (1) set up their own programs, (2) purchase existing organizations outright, or (3) contract for services. In 1996, in anticipation of a potential role as a subcontractor under Medicaid mandatory managed care, the Healthy Start Consortium developed by-laws to set itself up as an entity separate from the Health Department. Potentially such a body could serve either as a credentialing and standard-setting body (granting accreditation like the Joint Commission on Accreditation of Healthcare Organizations) or as an umbrella contractor of services with health providers and health plans. Even in the early stages of Philadelphia's Healthy Start effort, some expressed a need to create some greater permanence for the loosely structured coalition.

If Healthy Start is to survive, it will need to adapt to rapid changes in the provision of health services. Fragmented individual providers have been progressively linked into more organized networks. The growing excess capacity in the region and the increased competition to fill that capacity has created a buyer's market. The growing attention to community-based alternatives as a way of more effectively using fixed or shrinking health and social services dollars plays to the strength of the Healthy Start effort. Consumers, even Medical Assistance consumers, have growing leverage. The more Healthy Start can assert an independent, cohesive organizational identity, beyond simply a City Health Department program loosely connected to a diverse collection of contractors and community-based organizations, the more it will be able to shape the evolution of a rapidly changing health and social service delivery system.

3. *Overcoming racial divisions and distrust:* None of this will happen, however, without overcoming a pervasive, persistent, almost overwhelming legacy of distrust of a divided health system. Race matters most in determining the plight and predicaments faced by mothers and their infants. It most vividly underscores the stark divisions in wealth and power. These divisions and distrust are the land mines hidden just below the surface of the road ahead for Healthy Start and remain part of the legacy of a divided system. The Healthy Start program broke new ground in forging new coalitions between traditional established providers and more loosely structured community groups. Combining these lessons with those of the Title VI enforcement efforts described in chapter 6 will be a key focus of the final chapter.

Conclusion

The all too frustrating history of similar efforts by private foundations and public initiatives to address racial disparities appears to be unfortunately repeating itself with the Healthy Start program. Federal funding was drastically reduced in fiscal year 1998 and is likely to end. In spite of the assurances to the contrary, the evaluation of the program Healthy Start focused narrowly on birth outcomes rather than assessing the impact of community development efforts that many of the fifteen Healthy Start sites nationwide had emphasized. Locally and nationally the five years and $530 million invested in the program could show little convincing impact in reducing infant mortality rate in the targeted neighborhoods.[56] Infant mortality declined in the fifteen Healthy Start program sites nationally, but these declines mirrored overall declines in infant mortality. In the United States infant mortality declined 8.9 per 1,000 births during this period to 8.0. In Philadelphia's Healthy Start area, infant mortality declined from 19.8 to 17.5, almost identical to the national rate of decline and far short of the 50 percent infant mortality reduction goal set at the onset of the program.[57]

Given all the difficulties described in this and related efforts to address the "broader social and economic issues" inherent in disparities in birth outcomes, is it worth it? Is it worth expending the time, political capital, income from private endowments, and tax dollars to preserve and expand Healthy Start–type initiatives focused on health outcomes? Community members and their neighborhood organizations did not define infant mortality as the top priority problem. Housing, employment, and safety from crime were their major concerns, as they had been one hundred years earlier when Du Bois studied the problem in *The Philadelphia Negro*. As one West Philadelphia community organizer observed, "Part of the problem is that there are too many people in programs for whom it is just a 'job.' They don't want to deal with the presenting problem. For example, they go door to door canvassing for a project and the person might say, 'Philadelphia Electric is going to shut off my electricity.' But the program doesn't deal with that problem."

Somehow, however, infant mortality has become the fragile cord that ties us together across deepening divisions of race, class, and politics. It links all the participants in the struggle in Charleston. It is a cord that ties the supposed wealthy Pittsburgh Republican dowager by a presidential phone call to a pregnant inner-city crack addict. If that is all that ties us together, then that is where we have to start. But it cannot end there.

CHAPTER 9

Healing a Nation

> Researchers sometimes do not know, forget, or are unimpressed that Dante reserved the seventh level of hell for those who recognize a problem and do not attempt to do anything to solve it.[1]

The literature documenting the persistence of racial disparities in health services grows, as does national impatience. Race continues to matter to those being born and those growing old. Persistent racial disparities in opportunities that result from unequal health care are the legacy of a racially divided health system. Embedded in the story of the effort to overcome this legacy are many lessons that could lead to solutions. This final chapter struggles, as so many dedicated health care professionals, policymakers, program managers, and community advocates have struggled for decades, to avoid the fate of those who recognize a problem but do nothing to try to solve it.

The next decade will be a key turning point in the organization of health services in the United States, perhaps more profound than the one that coincided with the passage of the Civil Rights Act and the implementation of the Medicare program in the 1960s. The transformation currently taking place in the way health care is organized offer both threats to the progress that has been achieved and new opportunities to finally get it right. Just as the civil rights era offered a window of opportunity to end a divided system, so does the current period. Key to taking advantage of this new period of opportunity is understanding the lessons of this previous era. This chapter will (1) briefly summarize those lessons and (2) suggest how they can be applied.

The Lessons of the Civil Rights Era

There are six obvious yet largely overlooked lessons from the story presented in this book. They emerge from the many personal stories and the statistics pulled together in the previous chapters.

1. *The advocacy of independent health practitioners was one of the keys*

*to the emergence of the civil rights movement: the largest threat embedded in
the current transition is the elimination of their ability to serve as advocates.*

In racially segregated southern communities, few could afford to push
against the system. Before the civil rights era, farmers, tradespeople, and
shopkeepers had their loans called and their businesses boycotted by purchasers and suppliers. Those who were employed by white-controlled organizations were fired. Most of the resistance was driven underground. Black
teachers and many others paid their dues to local chapters of the NAACP
in cash to protect their anonymity and their livelihoods. Black physicians,
dentists, and ministers were comparatively insulated from such retaliation.
Since they relied on the black community for their livelihood, they were
harder for the white establishment to control. The physicians and dentists
were solo, fee-for-service practitioners relying mostly on the out-of-pocket
payments of their patients for their income. Payments from health insurance plans contributed little to their income. Their exclusion from staff
privileges at the white-dominated hospitals made retaliation more difficult.
Black dentists in particular were well insulated. Their practices were more
self-contained. In comparison to black physicians they were less likely to
need the help of white specialty physicians and the diagnostic services of
white hospitals in caring for their patients. Black dentists and doctors could
make a comfortable living, particularly in communities with a relatively
affluent black population. The backbone of the civil rights movement in the
South was drawn from their ranks. Few black practitioners became active,
sustained participants in the civil rights movement, but their courage and
persistence made a difference. In Fort Lauderdale, Greensboro, Atlanta,
Mobile, and many other communities where there were persistent local
efforts, the names of black physicians and dentists abound on the letter-
heads of local chapters of the NAACP and in the court suits brought
against discrimination in education, public accommodations, and employment opportunities in the 1940s and 1950s. The alliance these leaders fash-
ioned with northern physician groups such as the Medical Committee for
Human Rights set in motion the approach that would later be adopted by
the Department of Health, Education and Welfare in enforcing Title VI of
the Civil Rights Act for hospitals participating in the Medicare program.

Medical practice is now organized much differently. Most physicians,
at least in urban areas, have been absorbed into integrated delivery systems and rely increasingly on the payments of large health plans for their
livelihoods. State medical societies now fight for legislation to prohibit
"gag rules" in physician contracts with HMOs. Gag rules prohibit physicians from criticizing or even explaining to their patients the incentive systems imposed on physicians by these plans. Legislation against gag rules

does little, however, to stem the broader chilling effect of large managed-care systems on dissent. The system may choose not to contract with "uncooperative" practitioners, just as white-controlled local communities disciplined dissenters during segregation. What if such integrated delivery systems and managed-care financing of services had existed before the civil rights era? Would these activist practitioners have been able to act as civil rights advocates in their communities? One could make a convincing case that there would have been no civil rights era and that most of the Jim Crow barriers would have remained unchallenged. It would seem equally important today to protect the role of the health practitioner as an independent advocate for their patients and communities.

2. *Voluntary health care organizations, insulated from public accountability, contributed to both the perpetuation of segregation and to its elimination.* In summarizing the distinctive character of hospitals in the United States in the twentieth century, historian Rosemary Stevens concluded that voluntary hospitals have been central because they "carry the burden of unresolved and perhaps unresolvable contradictions—and because they make those contradictions visible."[2] Voluntary institutions are the dominant form of organization of health care in the United States. About 60 percent of the acute hospitals accounting for 71 percent of the beds in the United States are voluntary, not-for-profit institutions. They are an almost distinctively American institution. In most other countries the dominant form of ownership is public. The typical pattern in developed countries is that of large, public-owned teaching institutions with a scattering of private clinics and hospitals owned and operated by physicians.

Race and ethnic divisions contributed to the emergence of this distinctive form of ownership, insulated from both the political controls of government ownership and the market controls of privately operated businesses. Most nineteenth-century voluntary hospitals were created to care for the "deserving poor," as an alternative to the public poor farms and poorhouses. The deserving poor were those who deserved more compassionate care than the more stigmatizing if not punitive treatment provided by public facilities. Their needs for care resulted from misfortunes that were seen as beyond their own control and not as a result of their own moral failings. An affinity between donors to and recipients of charity was a key to making such operations financially viable. There were no voluntary institutions created to care for those suffering from sexually transmitted diseases or drug addiction. There were plenty created for children, and children's hospitals continue to receive a disproportionate share of private charitable dollars flowing into the provision of health care. The affinity between the donor and the recipient of charity that was necessary to create and assure a continued flow of voluntary charitable contributions was inevitably shaped by racial and ethnic prejudices. It resulted in taking care of one's own religious, ethnic, and racial group. In the United States, it also resulted in either rigidly segregated care or the total exclusion of blacks.

As hospitals became more central to the viability of medical practices in the twentieth century, and as control of these institutions shifted to the organized medical staff, the burden of the contradictions of these patterns of ownership grew. Voluntary ownership exacerbated racial and ethnic divisions. Prolonged battles over staff privileges began to take place. New institutions, including ones for black physicians, were created to accommodate racial and ethnic groups largely excluded from the staffs of other hospitals. The first nonblack facilities at which black physicians were able to gain staff privileges were publicly owned institutions. The black vote became increasingly important to urban politicians, and resulting political pressures began to bring about medical staff integration of public hospitals in New York City in the 1920s. Similar political pressures began to open the staffs of public hospitals in many northern cities to blacks. The voluntary hospitals, however, remained aloof and insulated from such pressures.

The *Simkins* case was the culmination of a prolonged battle to end that insulation. While free from accountability to publicly elected officials, voluntary hospitals did assume many of the responsibilities and benefits of public ownership. They were tax exempt and received local and state government funds for the care of the indigent, and, after 1946, Hill-Burton funds for construction. An invisible boundary had been crossed. Enacted as a part of Reconstruction after the Civil War, the Fourteenth Amendment had prohibited any state from denying to any person within its jurisdiction the equal protection of the laws. The *Brown v. Board of Education* decision in 1954 had concluded that separate state arrangements for education were by definition unequal. Separate state arrangements for the provision of health services could hardly be defined differently. The *Simkins* case did not hinge on proving discrimination; it hinged on proving "state action." In effect, the argument in the case went, the voluntary hospitals in Greensboro were so intertwined with public functions that they were an "arm of the state." Voluntary health care institutions receiving federal or state funds, at least in terms of the prohibitions of the Fourteenth Amendment, were public institutions. This conclusion was reached even before the massive infusion of public dollars to these institutions through the Medicare and Medicaid programs.

Yet any attempt to assess the civil rights track record of voluntary health care institutions in the United States confronts the most bewildering "burden of unresolved and perhaps unresolvable contradictions." The very insulation of this "arm of the state" that had held back integration efforts prior to the passage of Medicare worked to the advantage of subsequent integration efforts. Hospital integration in most communities, protected from the heat of local political passions, proceeded quickly, quietly, and smoothly. There was little of the divisiveness of the public-school integration process, which began long before that of the hospitals and has dragged on long afterward. The *Simkins* case and the related cases were actually settled. Remedies were hammered out. In contrast, more than forty years after the Supreme Court decision in *Brown vs. Board of Education,* litigation continues to seek acceptable remedies in all of the original cases of school segregation that were part of that decision.[3] As public sentiment increasingly turns against policies of affirmative action, the voluntary institutions have, perhaps ironically, done the most to blunt its impact. The American Association of Medical Colleges, which had in the early 1950s refused to take any position on the racially discriminatory admission practices of some of its members, now appears through its Project 3000 by Year 2000 initiative to be among the strongest advocates of affirmative-action policies.[4] Many voluntary health systems have formed innovative and productive partnerships with minority communities. The "interagency agreement" between the state-owned Medical University of South Carolina hospital and the local prosecutor, providing hospital assistance in the arrest of pregnant women who tested positive for cocaine (see chapter 8), suggests the hazard inherent in the lack of insulation of health care from state police powers.

3. *The purchasers of health care define the self-interests of providers and, in the process, narrow or widen its racial divisions.* The story in this book has focused on the importance of race in shaping the organization of health services in the United States. The most hopeful message of that story, however, is that race has always been a secondary consideration. Actions may be filtered through the distorted lens of racial perceptions, but those perceptions have never driven what individuals and institutions do. There is always something more important than race.[5] The trick is to find out what it is and make sure it works against, rather than as reinforcement to, a deeply ingrained history.

In short, individuals and health services organizations are by and large rational, and racial considerations don't take precedence over self-interest. In the late 1940s, the people of Greensboro, whose children were dying from a polio epidemic, worked together to erect almost overnight an integrated hospital within a rigidly segregated community in order to care for those children. More than a thousand acute-care hospitals, ignoring the trepidation of board members, physicians, and patients, within a few months broke down the walls that had racially divided their staffs and patients since their founding in order to become Medicare providers on July 1, 1966. State mental-health officials in Virginia, Alabama, and Mississippi eventually ignored the dire predictions made by state politicians warning of inmate riots and irreparable harm to their charges and proceeded to smoothly and uneventfully integrate their facilities. When hospital and program survival was contingent on the elimination of the visible signs of segregation, these signs were quickly and efficiently eliminated.

Unfortunately, however, the self-interest of individuals and institutions too often works to reinforce the effects of our deeply ingrained history. Concerned with losing the private paying white patients that are key to their profitability, nursing homes find ways to influence admission practices and room assignments. Hospitals track the suburban flight of their medical staffs and the declining profitability of the payer mix in their service area and choose to relocate or expand operations in the suburbs. Managed-care plans run their own numbers, cherry-pick practices in predominantly white, low per capita health insurance cost neighborhoods, and redline high per capita insurance cost, often predominantly black, neighborhoods. Health care, as a result, becomes more racially divided and more unequal.

One of the key lessons of the story presented here is the power of the purchasers of services to shape the behavior of providers. In 1966 Medicare required Title VI certification of hospitals as a condition of participation in the program, and hospitals did what was required of them. The power of purchasers has become even more dominant since then. Managed-care plans now impose requirements on medical practices and hospitals that the implementers of the Medicare program would never have dared to dream about. Purchasers, whether contracting for services for private employees or for public beneficiaries in the Medicare or Medicaid programs, now call the shots. They set the rules of the game that define the self-interest of providers. Those rules can both widen or narrow the racial divisions in the organization of services. Changes in conditions of participation, methods of payment, and reporting requirements can broaden or diminish the divide. Civil rights compliance in the absence of a direct and self-conscious connection to the purchase of services is a hollow ritual.

4. *The selective enforcement of Title VI of the Civil Rights Act of 1964 exerted a profound, unintended, and unacknowledged influence on the organization of health services in the United States.* No purchaser exerted a more profound influence on the racial divisions in health care than Medicare. Compliance with Title VI of the Civil Rights Act was a condi-

tion of participation in the program. Yet enforcement was selective, reflecting the administrative and political realities faced by the Johnson administration in launching this ambitious new program. Providers responded selectively, accommodating these requirements but moderating their impact on the communities they served.

Prior to Medicare, segregation, even in the Deep South, had never implied absolute separation of the races, but only separation in circumstances that implied a degree of equality. Blacks were free to stand, but not to sit, next to whites. Lying in beds next to each other in a shared hospital room implied the greatest degree of equality and, hence, generated the most resistance. The random room assignment of patients to hospital rooms became the easily documented acid test of Title VI compliance.

However, the political and administrative realities faced in assuring Title VI compliance in the Medicare program forced the Office of Equal Health Opportunity to pick its battles carefully. Hospitals were the only part of the health system subjected to field audits by federal inspectors, and a strong working relationship had developed between the federal civil right regulators and local civil rights activists. Nursing homes were subjected to only pro forma paper compliance reviews, and private physician practices were specifically exempted. Elegant adaptations to these new constraints by health care providers muted their impact. In summary, these adaptations included

- A massive expansion of private room accommodations in acute-care hospitals, combined with increasing pressure to increase the acuity of patients in those facilities and to reduce their length of stay.
- A more than doubling of nursing-home bed capacity, as nursing homes increasingly substituted for acute-hospital care in a completely separate and segregated system.
- An increased emphasis on ambulatory-based services, including diagnostic, surgical procedures, rehabilitation, drug and alcohol treatment, and mental health.

The result was a health care system structured differently from that of any other country in the world. The United States has the shortest length of stay and the fewest number of general hospital beds per one thousand population of any developed country in the world. It has an organizationally separate long-term care system that is unique, and it claims an almost virtual monopoly of private-room, acute-hospital accommodations. Certainly other factors more commonly used to explain this transformation played a role. Changes in medical technology, the influence of private-practice physicians over inpatient settings, and the efforts of a complex array of insurers to control or shift the costs all contributed. Yet those who argue that it is more rational and cost effective to reduce inpatient stays and expand the provision of services on an ambulatory basis still have difficulty explaining why inpatient hospital care is so much more costly on a per capita basis in the United States than in any other developed country. The adaptation to the selective Title VI enforcement provides the most parsimonious, if troubling, explanation.

5. *A divided health system persists, both exacerbating and distorting racial disparities.* In spite of the federal efforts to end segregation, health care remains, at best, more than half the distance between a fully separate and an integrated system. The Northeast and Midwest rather than the South now provide the most racially segregated health care. Nursing-home care tends to be the most segregated, and ambulatory care remains highly segregated as well. In part, this racially divided care reflects patterns of geographic and residential segregation. These racial divisions do not always work to the disadvantage of blacks. Blacks, for example, are more likely to receive care at teaching hospitals and clinics that set the standards for private medical practice. Yet many of the changes in the organization of care, ironically set in motion in part by the accommodation of providers to selective civil rights enforcement, do work to the disadvantage of blacks. For example, the shift away from acute-hospital care toward more emphasis on outpatient, home, and long-term care has a disparate impact on blacks located in neighborhoods where such resources are in shorter supply. The central issue is not so much that care provided to blacks is bad or even that a separate health care system is inherently unequal. The issue is that, since health care remains substantially divided along racial lines, changes in health care financing and organization should not be evaluated with an eye blind to this division.

Perhaps the most perverse consequence of the failure to acknowledge these racial divisions in the organization and financing of health care is the tendency to attribute characteristics of these systems to the people that use them. The more fragmented, less preventive, and episodic use of health care by blacks is translated as a lack of personal responsibility rather than as a reflection of the differences in the nature of the institutions providing care and their relationships with their patients. At least some of the reported differences in rates of drug addiction, sexually transmitted diseases, and possibly even infant mortality reflect differences in the screening and reporting practices of the settings in which care is provided to blacks as opposed to those catering to whites. Such screening and reporting is more likely to be a part of the standard operating procedures of the more urban clinic settings where blacks disproportionately receive their care. In effect, these differences in procedures amount to an institutionalized form of racial profiling. Unlike the racial profiling that has been used by state police to search drivers on interstate highways for drugs, there is nothing unconstitutional about it, but the effect is similar. The differences in procedures contribute not just to exaggerating racial differences in incidence rates, but to a qualitative difference in the relationship between providers and their patients. That relationship is more likely to be one in which there is a higher level of distrust, where the provider is less of a patient advocate, and where, as a consequence, there is a lower level of patient compliance.

6. *Health care settings can close racial divisions.* Yet, however incomplete and however discouraging the longer-term outcomes, there was something profound and almost magical about the quiet disappearance of seemingly intractable barriers. The most powerful part of the story presented in this book were the events that didn't happen. On a night in June 1965 Grady Hospital's twin patient towers in Atlanta were integrated. The nurses, speaking with a confident reassurance that none of them felt, informed their patients that their rooms had been reassigned. There was not a single protest. Similar events took place in almost one thousand hospitals in the United States that year. The signs on entrances and waiting areas changed. Room and floor assignment policies changed. Physicians long excluded received hospital privileges. Most of these changes were nonevents escaping the notice of local news media. It was almost as if, as one black physician observed, it had always been that way.[6] Contrary to the predictions of alarmed state officials, there were no riots on the wards of state psychiatric hospitals in Virginia, Alabama, and Mississippi following integration. Southern legislators, concerned about the trauma that would be inflicted by random room assignment, got changes in the Title VI regulations permitting attending physicians to certify in individual cases that the health and recovery of a patient was threatened by a racially mixed room assignment and to have them stay in an unmixed room. It was, however inadvertently, a powerful social statement. It said that racism was not an imbedded part of the structure of American society but a disease that could be cured, or at least managed. This newly defined complicating medical condition was almost never diagnosed. A seemingly instantaneous and miraculous cure resulted. Physicians and health care institutions had been delegated great latitude and trust in the cure and management of that disease. The lack of protest that made the integration of hospital settings the quietest and smoothest transition of the civil rights decade is testament to the effectiveness of that delegation. It is a power that cries out for broader application.

Applying the Lessons

What *Not* to Do

> We had diversity training. We had a black facilitator. The people were
> mad from the time they came in the room. Afterward there was a girl
> crying because it made her realize how racist she was. But she wasn't
> ready to make any changes. The result of the training was nothing.
> Token steps. Blacks think it won't be effective. Whites don't want to
> be there. Both sides leave a little angrier than before.[7]

Both have a right to be angry. The often-implicit assumption of such
workshops in health care settings is that the people in the training group
have the power to fix the problem. It assumes that the problems are primarily ones of communication, of understanding, and of respect for cultural differences, and all that's needed is to grease the wheels a bit so that
everybody can work more effectively together. The most basic and
irrefutable lesson of the story of health care's civil rights struggle is that the
problem is much more institutional than individual. Such problems are
beyond anything that can be resolved through training groups. They
require far more profound commitments—in time, in redirection of
resources, and in reallocation of power—than is possible for individuals,
groups, or even the organizations they work for to do by themselves. Institutional problems require institutional changes to correct.

Yet, it was precisely in the crafting of such institutional solutions that
failure was guaranteed. This history of the evolution of health care and the
monitoring of civil rights compliance offers little assurance that discrimination does not continue to play a role in accounting for some of the racial
discrepancies in use and outcomes. In effect, there is no monitoring. The
application of Title VI of the Civil Rights Act to health care was described
at the time of the implementation of the Medicare program as a "potentially powerful engine of social change."[8] It never realized its potential and
ran out of steam. Institutional change and regulatory processes are, in a
democracy, imprecise and messy. This one, however, seemed overdesigned
to fail. That failure hinged on four fatal flaws.

1. *The standards have never been defined or agreed upon.* Title VI of the
1964 civil rights legislation, as its southern legislative opponents were correct in pointing out during the debate over its passage, never defined discrimination. It failed to specify in any measurable way what would cause
the termination of federal funding. Removing that definition from the
political bargaining process presented the agency with an almost impossi-

ble problem in developing regulations and enforcing them. Once the most obvious and transparent symbols of Jim Crow were eliminated, the process inevitably floundered. Gaining access and receiving medical treatment is a complex process not easily reducible to simple standards to prevent unequal treatment. There was no simple way of untangling more subtle forms of racial discrimination from economic discrimination. Adding to the difficulties, this flawed and leaky vessel was soon overloaded with new occupants. Other groups that had historically been discriminated against—women, the disabled, and other ethnic minorities—now, in the language of the civil rights era, demanded government protection. The Office for Civil Rights faced expanding enforcement responsibilities through successive waves of legislation prohibiting discrimination by sex, age, and disability in a period during which staffing and funding continued to decline.[9] Thus the agency could, perhaps quite consistently, be accused by its critics of being a "hotbed of regulatory zealots obsessed with vast social engineering schemes" and by its constituents of being a "lumbering bureaucracy, addressing its obligations in the most timid, halfhearted, and ineffectual manner."[10]

2. *The regulatory process produces no information.* Perhaps, as some would argue, the issue is moot. Perhaps it is not really the regulatory process that is vestigial, but the need for it. Have we won the war to end a racially divided and discriminatory health system? If so, knowing this would be helpful. If not, it would be helpful to know where to best use scarce resources to correct the remaining disparities. In the absence of such information, only impossible-to-conceal events such as hospital relocations invite more careful review. Title VI certification and compliance involves essentially the completion and filing of a form. There are no standard forms or procedures adopted by the state agencies responsible for Title VI certification. No analysis or summary reports are routinely completed from these efforts. While OCR conducts its own compliance reviews of facilities, budget limitations make it possible to do only a few each year in each region. Yet even for these limited federal compliance reviews, investigators have no data resources other than census figures. In the age of the information superhighway, investigators must often rely on hand tabulation from facility records.

Identified as a major weakness of civil rights monitoring efforts almost from their inception, efforts to improve the information available have produced little.[11] In 1979 OCR worked with Health Resources Administration to design a common survey to fulfill Hill-Burton requirements and OCR needs for information from hospitals. OCR also worked with Health Care Financing Administration to include racial data on the proposed Uniform Discharge Data System. Both initiatives combined the advantages of supplying basic essential information while reducing the burdens on providers. The Hill-Burton surveys have apparently not been translated through analysis into information that can be used in compliance reviews. Fifteen years later in 1994, the proposed uniform claim forms, likely to become industry standards (UB-92/HCFA-1450 claim form for hospitals and the HCFA-1500 claim form for other providers), excluded race/ethnicity information. A suit supported by many advocacy groups attempted to prevent the exclusion of this information from the forms and to require DHHS to collect and report more information on how federally subsidized health care providers were serving minority Americans.[12] HCFA argued that it would be more appropriate to obtain such information from Social Security enrollment files, and the suit was eventually dismissed. DHHS, in response to these criticisms, however, did initiative efforts to improve the level of detail and completeness of information on minorities served by federal health programs. Yet as a lawyer representing the plaintiffs in the suit observed, the failure to routinely include such a data element could "permanently relegate minority health research and civil rights enforcement to the breakdown lane of the electronic information highway."[13]

3. *The process is not embedded in operations.* Secretary Gardner during the Johnson administration wanted the civil rights enforcement function embedded in the Department of Health, Education and Welfare's operational divisions. This was both a statement of philosophy about its central importance to the mission of the agency and a calculated strategy to circumvent control of these activities by legislative budget committees controlled by southern opponents of the Civil Rights Act. That battle was lost in 1967. After 1968, federal efforts to monitor civil rights compliance faced diminishing effectiveness and influence. They (1) became insulated from the operational divisions that could have greatly helped their efforts, (2) were ignored by their own agency, which was preoccupied with assuring civil rights compliance in the schools, and (3) were increasingly disengaged from direct monitoring and certification through delegation to state agencies.

Delegating monitoring to the states added to the insulation from operations. Given the insulation from the operational health agencies, the lack of priority attention given to health care in the more formative years of the Office for Civil Rights, and its lack of resources, it made sense to fold Title VI certification in with state Medicare and Medicaid provider certification efforts. OCR could then limit its focus to (1) requiring and filing Title VI assurances from health facilities certified as participating providers in the Medicare program, (2) requiring state agencies to submit Title VI compliance plans describing state certification and enforcement activities, and (3) investigating complaints and noncomplying recipients identified by assurance documentation. Certification of health facilities as providers in the Medicare and Medicaid programs has involved complicated arrangements with traditional state licensing and private accreditation bodies such as the Joint Commission on Accreditation of Health Care Organizations. There was little resulting uniformity in how different states handled the Title VI requirements, little guidance, little analysis of the information collected by this process, and no research and development. The on-site surveys typically combined state licensure, reviews of compliance with Medicare and Medicaid conditions of participation, and Title VI. Some states have done a good job and taken these responsibilities seriously. Yet for most state inspection programs, Title VI certifications became just another form and set of boxes to check off. From the perspective of the state inspectors, whose major responsibilities dealt with protecting the health and safety of patients in facilities, Title VI reviews were probably seen as the least important of their responsibilities and the one they were least likely to get in trouble about if something were overlooked.

4. *The process failed to adapt and take advantage of newly emerging resources.* One of the predictable consequences of the insulation of health care civil rights monitoring from operations was a failure to adapt to changes in that operational environment. Health care civil rights efforts became absorbed as a result into the broader growing inertia over civil rights.[14] The larger environment was not as conducive to bold action. Most of the easy, visible gains toward the elimination of Jim Crow symbols had been achieved. The more difficult ones now had to be achieved with (1) a less activist civil rights executive branch, (2) an increasing preoccupation with controlling health care costs and reducing federal bureaucracy, (3) an increasing, diverse array of ill-defined "civil rights" responsibilities, and (4) a generally less sympathetic public. These changes created myriad interrelated difficulties for monitoring compliance with civil rights law in the field of health care.

Health care, however, has also changed. It has changed in many ways that potentially make civil rights monitoring far easier. Health care is now a far different world than the private, fragmented, insulated one the civil servant "volunteers" to OEHO entered in 1966. The computer-information revolution, the explosive growth of managed care, the massive consolidation and integration of health-related services, and the growing purchaser-driven demand for accountability offer promising new resources and alliances.

What to Do

Routine and ongoing examination of racial disparities in the use of services and in the choices of diagnostic and therapeutic alternatives should be part of the quality assurance protocols of every hospital, every health maintenance organization and every other system of care.[15]

As advocated by this editorial in the *New England Journal of Medicine,* and given the lessons of the civil rights era and the weaknesses of existing civil rights monitoring efforts, it would seem a simple problem to solve. The growing research literature that documents significant racial disparities in patterns of use and outcomes make it an increasingly difficult problem to ignore. For example, a review prepared for the American Medical Association's Board of Trustees restricted to the literature appearing only in the *New England Journal of Medicine* and the *Journal of the American Medical Association* between 1984 and 1994 filled sixty-six pages.[16]

In attempting to address the problem, however, it is important to acknowledge two key changes in the context in which such monitoring now takes place. First, whatever racial discrimination (separate and/or unequal treatment unrelated to insurance status or the ability to pay) is currently taking place in the provision of health services is different from that which took place before the 1964 Civil Rights Act and the implementation of the Medicare program. It is subtler and more difficult to untangle from the economic imperatives faced by providers. At a structural level, it is shaped by residential segregation and the limitations of the health-related resources in predominantly minority communities as opposed to more affluent, predominantly white communities. At the interpersonal level it is shaped by the level of trust, affinity, and expectations that both providers and patients bring to their encounters. In many cases neither the provider nor the patient leaves such encounters consciously aware of how race mattered. Second, it is important to place the conclusions about the limitations of existing civil rights monitoring within a broader context. Until recently, the organization of health care has remained well insulated from almost *all* forms of external monitoring. External quality assurance efforts, such as those of the Joint Commission on Accreditation of Health Care Organizations (JCAHO), which is responsible for certifying most hospitals for Medicare participation, focused almost exclusively on structure. That is, it focused on the credentials of staff, the bylaws and committee structure, record-keeping systems, and physical plant. Little attention was given to the other generally recognized major approaches to quality assessment, to "process" (assessing the treatment patients actually received), or to "outcomes," in terms of survival rates, complication rates, and so forth.[17] Similarly, civil rights compliance efforts have focused on structure. That is, they have looked at documentation of civil rights assurances by the board and management of health services organizations and at physical evidence of racial segregation. Assessing structure is the least costly and least intrusive form of external assessment. It also provides the least assurance to the individual patient or third-party purchaser of care.

Major structural changes in the organization of health care, however, have produced substantial changes in the way medical care is monitored. Power has swung increasingly away from providers and into the hands of large health plans and major purchasers of care.[18] In addition, as methods of payment shift to managed care and risk-sharing arrangements, and given the shift of incentives to providers, there is a greater need for external monitoring of process and outcomes. In response to these changes, a massive consolidation and integration of physicians, hospitals, and other service providers is taking place. Increasingly, integrated and computerized clinical and financial information systems serve as the essential backbone of these delivery systems and health plans.

These changes are reflected in the nature of the information collected by providers and purchasers of health care. Different "report cards" have been developed to assure accountability, consumer choice, and goal-directed action. Most have undergone extensive review and development. Only minor changes in the reporting formats would be necessary for civil rights monitoring purposes.

The existing report card strategies need only to be expanded to include comparisons of the recently revised Office of Management and Budget standard racial categories.[19] The OMB categories provide the common racial classification scheme for data collected by all federal agencies, and that classification scheme is also used by most state agencies, hospital discharge abstracts, and clinical record-keeping systems. A standard for communities, health plans, and accredited health institutions would be to bring all discrepancies by race on the indicators to within 80 percent, the commonly used legal standard for measuring disparate impact. The indicators, the racial categories, and the statistical adjustments for income and insurance, which might explain racial discrepancies, would be continuously refined.

Table 9.1 presents examples of such consensus indicators that have evolved out of the extensive efforts of public-private professional partnerships spanning several decades. There is nothing magical about any of these specific indicators. They are presented here simply for illustrative purposes. Twelve have been selected from each of three efforts. Other indicators, developed in parallel efforts, could be added to this list. The first twelve are consensus indicators routinely collected and reported by the national vital statistics reporting system designed to focus on the comparative evaluation of the health of geographically defined populations. They are a part of the larger Healthy People 2000 monitoring effort conducted at the national, state, and local levels. The indicators were selected because they are readily available, measure the health status of the population, and lend themselves to modification through specific public-health and preventive efforts. The second twelve measures are ones developed from efforts to provide major purchasers and consumers with good comparative information on managed-care plans. Six of the indicators come from the basic Health Plan Employer Data Information Set (HEDIS), developed by the National Committee for Quality Assurance to assess the relative success of health plans in meeting preventive-care standards. The other six are selected from a similar effort to develop a uniform consumer assessment of such plans by the Agency for Health Policy Research from their adult survey proposed core data set.[20] The third set of measures is selected "beta indicators" proposed by the Joint Commission on the Accreditation of Health Care Organizations in 1993 to monitor inpatient hospital performance. The commission chose to give hospitals latitude in selecting among a variety of standardized approaches but to require process and outcome assessments as the focus of future accreditation.[21] Four indicators for obstetrical care, cancer, and cardiovascular care were selected for illustrative purposes here, because studies have reported large racial discrepancies and they represent major health problems.

This use of such monitoring indicators has the advantage of (1) using broadly accepted methods that have undergone considerable research and development, (2) using data that for the most part is already routinely collected, and (3) providing a way to accomplish goals already embraced in the mission statements of all health professional organizations, health plans, and health services organizations. It substitutes public and peer pressure for litigation and harnesses competing initiatives in a common purpose.

These types of indicators could play a small but constructive part in a larger improvement process, just as similar indicators do in the continuous quality improvement processes adopted by many integrated delivery systems. There are, however, two general objections that will be raised about their use.

From a methodological viewpoint, many indicators reflect outcomes beyond the direct control of health services providers. There remain stark racial discrepancies in income, wealth, insurance, housing, and environ-

TABLE 9.1.　Examples of Report Card Indicators

Unit of Analysis	Indicators
Geographically defined population	1. Total Age-Adjusted Death Rate 2. Automobile Death Rate 3. Suicide Death Rate 4. Lung Cancer Death Rate 5. Breast Cancer Death Rate 6. Cardiovascular Death Rate 7. Homicide Death Rate 8. Teen Births 9. Inadequate Prenatal Care 10. % Low Birth Weight Births 11. Infant Death Rate 12. Children in Poverty
Health plan covered lives	1. % women for whom prenatal care began in the 1st trimester 2. % children who by 24 months received all childhood immunizations 3. Cholesterol screening once in 5-year period for those 40–64 4. % women 51–64 continuously enrolled for 2 years who received mammogram breast cancer screening 5. % women 21–64 continuously enrolled for 3 years who received pap test 6. % of members 2–19 with one or more asthma admissions 7. % diabetics 31–64 who had retinal exam during the preceding calendar year 8. % members 23–39 who visited a health practitioner in the last three years 9. % rating how well the doctor listened as excellent 10. % for whom last visit to doctor fully met their needs 11. % choice of doctors not a problem 12. % satisfied with overall plan
Hospital patient clinical population	1. % low birth weight infants 2. % term infants admitted to NICU within one day of delivery 3. % neonates with an apgar of 3 or less at 5 minutes and a birthweight > 1,500 grams 4. % neonates with a discharge diagnosis of significant birth trauma

TABLE 9.1—*Continued*

Unit of Analysis	Indicators
Oncology indicators	
	5. Survival of patient with primary cancer of the lung, colon/rectum, by state and histologicity
	6. Use of tests critical to diagnosis, prognosis, and treatment
	7. Use of treatment approaches that impact quality of life
	8. Interdisciplinary treatment and followup
Cardiovascular indicators	
	9. Intrahospital mortality as a means of assessing multiple aspects of CABG care
	10. Extended postoperative stay as a means of assessing multiple aspects of CABG care
	11. Intrahospital mortality as means of assessing multiple aspects of PTCA care
	12. Intrahospital mortality as means of assessing multiple aspects of acute myocardial infarction care.

Source: David B. Smith, "Addressing Racial Inequities in Health Care," *Journal of Health Politics, Policy and Law* 23, no. 1 (1998): 96–97, with permission. The specific indicators were adapted from the following sources: (1) Geographically Defined Populations: National Center for Health Statistics, *Healthy People 2000 Review,* (Hyatsville, Md.: Public Health Service, 1994); (2) Health Plan Covered Lives: HEDIS 3.0, Washington, D.C.: National Committee for Quality Assurance, January, 1979, and Research Triangle Institute, *Design of a Survey to Monitor Consumer's Access to Care, Use of Services, Health Outcomes and Patient Satisfaction: Final Report* (Rockville, Md.: Agency for Health Policy Research, DHHS, 1995); and (3) Hospital Patient Clinical Population: Joint Commission on the Accreditation of Health Care Organizations, *The Measurement Mandate* (Chicago: JCAHO, 1993), 197–209.

mental risk exposures that play more of a role than the provision of health services in affecting outcomes. These can be directly addressed or adjusted for. Most not-for-profit integrated delivery systems, mindful of preserving their tax-exempt privileges, pay at least lip service to community benefits, and a few actually invest real effort in providing adequate housing, improved access to primary care, screening, and prevention programs. Methodologically, it may also be that many of the existing racial discrepancies are artifacts created by the lack of uniform reporting, or by census undercounts that go into the calculation of ratios, or by the failure to adjust for factors such as income and occupational group. This would indeed be reassuring. There is a wonderful tyranny about measurement in that what is measured becomes important and that importance makes its measurement more precise.

From a political perspective, some would question the feasibility of collecting and analyzing such data. They would argue that it will not happen in the current environment and that, even if it does, the data would be either attacked or ignored. That may be the case. It is, however, instructive to look at the example of the banking industry, which has an insulated, powerful institutional subculture of its own. Since 1990 amendments to the Home Mortgage Disclosure Act (HMDA) have required residential mortgage lenders to reveal the deposition of each residential loan application, the census tract location of the subject property, the loan amount, the loan type, and the race and income of the applicant. Reports based on these disclosures have found significant racial disparities that cannot be explained by other variables. This produced the predictable cycle of uncomplimentary headlines, indignant scathing industry critiques of the methodology and accuracy of the data, and subsequent refinements in response to these criticisms that left the conclusions essentially unchanged.[22] The banks concerned about regulatory approval of the many mergers and consolidations currently taking place, however, appear to have responded to the harsh light of these disclosures. In 1994, according to HMDA data, the number of mortgages approved for blacks jumped 55 percent.[23] A similar process of merger and consolidation is taking place in health care in most medical markets in the United States. The implications of these mergers in view of antitrust laws, local tax exemptions, appropriate use of the combined charitable endowments, and so on, are undergoing similar public scrutiny.

The final and perhaps most telling objection, however, is that the process of providing health services, particularly in a rapidly changing managed-care environment, is so complex and so poorly understood that it defies useful objective measurement.[24] Many critics fear that such complexity and lack of knowledge will result in "report cards" that inevitably become the innocuous captive products of the industry. As such they serve as public-relations fluff, a smokescreen behind which cherry picking, risk shifting, and more subtle forms of access restrictions and cost cutting can go on undetected, financially benefiting the managed-care plans at the expense of their subscribers and the private employers and taxpayers who pay most of the bills. Certainly, as some have suggested, the failure to include satisfaction measures for those with serious acute illness episodes or chronic health problems, or on those whose care seriously stress-tests the system, raise questions.[25] The failure of the HEDIS indicators to include a measure of referral rates to specialists (an often closely guarded competitive secret), which are of great interest to consumers and something that early research in managed-care plans showed to be significantly related to race, raises questions.[26] In the absence of more qualitative insights and external pressures, its inclusion is unlikely to occur.

Report cards, of course, will only be effective if they are the tip of the iceberg of a much larger process. The brief period of aggressive enforcement of civil rights compliance between 1964 and 1968 is instructive of what is required. It suggests that the indicators themselves are the least important ingredients. Civil rights inspection teams during this period did not rely solely upon the reports of hospitals and the routine collection of statistical information, or even upon on-site inspections. Data resources were far inferior to what exist today, and the inspectors were usually pulled on temporary assignments from unrelated parts of the federal bureaucracy and often lacked any familiarity with the institutions they were reviewing. They often faced far more determined and hostile adversaries, willing to go to extensive lengths to conceal their actual operations and to circumvent compliance. Yet to a surprising extent they were successful. They were successful for two reasons. First, a network of local civil rights organizations and health services workers, intimately familiar with the operations of local hospitals, did the "real work." Periodic telephone contacts between the president of the NMA, hired as a part-time consultant to the Office for Equal Health Opportunity, and local physicians helped target problem areas. Local hospital employees, often meeting in secret locations with inspectors the evening before site visits in order to avoid retaliation, would review the floor plans and instruct inspectors about the problem areas. The knowledge that this was part of the procedures circumvented much obfuscation. Second, there was a commitment to use the information in certifying providers for Medicare participation. The proposals of the Coalition for Health Care Choice and Accountability and other groups for standards and certification of health plans could produce similar conditions.

In short, rather than cutting across the grain of a long tradition of professional self-governance and autonomous voluntary institutional structures, report card accountability builds on that process. It is also in the self-interest of providers. Report cards that do not adjust for race, a proxy for all of the unfinished civil rights agenda, much of which is beyond the capacity of individual health providers to influence, will unfairly grade health plans and delivery systems. One could even offer it as an alternative to the current inspections of civil rights compliance that health facilities and integrated delivery systems currently undergo by state-designated Civil Rights agencies. It could serve a function similar to the "deemed status" offered Medicare providers for JCAHO accreditation, exempting them from state Medicare certification inspections. Packaged (quite accurately, given the limited resources and attention current given to civil rights inspections) to reflect a higher level of commitment/compliance by the provider, voluntary compliance would be assured, given the sensitivities of major purchasers and the providers themselves in an increasingly competitive market.

The rapid growth of integrated delivery systems, driven by risk-based population financing, presents new opportunities for more effective monitoring. It also presents new risks. Without concerted effort the external paper trail of fee-for-service billing that has been used to document most of the racial discrepancies in the use of health services will disappear with nothing to replace it.

The history of civil rights efforts in health care clearly suggests that the bulk of the gains have come from the voluntary efforts of providers concerned about "doing the right thing." Many providers, not unmindful of their own self-interest in an increasingly competitive market with changing demographics, have recently developed their own "diversity" initiatives. Every Medicare and Medicaid provider has signed a civil rights assurance form and posted the appropriate notices. Why not act on those assurances? Ultimately, it is the lack of imagination, as well as the lack of will that underlies that lack of imagination, rather than the lack of methodological sophistication or resources, that represents the major impediments. It is time to translate the assurance into action.

Recovering a Lost Vision

> As far as gangs are concerned, if you are on your own you can get robbed or beaten up. But nobody's going to mess with you if you are in a gang. It's called "slippin." If you are by yourself, they say you're "slippin." They're going to get you, you know? It's like wearing a sign that says, "I'm alone."[27]

In Broward County, South Florida, teen gangs don't fit the conventional stereotypes. Race and geographic areas have little meaning in a rapidly changing community where there are no neighborhoods, where everyone has become an ethnic minority, and where there is no history. The gangs are loosely connected groups that cut across geography, class, race, and ethnicity. College-bound kids of professionals are connected through these affiliations to dead-end kids; skin color and language mean little. They are linked for self-preservation and reflect, perhaps, for all their more troubling aspects, the powerful natural human capacity for creating community.

In the nineteenth century, freed slaves and new European immigrants joined mutual-aid societies for similar protection. These associations gave birth to health insurance and other arrangements for caring for members who became ill or incapacitated. The logic of solidarity, the purpose for joining such groups in the first place, dictated that the costs of such care be spread across all members. In other developing nations, more homogeneous and less fragmented by racial and ethnic divisions, this led eventually to the creation in the twentieth century of some form of universal protection through a national health service or health insurance. In the United States, it produced a divided and fragmented system of private insurance and reluctant public subsidies of a system of care for those at the bottom of the American caste system.

Only during the civil rights era in the 1960s did the logic of solidarity begin to break down these divisions. It was here that some measure of equality in access to health care began to be viewed, through the passage of the Medicare and Medicaid legislation, not so much as an individual right, but as a collective responsibility. The force of a grassroots movement and a ragtag army composed mostly of children swept through the lunch counters, fire hoses, and jails into legislation. That legislation said that public funds raised for collective purposes must assure equal protection for all citizens and that nowhere was such a principle more appropriately applied than in the provision of health care. It is that same logic, that same simple idea, that now drives the efforts to expand insurance coverage for children. The Balanced Budget Act of 1997 emerged out of bitter partisan battles over the federal deficit and found common ground in expanding the coverage of health care costs for children.[28] The act potentially will produce the largest expansion in coverage of health care costs since the passage of the Medicare program and could provide something close to universal health care coverage for all children in the United States up to the age of eighteen.

Yet even with such expansions in health care coverage, we are, in the words of the South Florida teen gang member, "slippin." Such efforts will face an uphill battle in an era that has increasingly embraced the language of individual responsibility. That language assumes that one can shift the cost of collective protection back onto individuals. No one wants to pay for "those other people's" cost.

There are, of course, many rational arguments that could be made for the assumption of greater collective responsibility. The higher rates of morbidity and hospitalization in uninsured and uninsurable populations translate for everyone else into either (1) higher premium rates to subsidize providers for these costs, (2) higher taxes to provide for their care under public programs, or (3) a degradation in the care they themselves receive. Even for drug and alcohol abuse, where individual responsibility might temper compassion, it is impossible to wall off the impact on others. The decline in support for inpatient treatment for drug and alcohol and mental health problems in the last decade has been matched by a corresponding increase in the prison incarceration rates. These rates in the United States almost doubled between 1985 and 1995, and the racial disparities increased.[29] The "urban plagues," teen pregnancy, drug addiction, crime, AIDS, and whatever new infectious diseases appear in an increasingly drug-resistant, interconnected world, cannot be contained in urban ghettos. They spread across boundaries of race and municipalities, along major transportation routes like cancers against which individuals or even local municipalities, alone and divided, are powerless to defend.[30] Those individuals and municipalities are, indeed, "slippin."

Finishing the Story

The plea for a National Health Service by the president of the Medical Association of South Africa in 1931 was echoed by the government-appointed National Health Service Commission in 1944. The rejection of this proposal, the subsequent election of a Nationalist government in 1948, and the institution of apartheid were associated with the development of a health service characterized by racial discrimination, fragmentation, poor coordination, duplication of services, and a predominant focus on hospital-based care rather than primary care.

Privately financed medicine flourished providing excellent primary and community-level care for patients (predominantly white) who had health insurance through more than 200 private insurance companies. Primary care and community facilities for poor patients (predominantly black) remained woefully inadequate.[31]

The United States and South Africa share the distinction being the only developed nations that lack universal health insurance coverage for their citizens. Much of the outline of the evolution of the South African health system parallels developments in the United States. Despite the parallels, the task of health care reform in South Africa is daunting in contrast to that of the United States. Black and white infant mortality differs by a factor of almost sevenfold rather than the twofold difference that exists in the United States. Per capita health expenditures are one-fifteenth that of the United States and far more inequitably distributed by race. Yet South Africa's overwhelming black majority and the recognition that national survival depends on reconciliation has fostered instructive innovation. The Truth and Reconciliation Commission heard the stories of the apartheid era. It was created in the hope that the truthful telling of the stories by both its victims and perpetrators would help heal its wounds. In an historically unique accommodation to conflicting political pressures, amnesty to apartheid's more brutal perpetrators is offered in exchange for truth.[32]

Little of the parallel story in the United States has been told about health care, and far less has penetrated the consciousness of policymakers, providers, and the general public. Yet the details are less important than the celebration of the lives that deprived this largely private world of some of the inertia and cynicism necessary to continue to be "just the way things were." Each of the individuals that helped change things could have made other choices and led more comfortable and, at least in financial terms, more rewarding lives. Yet they made choices that exposed them to many risks. Some were motivated by a broader passionate vision of a better world. For others, it was just a personal statement reflecting remarkable inner strength and stubbornness. The lives worth celebrating include those of early pioneers such as Louis Wright, who began the process of medical staff integration at Harlem Hospital after World War I and remained an activist in the NAACP throughout his career; Dorothy Ferebee, a pediatrician whose volunteer work in the 1930s in the Mississippi Delta created a network that persists to the present; and Mabel Staupers, whose vision and persistence with other nurses in the leadership of the National Association of Colored Graduate Nurses and American Nursing Association led to the closing of their ranks in 1951, long before the rest of the world of health care had begun to think about what Jim Crow meant in health care. It includes an anatomy professor, W. Montague Cobb, who orchestrated a sustained and successful strategy of hospital integration and flailed with a sharp and pointed pen those who would compromise. It includes John Holloman, who would eventually head the National Medical Association and New York Hospital Corporation, and Paul Cornely, Cobb's public-health colleague at Howard, who stood self-consciously next to the sandwich board on the boardwalk at Atlantic City with other colleagues at the convention of the American Medical Association in 1963, ushering in a new era of medical activism. The list must certainly include Hubert Eaton, who first pushed and continued to push for medical staff integration against overwhelming odds, and George Simkins, the Greensboro dentist who got his back up in the cause of democracy and never backed down. The names of Thurgood Marshall, Jack Greenberg, Jim Nabrit, Michael Meltzner, and all the other NAACP Legal Defense Fund lawyers who patiently paved the way through the courts, making the groundswell of change possible, should also appear on the list. The list should include the many physicians and nurses of the Medical Committee for Human Rights, volunteers whose summer campaign in the South in 1965 became the blue-print for the Medicare certification process. The list should most certainly include Lyndon Baines Johnson, the complex and driven backbone of the federal civil rights initiatives, who, with the implementation of the Medicare program, stiffened his resolve in a way that no president had done previously or has since. It should also include Robert Nash, the pro-totypical faceless career federal bureaucrat who commanded the army of volunteer transfers to the Office of Equal Health Opportunity with an understated, quiet ferocity. It should include Marilyn Rose, Counsel to OEHO who commanded that office in exile after its elimination. It should include all the members of OEHO's original invisible underground volun-teer army, who kept the Title VI certification process honest, and all of those who continue to struggle to keep it so.

Most importantly, however, it should include the names of all of those hospital workers and health professionals who risked their liveli-hoods and as perhaps in the case of Dr. Jean Cowsert of Mobile, their lives to keep Title VI certification honest by serving as the eyes and ears of this effort.

The forty names of persons who died in the larger civil rights move-ment are engraved on a monument designed by Maya Lin, the architect who designed the Vietnam War Memorial in Washington, D.C. It stands outside the offices of the Southern Poverty Law Center in Montgomery, Alabama, a few blocks from the White House of the Confederacy and a block from the Dexter Avenue Baptist Church where Martin Luther King helped organize the Montgomery bus boycott. Water flows over the names. Those whose names appear on that monument and those who have been mentioned here wait, as the monument's inscription proclaims, UNTIL JUSTICE ROLLS DOWN LIKE WATERS AND RIGHTEOUSNESS LIKE A MIGHTY STREAM (AMOS 5.24). Until then, it will be the celebration of their lives and the small victories they made possible that sustains the hope of a health system that can heal a nation.

Notes

Preface

1. This perspective reflects the influence of the "Population Ecology" school of organizational theory and behavior. At its best, it is an inventive blending of many ideas and disciplines that tries to explain the shift in organizational forms over time as a reflection of the changes in their environment. See Howard Aldrich, "New Paradigms for Old: The Population Perspective's Contribution to Health Services Research," *Medical Care Review* 44, no. 2 (1987): 257–77; Jeffrey Alexander, Arnold Kaluzny, and Suann Middleton, "Organizational Growth, Survival, and Death in the U.S. Health Care Industry: A Population Ecology Perspective," *Social Science and Medicine* 22, no. 3 (1986): 303–8; and Glenn R. Carroll, "Organizational Ecology," in *Annual Review of Sociology,* vol. 10, ed. Ralph H. Turner and James F. Short (Palo Alto, Calif.: Annual Reviews, 1984), 71–93.

2. The comparison has been proposed as a productive paradigm for epidemiology. See Mervyn Susser and Ezra Susser, "Choosing a Future for Epidemiology: II. From Black Box to Chinese Boxes and Eco-Epidemiology," *American Journal of Public Health* 86, no. 5 (1996): 674–77.

Chapter 1

1. Office of Management and Budget, "Revisions to the Standards for Classification of Federal Data on Race and Ethnicity," *Federal Register* 62, no. 210 (October 30, 1997): 58789.

2. See, for example, Jill Quadagno, *The Color of Welfare: How Racism Undermined the War on Poverty* (New York: Oxford University Press, 1996).

3. National Center for Health Statistics, *Health in the United States, 1996–97, and Injury Chartbook* (Hyattsville, Md.: Public Health Service, 1997), 104, 105, and 249.

4. For a useful review see David R. Williams, Risa Lavizzo-Mourey, and Rueben Warren, "The Concept of Race and Health Status in America," *Public Health Reports* 109, no. 1 (1994): 26–41. In addition, see the issue of *Health Services Research* devoted to "The Role of Race and Ethnicity in Health Services Research," *Health Services Research* 30, no. 1, pt. 2 (1995): 145–273.

5. Douglas S. Massey and Nancy A. Denton, *American Apartheid: Segregation and the Making of the Underclass* (Cambridge: Harvard University Press, 1993), 1.

6. Philip Slater, *The Pursuit of Loneliness* (Boston: Beacon Press, 1970), 15.

7. For a fascinating synthesis of these issues see Madison Powers, "Efficiency, Autonomy, and Communal Values in Health Care," *Yale Law and Policy Review* 10, no. 2 (1992): 316–61.

8. See David Smith, *Partners for a Healthy Community: Health Assessment for Northwest Philadelphia and the Adjoining Suburbs* (Philadelphia: Germantown and Chestnut Hill Hospitals, 1994), 35.

9. See, for example, Vanessa N. Gamble, *Germs Have No Color Line: Blacks and American Medicine, 1900–1940* (New York: Garland, 1989), and the subsequent discussion in this chapter.

10. Rodrick Wallace and Deborah Wallace, "The Coming Crisis of Public Health in the Suburbs," *Milbank Quarterly* 71 (1993): 543–64.

11. David M. Lang and Marcia Polansky, "Patterns of Asthma Mortality in Philadelphia from 1969 to 1991," *New England Journal of Medicine* 331 (1994): 1542–85.

12. Asthma-related hospital admissions are one of many conditions that could be preventable or greatly reduced through adequate primary-care management. A collection of such conditions has been pooled into an "Ambulatory Sensitive Condition" rate of hospitalization, which appears to be a good indicator of lack of access to primary care in a geographic area. See John Billings et al., "Impact of Socioeconomic Status on Hospital Use in New York City," *Health Affairs* 12, no. 1 (1993): 162–73. In these North Philadelphia neighborhoods, the ambulatory sensitive condition rates are more than three times the age-adjusted regional rate. The costs involved in that difference in rates could easily finance private office care in the style offered to the region's most affluent.

13. See Daniel Haney, "A Creepy Cause of Asthma: The Roach," *Philadelphia Inquirer,* June 17, 1996, F1.

14. See, for example, Norman Daniels, *Just Health Care* (New York: Cambridge University Press, 1985).

15. Confidential interview by the author, tape recording, April 17, 1996.

16. Harold F. Dorn, "The Health of the Negro, a Research Memorandum," Carnegie-Myrdal Study, Schomburg Center for Research in Black Culture, New York, 1940.

17. Ibid., 125.

18. Fred B. Rogers and A. Reasoner Sayre, *The Healing Art: A History of the Medical Society of New Jersey* (Trenton: Medical Society of New Jersey, 1966), 51.

19. Mitchell F. Rice and Woodrow Jones Jr., *Public Policy and the Black Hospital: From Slavery to Segregation to Integration* (Westport, Conn: Greenwood Press, 1994), 1.

20. See Rosemary Stevens, *In Sickness and in Wealth: American Hospitals in the Twentieth Century* (New York: Basic Books, 1989), 18–51.

21. Mark Lloyd, *A History of Caring for the Sick since 1863* (Philadelphia: Germantown Hospital and Medical Center, 1981).

22. See, for example, Charles Perrow, "Goals and Power Structures: A Histor-

ical Case Study," in *The Hospital in Modern Society,* ed. E. Freidson (New York: Free Press of Glencoe, 1963), 112–46.

23. For origins of the still-debated argument over the degree of segregation after the Civil War, see C. Vann Woodward, *The Strange Career of Jim Crow* (New York: Oxford University Press, 1955).

24. Robert Martensen, "Sundown Medical Education: Top-Down Reform and Its Social Displacements," *Journal of the American Medical Association* 273 (1995): 271.

25. Abraham Flexner and Henry S. Pritchett, *Medical Education in the United States and Canada,* Carnegie Foundation for the Advancement of Teaching Bulletin No. 4 (New York, 1910), 180.

26. Vanessa Gamble, *Making a Place for Ourselves: The Black Hospital Movement, 1920–1945* (New York: Oxford University Press, 1995), 124.

27. Ibid., 22.

28. Ibid.

29. Rice and Jones, *Public Policy,* 16.

30. Gamble, *Making a Place,* 35–69.

31. Julius Rosenwald Fund, *Negro Hospitals: A Compilation of Available Statistics* (Chicago: Julius Rosenwald Fund, February 1931), 2–3. The hospitals provided assistance by the fund included St. Agnes Hospital at Raleigh, N.C., L. Richardson at Greensboro, N.C., Good Samaritan Hospital at Charlotte, N.C., Spartanburg General Hospital at Spartanburg, S.C., Toomy Hospital at Sumter, S.C., a projected hospital at New Bern, N.C., Flint-Goodridge Hospital in New Orleans, Charity Hospital in Savannah, Ga., Knoxville General Hospital, Knoxville, St. Phillips Hospital, Richmond, Va., a new TB sanatorium in Little Rock, Ark., Provident Hospital, Chicago, Mercy Hospital, Philadelphia, and Provident Hospital, Baltimore.

32. Charles Watts, M.D., interview by the author, tape recording, August 28, 1996.

33. Susan L. Smith, *Sick and Tired of Being Sick and Tired: Black Women's Health Activism in America, 1890–1950* (Philadelphia: University of Pennsylvania Press, 1995), 149–67.

34. John Hatch, interview by the author, tape recording, August 29, 1996.

35. K. Oliver, "Illnesses of Bodies and Minds: Early Black Doctors Faced Both," *Miami Herald,* October 7, 1985, C1, C3.

36. Charles Watts, interview by the author, tape recording, August 28, 1996.

37. Gamble, *Making a Place,* 58.

38. John S. Haller, Jr. "The Physician versus the Negro," in *Outcasts from Evolution: Scientific Attitudes of Racial Inferiority, 1859–1900* (Urbana: University of Illinois Press, 1971), 40–68.

39. Discussion on the paper of Dr. Jones, *Transactions of the Tennessee State Medical Association,* 1907, 180, as reproduced in Gamble, *Germs,* 25.

40. C. E. Terry, "The Negro, a Public Health Problem," *Southern Medical Journal* 5 (1915): 462–63, as reproduced in Gamble, *Germs,* 49–58.

41. E. Mayfield Boyle, "A Comparative Physical Study of the Negro," *Journal*

of the National Medical Association 4 (1912): 344–48, as cited in Gamble, *Germs,* "Introduction," 3.

42. Gamble, *Germs,* "Introduction," 1.

43. Keith Wailoo, *Drawing Blood: Technology and Disease Identity in Twentieth-Century America* (Baltimore: Johns Hopkins University Press, 1997).

44. Aubre L. Maynard, *Surgeons to the Poor: The Harlem Hospital Story* (New York: Appleton-Century-Crofts, 1978), 3.

45. Clovis E. Semmes, *Racism, Health, and Post-industrialism: A Theory of African-American Health* (Westport, Conn: Praeger 1996), 110–11.

46. W. Montague Cobb, "Surgery and the Negro Physician: Some Parallels in Background," *Journal of the National Medical Association* 43 (1951): 148.

47. James H. Jones, *Bad Blood: The Tuskeegee Syphilis Experiment* (New York: Free Press, 1981).

48. No one directly involved in the project has ever acknowledged that anything about it was unethical. All became ensnared in the web of deceit, not only of the subjects of the experiment, but of themselves. In May 1997 at a White House ceremony, President Clinton apologized on behalf of the nation to the remaining survivors and their relatives. Five of the eight remaining survivors, all over ninety years of age, attended the ceremony (Allison Mitchell, "Clinton Regrets 'Clearly Racist' U.S. Study," *New York Times,* May 17, 1997, A1).

49. Paul Cornely, interview by the author, tape recording, July 8, 1990.

50. See, for example: Vanessa N. Gamble, "Under the Shadow of Tuskegee: African Americans and Health Care," *American Journal of Public Health* 87, no. 11 (1997): 1773–78.

51. Philip M. Boffey, "U.S. Drops AIDS Study in Community Protests," *New York Times,* August 17, 1988, A14.

52. Quentin Young, interview by the author, tape recording, June 14, 1997.

53. Deborah Stone, "The Struggle for the Soul of Insurance," *Journal of Health Policy Politics and Law* 18, no. 2 (1993): 287–318.

54. David T. Beito, "The Lodge Practice Evil Reconsidered: Medical Care Through the Fraternal Societies 1900–1930," *Journal of Urban History* 23 (1987): 569–600.

55. Stone, "Struggle for Soul," 296.

56. Isadore Sydney Falk, Margaret Klem, and Nathan Sinai, *The Incidence of Illness and the Receipt and Costs of Medical Care among Representative Families,* Committee on the Cost of Medical Care Report No. 27 (Chicago: University of Chicago Press, 1933), 5.

57. Rufus Rorem, "Scope and Significance of Hospital Care Insurance," summary of remarks at luncheon meeting, Palmer House, April 18, 1938, for announcement of hospital care insurance plans approved by the American Hospital Association and for presentation of approval certificate to Plan for Hospital Care, Chicago, in *Claude A. Barnett Papers: Associated Negro Press, 1918–1967.* Microfilmed from holdings of Chicago Historical Society (Fredrick, Md.: University Publications of America), part 3, series E, 9.

58. L. Abbott, *The Story of NYLIC: A History of the Origin and Development*

of New York Life Insurance Company 1845 to 1929 (New York: New York Life Insurance Company) 279, as quoted in Stone "Struggle the Soul," 299.

59. Interdepartmental Committee to Coordinate Health and Welfare Activities, *Proceedings of the National Health Conference, July 18–20, 1938,* 87.

Chapter 2

1. Confidential interview by the author, tape recorded, June 27, 1996.

2. David Levering Lewis, *W. E. B. Du Bois: Biography of a Race* (New York: Holt, 1993), 174–75.

3. See Gamble, *Making a Place,* esp. 35–69.

4. Ibid., 66–68.

5. Maynard, *Surgeons to the Poor,* 76.

6. Cited in Gamble, *Making a Place,* 64.

7. Maynard, *Surgeons to the Poor,* 77.

8. "20-Year Drive Opens for Negro Hospitals," *New York Times,* February 24, 1934, 11.

9. Letter to Claude Barnett from E. H. Perry, February 10, 1936, *Claude A. Barnett Papers,* part 3, series E, 1.

10. Letter to Claude Barnett from W. Harry Barnes, February 10, 1936, *Claude A. Barnett Papers,* part 3, series E, 1.

11. Amos H. Carnegie, "Washington Proposal for Self-Help," *Modern Hospital* 76 (August 1952): 76–77.

12. W. Montague Cobb, "The Future of Negro Medical Organizations," *Journal of the National Medical Association* 43 (1951):323.

13. T. M. R. Howard, annual message presented to the convention of the National Medical Association, Chicago, in *Claude A. Barnett Papers,* part 3, series E.

14. Carl T. Rowan, *Dream Makers, Dream Breakers: The World of Justice Thurgood Marshall* (Boston: Little, Brown, 1993), 237. At least once, however, Marshall's car wasn't fast enough. He himself barely escaped lynching by the Klan in Maury County, Tennessee, in 1946. Marshall was rescued only at a last-minute standoff by a local group of black ex-GIs armed with automatic weapons. The lynch rope and noose, still hanging by the Duck River the next morning, was cut down by his rescue party as a souvenir (ibid., 111).

15. Gamble, *Making a Place,* 58.

16. Correspondence included in *Papers of the NAACP, part 15, Segregation and Discrimination Complaints and Responses 1940–1955,* series A, Legal Department Files, ed. John H. Bracey, Jr. and August Meic (Bethesda, Md.: University Publications of America) (microfilm).

17. Ibid.

18. Ibid.

19. The material on nursing has been extracted from a previous publication, David Smith, "The Racial Integration of Medical and Nursing Associations in the

United States," *Hospitals and Health Services Administration* 37, no. 3 (1992): 387–405 and is used with permission of Health Administration Press.

20. Robert M. Cunningham, "Jim Crow, M.D.," *Nation,* June 7, 1952, 548–51.

21. D. Reitzes, *Negroes in Medicine* (Cambridge: Harvard University Press, 1957).

22. "Nurses Walk Out in Race Protest," *Modern Hospital* 76, no. 6 (1951): 65.

23. Ibid.

24. "Nurses Unit Votes to Admit Negroes," *New York Times,* September 28, 1946, 5.

25. "Democracy Is Color-Blind," *New York Times,* January 28, 1951, 2.

26. Ibid.

27. While a NACGN representative was appointed to the ANA board at the time of the merger, no additional black appointments to the board were made for another eighteen years. Some twenty years later, in 1971, a new group representing the concerns of black nurses, the National Black Nurses Association, was formed. However, concerns of this group focused on the issues of access and the nature of health care provided black Americans and the ANA's inattention to these issues, rather than issues of discrimination in employment within the profession.

28. Mary Elizabeth Carnegie and Josephine A. Dolan, *The Path We Tread: Blacks in Nursing, 1854–1984* (Philadelphia: Lippincott, 1986), 100.

29. *Journal of the National Medical Association* 31 (1939): 150–53.

30. *Journal of the National Medical Association* 32 (1940): 172.

31. *Journal of the National Medical Association* 38 (1946): 35.

32. Maynard, *Surgeons to the Poor,* 118.

33. Ibid., 120.

34. Ibid., 119.

35. "The Henry Wisdom Cave Testimonial Dinner," *Journal of the National Medical Association* 43 (1951): 191.

36. *Hospital Survey and Construction Act, U.S. Code,* vol. 42, sec. 291e; emphasis added.

37. Virginia Vanderveer Hamilton, *Lister Hill* (Chapel Hill: University of North Carolina Press, 1987).

38. See *Cook v. Ochsner Hospital Foundation et al.,* 61 F.R.D. 354 (E.D. La. 1972).

39. *Bulletin of the Medico-Chirugical Society of the District of Columbia* 4, no. 7 (August–September 1947): 3, 9, 10, in *Claude Barnett Papers..*

40. W. Montague Cobb, "The Seventeenth of May," *Journal of the National Medical Association* 46 (1954): 269.

41. The Memphis NAACP branch had originally supported the construction of a separate public hospital, known as the McLean Plan after its author, Dr. Basil McLean. See "Memphis NAACP Branch Rescinds Endorsement of Negro Hospital," *Journal of the National Medical Association* 44 (1952): 314.

42. W. Montague Cobb, "The National Health Program of the N.A.A.C.P.," *Journal of the National Medical Association* 45 (1953): 333–39.

43. Robert M. Cunningham, "Are Hospitals for the Sick—or Just Some of the Sick?" *Hospitals* 76, no. 6 (1951): 51.

44. Discrimination in Hospitals: Extension of Remarks of Hon. Barratt O'Hara of Illinois in the House of Representatives, February 7, 1955, *Congressional Record,* 84th Cong., 1st sess.

45. Young, interview.

46. Ibid.

47. "Chicago Physicians Sue for Admission to Hospital Staffs," *Journal of the National Medical Association* 55 (1961): 198–99.

48. Arthur Falls, interview by Walter Lear, tape recording, January 9, 1988.

49. Young, interview.

50. Ibid.

51. "Conference on Hospital Integration: Preliminary Announcement," *Journal of the National Medical Association* 48 (1956): 348.

52. Responding to Howard University's concerns about the potential impact on federal appropriations in an increasingly tense political environment, the conference moved from its original site at Howard University. "Proceedings of the Imhotep National Conference on Hospital Integration," *Journal of the National Medical Association* 49 (1957): 189–201.

53. Paul Cornely, interview by the author, tape recording, August 7, 1990.

54. "An Appraisal of the Imhotep Conference," *Journal of the National Medical Association* 49 (1957): 182.

55. "Proceedings of Imhotep Conference," 192.

56. "History of the Imhotep National Conference on Hospital Integration," *Journal of the National Medical Association* 54 (1962): 116–19.

57. "Hill-Burton Faces a Civil Rights Challenge," *Medical World News,* November 10, 1961, as excerpted in "Integration Battlefront," *Journal of the National Medical Association* 54, no. 1 (1962): 123.

58. Watts, interview, August 28, 1996.

59. "Executive Procedure without Effect in Hospital Area," *Journal of the National Medical Association* 54 (1962): 259.

60. "Hospital Discrimination and the Sixth Imhotep Conference," *Journal of the National Medical Association* 54 (1962): 254.

61. James Quigley, memorandum to Harris Wofford, July 6, 1961, Harris Wofford Papers, John F. Kennedy Library.

62. Memorandum from Parks M. Banta, General Counsel, DHEW to the Secretary, September 17, 1960, Harris Wofford Papers, John F. Kennedy Library.

63. Quigley, memorandum to Wofford, 7.

64. *Second Morrill Act,* (26 Stat 417, 7 USC 321–29).

65. Roy Wilkins and Arnold Aronson, "Proposals for Executive Action to End Federally Supported Segregation and Other Forms of Discrimination," submitted to the White House, August 29, 1961, White House Central Files, JFK Library.

66. Wilkins and Aronson, "Proposals for Executive Action," 53.

67. James Quigley, memorandum to the Honorable Harris Wofford, November 15, 1961, Wofford Papers, 3.

68. Taylor Branch, *Parting the Waters: America in the King Years, 1954–63.* (New York: Simon and Schuster, 1988), 399.

69. Burke Marshall, memorandum for the Attorney General, Monday Report, April 9, 1962, Burke Marshall Papers, JFK Library.

70. "Sixth Imhotep Conference Confident of Results from United Broad Effort," *Journal of the National Medical Association* 55 (1962): 501.

Chapter 3

1. C. Richardson Preyer, interview by the author, June 28, 1996.

2. For a detailed description of South before the civil rights era, see John Egerton, *Speak Now against the Day: The Generation before the Civil Rights Movement in the South* (New York: Knopf, 1994).

3. Several editorials appear, for example, in the *Greensboro News* on October 12, 1926, and May 16, 1929, and in other North Carolina papers during this decade protesting the conditions that permitted such events, usually in other states. See *Papers of the NAACP,* part 7, series A, Anti-Lynching Investigative Files, 1912–53, group 1, (Fredrick, Md.: University Publications of America), microfilm.

4. Ibid., 129–34.

5. Conrad Pearson, William A. March, and Floyd McKissick and other black lawyers had found more profitable business pursuits. C. C. Spalding founded North Carolina Mutual Insurance Company in Durham, and John Wheeler served as president of the Mechanics and Farmers Bank in the same city. See Jack Greenberg, *Crusaders in the Courts* (New York: Basic Books, 1994), 37–41.

6. Ibid., 40.

7. North Carolina Advisory Committee to the U.S. Commission on Civil Rights, *Equal Protection of the Laws Concerning Medical Care in North Carolina,* November 9, 1961, table 1, North Carolina Archives, University of North Carolina.

8. North Carolina Advisory Committee, *Equal Protection of Laws.*

9. Watts, interview, August 28, 1996.

10. For a detailed chronicling of these events see Robert L. Phillips, M.D., *The History of Integration of Medicine in Greensboro, North Carolina: Chronological Documentation* (Greensboro, N.C.: Greensboro Medical Historical Library, November 1990).

11. Robert Phillips, M.D., interview by the author, tape recorded, June 25, 1996.

12. Louis deS. Shaffner, "Racial Integration in the North Carolina Medical Society," *North Carolina Medical Journal* 51, no. 1 (1990): 43.

13. "Resolution on Restrictive Membership Provisions," *Journal of the American Medical Association* 143 (1950): 1086; emphasis added.

14. A. L. Terence, "NMA Activities: Impressions of the NMA Convention in Detroit," *Journal of the National Medical Association* 41 (1949): 233.

15. Phillips, *Integration of Medicine,* 16.

16. Confidential interview by the author, June 25, 1996, tape recorded.

17. Phillips, *Integration of Medicine,* 16.

18. Transactions 1955, *North Carolina Medical Journal* 1955:16–376.

19. Shaffner, "Racial Integration," 44.

20. Phillips, *Integration of Medicine,* 25–26.

21. Shaffner, "Racial Integration," 45.

22. Ibid., 45–46.

23. Watts, interview, August 28, 1996.

24. Ibid.

25. Shaffner, "Racial Integration," 45.

26. Hubert A. Eaton, *Every Man Should Try* (Wilmington, N.C.: Bonaparte Press, 1984), 225.

27. Ibid., 224.

28. "AMA 1966 Action on Discrimination," *Journal of the National Medical Association* 58 (1966): 383.

29. Shaffner, "Racial Integration," 46.

30. *The Carolinas and Georgia Coast* (New York: Fodor's Travel Publications, 1996), 107.

31. Watts, interview, August 28, 1996.

32. Schaffner, "Racial Integration," 46.

33. Eaton, *Every Man Should Try,* 3–4.

34. Ibid., 55.

35. *Eaton v. Board of Managers of James Walker Memorial Hospital,* 4 Cir., 261 F.2d 521, affirming 164 F. Supp. 191 (E.D.N.C. 1958), Cert. den. 359 U.S. 984, 79 S.Ct.941, 3 L.Ed.2d 934.

36. Eaton, *Every Man Should Try,* 55.

37. *Greensboro Daily News,* June 16, 1990, 1.

38. A bill was introduced to the state legislature that would let all licensed dentists vote for the State Board of Medical Examiners instead of having them chosen by the all-white North Carolina Dental Society. Hawkins attacked this proposal as a stratagem on the part of the society (*Charlotte Observer,* February 23, 1961).

39. See William H. Chafe, *Civilities and Civil Rights: Greensboro, North Carolina, and the Black Struggle for Freedom* (New York: Oxford University Press, 1980).

40. See Hal Sieber, *Holy Ground: Significant Events in the Civil Rights Related History of the African American Communities of Guilford County, North Carolina, 1771–1996* (Greensboro, N.C.: Simkins-Smith Center, 1995).

41. Tourgee in the *Plessy* case had attempted to turn the contorted logic of race against the segregationists, arguing that the case represented not a defense of a colored man against discrimination by whites, but a defense of the "nearly" white man against the penalties of color. In a property-conscious culture, the holder of the smallest bit of property (e.g., one drop white blood) was entitled to the same rights as those with the largest proportion of white blood, a fact he hoped would turn the enforcement of segregation into an administrative nightmare that would collapse of its own weight. See Otto H. Olsen, *Carpetbaggers Crusade: The Life of Albion Winegar Tourgee* (Baltimore: Johns Hopkins University Press, 1965).

42. Preyer, interview.

43. Moses Cone's father was Herman Cone, a German Jewish immigrant who

arrived in the United States at the age of seventeen in 1846. By the 1870s he was the owner of a thriving dry goods business in Baltimore. His two sons, Moses and Ceasar, served as traveling salesmen through the Carolinas. By the 1890s the Cone brothers had struck out on their own, constructing three textile mills in Greensboro, transforming its landscape, and amassing a fortune. In 1908 Moses died without a will, leading to an agreement signed in 1911 under which Bertha Cone, Moses' window, conveyed all her stock to a proposed hospital. During her lifetime she would receive income from the stock, and when she died, the assets would be used to build the hospital. It was not an elegant arrangement for Greensboro's medical community, for Bertha outlived Moses by forty years, dying in 1947—at which point the endowment for the construction of the new hospital at last became available. See Philip T. Noblitt, *A Mansion in the Mountains: The Story of Moses and Bertha Cone and Their Blowing Rock Manor* (Boone, N.C.: Parkway, 1996), 114.

44. Phillips, interview.

45. Phillips, *Integration of Medicine,* 1.

46. Alexander R. Stoesen, *A History of Guilford County* (1993) North Carolina Division of Archives and History.

47. Phillips, *Integration of Medicine,* 4.

48. Minutes of the Executive Committee, Moses Cone Memorial Hospital, October 12, 1950, 16, Moses Cone Hospital.

49. Ibid., March 13, 1952, 667–70.

50. Ibid., December 3, 1953, 759.

51. AFSC memorandum, March 10, 1954, January 19, 23, 1953, AFSC Papers, Philadelphia, as reported in Chafe, *Civilities and Civil Rights,* 49.

52. Harold Bettis, interview by the author, June 25, 1996, tape recorded.

53. George Simkins, interview by the author, May 3, 1996, tape recorded.

54. Minutes of the Board of Trustees, Moses Cone Memorial Hospital, December 11, 1952, 703.

55. Ibid., February 25, 1960, 1008.

56. John Harden, memorandum to Spencer Love on the Cone Hospital Survey, May 25, 1956, Moses Cone Hospital Historical Collection.

57. Letter to J. Spencer Love from Benjamin Cone, May 31, 1956, Moses Cone Hospital Historical Collection.

58. Phillips, interview.

59. Edward P. Benbow Jr., M.D., "Polio Epidemic," *North Carolina Medical Journal* 52, no. 6 (1991): 475–77; emphasis added.

60. S. Dubose Ravenel, M.D., "History of Polio in Greensboro," in *History of Medicine in Greensboro: A Series of Essays by Prominent Health Care Providers,* vol. 2 (Greensboro, N.C.: Greensboro Historical Medical Library, Printworks, 1991.

61. Chafe, *Civilities and Civil Rights,* 39.

62. Chafe, *Civilities and Civil Rights,* 111.

63. Jack Greenberg, *Crusaders in the Courts* (New York: Basic Books 1994), 363.

64. Letter to George Simkins from Thurgood Marshall, August 12, 1958, A&T Library Simkins Collection.

65. Letter to George Simkins from Jack Greenberg, September 18, 1958, A&T Library Simkins Collection.

66. Simkins, interview.

67. *Greensboro Daily News,* June 9, 1962, 1.

68. Correspondence in the Historical Collection of Moses Cone Hospital.

69. Correspondence to Charles E. Roth from Earl B. May November 29, 1963, Historical Collection of Moses Cone Hospital.

70. Bettis, interview.

71. Minutes of the Executive Committee, Moses Cone Memorial Hospital, March 11, 1964, 1048.

72. *New York Times,* March 2, 1964, 1.

73. "Historic Decision on Segregation," *Medical World News,* November 22, 1963, 54–56.

74. Arthur Krock, "A Court Ruling Extended to Pending Legislation," *New York Times,* March 4, 1964.

75. Note from Charles Roth to Harold Bettis, March 5, 1964, Moses Cone Hospital Historical Collection.

Chapter 4

1. John F. Kennedy, Special Message to Congress on Civil Rights and Job Opportunities, June 19, 1963, *Public Papers of the Presidents of the United States: John F. Kennedy, 1963* (Washington, D.C: Government Printing Office, 1964), 492.

2. "Vote Cast for President, by Major Political Party, 1936 to 1992," *The American Almanac* (Austin, Tex.: Reference Press, 1994), 269.

3. House Judiciary Committee, Subcommittee No. 5, Statement by the Southern Regional Council, Inc., Atlanta, June 25, 1963, *Civil Rights: Hearings Before Subcommittee No. 5,* 2587.

4. The AMA board of trustees executive committee refused to take action, claiming that membership in local societies was outside AMA jurisdiction and refusing to provide membership at large to those excluded on a local basis from membership because of race. Separate but equal Hill-Burton referred to the council on legislative activities and JCAH standards proposal referred to the Joint Commission. Ibid., 1846.

5. *Civil Rights: Hearings,* 1531–32.

6. Ibid., 1541.

7. Charles Whalen and Barbara Whalen, *The Longest Debate: A Legislative History of the 1964 Civil Rights Act* (Washington, D.C.: Seven Locks Press, 1985), 45.

8. Subcommittee No. 5, *Civil Rights: Hearings,* 2774–75.

9. Lyndon Baines Johnson, "Address before a Joint Session of the Congress," November 27, 1963, in *Public Papers of the Presidents of the United States: Lyndon B. Johnson 1963–64* (Washington, D.C.: Government Printing Office, 1965), 9.

10. Whalen and Whalen, *The Longest Debate,* 115–18.

11. Ibid., 140.

12. *Congressional Record,* Senate, March 3, 1964, 88th Congress, 2nd Session, 4183.

13. Ibid., 4185.

14. Ibid., June 10, 1964, A1332.

15. *Congressional Record,* Senate, April 21, 1964, 88th Cong., 2d sess., 8615.

16. Ibid., March 30, 1994, 6543–44.

17. Ibid., April 7, 1994, 7054.

18. Ibid., April 7, 1994, 7055.

19. Ibid., 7064.

20. Whalen and Whalen, *The Longest Debate,* 199–200.

21. Ibid., 213.

22. Ibid., 227–28.

23. "Celebrezze Testimony on Non-discrimination under Hill-Burton Law and Imhotep Type Conference," *Journal of the National Medical Association* 56 (1964): 286.

24. Nathaniel Wesley, "Struggle for Survival: Black Community Hospitals, 1961 to 1988," unpublished thesis prepared for Fellowship of the American College of Healthcare Executives, 1989, 20–21.

25. "H.E.W. Conference on the Elimination of Hospital Discrimination," *Journal of the National Medical Association* 56 (1964): 446.

26. Title 45—Public Welfare, Subtitle A—Department of Health, Education and Welfare, General Administration, Part 80, "Nondiscrimination in Federally-Assisted Programs of the Department of Health Education and Welfare—Effectuation of Title VI of the Civil Rights Act of 1964," *Federal Register* 29, no. 236 (December 4, 1964): 16298–305.

27. Ibid., 16301.

28. "National Conference on Title VI—Civil Rights Act of 1964," *Journal of the National Medical Association* 57 (1965): 164.

29. Robert L. Phillips, *History of the Hospitals in Greensboro, North Carolina* (Greensboro, N.C.: Printworks, 1996), 112.

30. Excerpted anonymous correspondence by the Administrator of Moses Cone Hospital, 1963, Moses Cone Memorial Hospital Historical Collection.

31. Draft questionnaire, undated, Moses Cone Memorial Hospital Historical Collection.

32. *Eaton v. Grubbs,* 329 F.2d 710, 715 (1964).

33. Eaton, *Every Man Should Try,* 60.

34. Charles Johnson, Jr., M.D., interview by the author, tape recording, June 24, 1996.

35. *Bell, et al. v. The Northern District Dental Society, et. al.* N.D. Ga., Civil Action No. 7966 Decided January 21, 1964).

36. J. William Pinkston, Jr., interview by the author, tape recording, June 10, 1996.

37. For a description of the continuing impact of the shift that took place in the

1964 election, see, for example, Thomas Byrne Edsall with Mary D. Edsall, *Chain Reaction: The Impact of Race, Rights, and Taxes on American Politics* (New York: Norton, 1991).

38. See, for example, Theodore Malmor, *The Politics of Medicare* (Chicago: Aldine, 1973); Richard Harris, *The Sacred Trust* (Baltimore, Md.: Penguin Books, 1969); Judith Feder, *Medicare: The Politics of Federal Health Insurance* (Lexington, Mass.: Lexington Books, 1977); David Blumenthal, "Medicare: The Beginnings," in *Renewing the Promise: Medicare and Its Reform,* ed. David Blumenthal, Mark Schlesinger, and Pamela Drumheller (New York: Oxford University Press, 1988), 3–19.

39. Walter Lear, interview by the author, tape recording, April 23, 1997.

40. "Third Meeting of the AMA-NMA Representatives," *Journal of the National Medical Association* 56 (1964): 104.

41. "NAACP Health Resolutions, 1964," *Journal of the National Medical Association* 56 (1964): 542.

42. Hubert A. Eaton, "Views of the North Carolina Negro Physicians on Medical Assistance for the Aged," *Journal of the National Medical Association* 57 (1965): 167.

43. "NMA President's Testimony in Support of H.R. 6675," *Journal of the National Medical Association* 57 (1965): 335.

44. Anthony Celebrezze to Senator Harry Byrd, April 27, 1965, Presidential Central Files, Lyndon Baines Johnson Library.

45. Lyndon Baines Johnson, "Statement by the President Following Passage of the Medicare Bill by the Senate," July 9, 1965, in *Public Papers,* 731–32.

46. Herman Somers and Anne Somers, *Medicare and the Hospitals: Issues and Prospects* (Washington, D.C.: Brookings Institution, 1967), 4–5.

47. Mary Holman, secretary of MCHR, memorandum to John Parham, September 9, 1965, Medical Committee for Human Rights Archives, Institute of Social Medicine and Community Health.

48. John Parham, memorandum to Ruth Hurwitz, September 9, 1965, Medical Committee for Human Rights Archives.

49. Legal Defense Fund, memorandum to John Gardner, December 16, 1965, Medical Committee for Human Rights Archives.

50. Statement by John Hollowman, December 16, 1965, Medical Committee for Human Rights Archives.

51. These five were the Office of Education, the Public Health Service, the Surplus Property Division attached to the Office of the Secretary, the Vocational Rehabilitation Administration, and the Welfare Administration.

52. DHEW and other executive agencies worked on a fiscal year running from July 1 to June 30. Budget requests were submitted to the Bureau of the Budget during the fall and then, after review, to Congress in January as a part of the president's budget for the executive branch. The budget committees in the House and Senate subsequently reviewed and heard testimony on the budget from DHEW officials, and allowed or disallowed parts of the request. Other legislative requests had to be factored into these negotiations.

53. John Gardner, memorandum to Executive Staff, December 14, 1965, in Elaine Heffernan, "OCR Historical Record, Title VI Implementation," DHEW, December 1968, LBJ Library, 163–64.

54. Lyndon Baines Johnson, "Statement to the Cabinet Affirming the Duty of Federal Employees to Respect the Constitutional Rights of Others," March 25, 1965, in *Public Papers,* 317.

55. Lyndon Baines Johnson, "Memorandum on Reassignment of Civil Rights Functions," September 24, 1965, in *Public Papers,* 1017. (The memorandum included one from the vice president supporting the reorganization, but drafted by the president's staff for Humphrey's signature. See Joseph A. Califano, *The Triumph and Tragedy of Lyndon Johnson* [New York: Simon and Schuster, 1991], 65–68.)

56. This meeting was a well-entrenched part of the folk wisdom among older staff in the Office for Civil Rights interviewed in this study. The exact nature of this conversation is important in interpreting subsequent events but must await the release of the presidential tapes.

57. James M. Quigley, "Hospitals and the Civil Rights Act of 1964," read to the Sixty-seventh Annual Meeting of the American Hospital Association, San Francisco, September 1, 1965, *Journal of the National Medical Association* 57 (1965): 455–58.

58. "Title VI and Hospitals," *Journal of the National Medical Association* 58 (1966): 212–13.

59. Ibid., 212.

60. Quigley, "Hospitals," 457–58.

61. Frank Weil, interview by the author, tape recorded, July 1995.

62. Ibid.

63. Ibid.

64. Peter Libassi, memorandum to Califano, Cater, and Katzenbach, Title VI Compliance—Hospitals, April 25, 1966, White House Central Files, LBJ Library.

65. Farris Bryand, memorandum for the president, May 23, 1966, White House Central Files, LBJ Library.

66. Weil, interview.

67. Confidential interview by the author, tape recorded, July 7, 1996.

68. Weil, interview.

69. Ibid.

70. Douglass Cater, memorandum to the President, Report on Hospital Civil Rights Compliance Efforts in the South, June 18, 1966, White House Central Files, LBJ Library.

71. Lyndon Baines Johnson, "Remarks to Members of the National Council of Senior Citizens," June 3, 1966, in *Public Papers,* 578–79.

72. Lyndon Baines Johnson, "Remarks at a Meeting with Medical and Hospital Leaders to Prepare the Launching of Medicare," June 25, 1966, in *Public Papers,* 605–6.

73. Douglass Cater, memorandum to the President, June 23, 1966, White House Central Files, LBJ Library.

74. Peter Libassi, memorandum to Douglass Cater, Hospital Compliance Program—Congressional Contacts, June 28, 1966, White House Central Files, LBJ Library.

75. Lyndon Baines Johnson, "Statement by the President on the Inauguration of the Medicare Program," June 30, 1966, in *Public Papers,* 676–77.

Chapter 5

1. Young, interview.

2. Peter Libassi, memorandum to Califano, Cater, and Katzenbach, July 28, 1966, White House Central Files, LBJ Library.

3. Attachment to memorandum from Peter Libassi to Califano, Cater, and Doar, November 18, 1966, White House Central Files, LBJ Library.

4. Confidential interview by the author, tape recorded, July 17, 1995.

5. Frank Weil, interview by the author, tape recorded, June 27, 1995.

6. C. E. Beardsley, "Good-bye to Jim Crow: The Desegregation of Southern Hospitals, 1945–70," *Bulletin of the History of Medicine* 60 (1986): 367–86.

7. *United States v. Medical Society of South Carolina,* 289 F. Supp. 145 (1969).

8. Marilyn Rose, memorandum to the author, November 20, 1997, 3.

9. Ibid.

10. Ibid., 4–5.

11. Ibid., 5–6.

12. Peter Libassi, memorandum to Douglass Cater, January 12, 1967, White House Central Files, LBJ Library.

13. Rose, memorandum, 8–9.

14. Governor Johnson owed his election to an unexpected opportunity to play the race card. Because of bad flying weather, his predecessor, Governor Ross Barnett, had been delayed in getting to Oxford to confront the federal marshals protecting James Meredith in his attempt to register at the University of Mississippi (James W. Silver, *Mississippi: The Closed Society* [New York: Harcourt, Brace and World, 1964], 44). As lieutenant governor, Johnson arrived with state troopers to block Meredith's second attempt to enter the front gate of the university. Johnson ran for governor in 1963 on the slogan, "Stand Tall for Paul, He Stood Tall for You" (Jason Berry, *Amazing Grace: With Charles Evers in Mississippi* [New York: Saturday Review, 1973], 42). Several years later, the former governor in an interview revealed an eerie familiarity with the circumstances surrounding the murder of three civil rights workers, James Chaney, Andrew Goodman, and Michael Schwerner, in June 1964.

One thing that is not known to people anywhere in this country is that these Klansmen—of course I knew them well; most of them had supported me when I ran for governor—did not intend to kill these people. What happened was that they had been taken from jail and brought to this spot. There were many people in the group besides the sheriff and deputy sheriff and that group. What they were going to do, they were going to hang these three persons up in a big cotton

352 Notes to Pages 152–56

sack and leave them hang in the tree for about a day or a day and a half, then come out there at night and turn them loose. They thought that they'd more or less scare them off. While they were talking this Negro [James], the Negro boy from over in Meridian, he seemed to be the ringleader of the three. He was acting kind of smart aleck and talking pretty big, and one of the Klansmen walked up behind him and hit him over the head with a trace chain that you use, you know, plowing and that sort of thing. And the end of it is about that large [two or three inches long] . . . The chain came across his head and hit him just above the bridge of the nose and killed him as dead as a nit. After this boy had been killed, then is when they determined, "Well, we've got to dispose of the other two."

Paul Johnson, interview, September 8, 1970, Interviewed by T. H. Baker, Oral History Collection, LBJ Library.

15. Derrick Bell, memorandum to David Rose, Special Assistant to the Attorney General, June 14, 1967, White House Central Files, LBJ Library.

16. Rose, memorandum, 10–11.

17. Derrick Bell, memorandum to David Rose, Special Assistant to the Attorney General, June 23, 1967, White House Central Files, LBJ Library.

18. "Mobile Physician Fatally Wounded," *Mobile Register,* January 30, 1967, 1, 1.

19. "Dr. Cowsert's Death Ruled Accidental," *Mobile Register,* February 1, 1967, 6, 8.

20. A fifth hospital, Doctor's Hospital, a for profit facility with 135 beds also provided care for whites only and was also refused Title VI certification for Medicare but played a secondary marginal role in the ensuing civil rights struggle.

21. Robert Gilliard, DDS, telephone interview, May 7, 1998.

22. DHEW, Title VI Decision, Mobile Infirmary, Mobile, Alabama, Part II (July 14, 1997): 1.

23. Letter to James Quigley, Assistant Secretary of DHEW, August 13, 1965 from J. L. Leflore Non-Partisan Voter's League Archives, University of Southern Alabama.

24. Susan Chapman, RN (Supervisory nurse Providence Hospital, Mobile during the 1960's), interview by author, September 29, 1995, tape recording. The drop in the census of Providence Hospital was also noted in Title VI Decision, Mobile Infirmary, Mobile, Alabama, Part II (July 14, 1967): 1.

25. Title VI Decision, Mobile Infirmary, section II (July 14, 1967): 1.

26. Quentin Young (Member of the Committee to End Segregation in Chicago's Hospitals) interview by author, June 14, 1997, tape recording and "Chicago Physicians Sue Admission to Hospital Staffs," *Journal of the National Medical Association* 55, no. 2 (March 1961): 198–99.

27. Such more subtle patterns persist and have been frequently documented in recent analysis on racial disparities in use. See, for example, Marion E. Gornick, Paul W. Eggers, Thomas W. Reilly, et al., "Effect of Race and Income on Mortality and Use of Services among Medicare Beneficiaries," *New England Journal of Medicine* 355 (1996): 791–99.

28. Mobile Physician Fatally Wounded," *Mobile Register,* January 30, 1967, 6, 3.

29. OEHO staff member, interview by author, July 17, 1995, tape recording.

30. Letter from J. L. LaFlore to James Quigley, October 6, 1966, Archives of the Non-Partisan Voters League. University of Southern Alabama.

31. Letter from J. L. LeFlore to Robert Nash December 20, 1966, Archives of the Non-Partisan Voters League, University of Southern Alabama

32. "Infirmary Has 100 Vacancies as HEW Stalls Medicare OK," *Mobile Register,* December 18, 1966, vertical files of the Mobile Register, Mobile Municipal Archives.

33. "HEW Discriminates" *Mobile Register,* December 18, 1966, vertical files of the Mobile Register, Mobile Municipal Archives.

34. "Wallace Joins Protest Over Medicare Okay Denial" *Mobile Register* December 21, 1966, vertical files of the Mobile Register, Mobile Municipal Archives.

35. This was believed to be common practice. For example, the Birmingham hotel switchboard calls of *New York Times* reporter Harrison Salisbury in 1960 had been monitored and all those, which he had contacted for the story he was writing, had been subpoenaed by a grand jury and publicly harassed. Even the calls by Byron White from the Maxwell Air Force Base in Montgomery, Alabama, to the president during the 1961 Freedom Rides had been monitored and transmitted to Alabama's governor providing key intelligence to assist in his negotiations with the federal government. See Don T. Carter, *The Politics of Rage* (New York: Simon and Schuster, 1995), 229–30.

36. Marilyn Rose, interview. An FBI investigation into the death was apparently requested by OEHO. A Freedom of Information and Privacy Act request of the FBI by the author revealed no records of such an investigation. Officials higher up in DHEW may have chosen not to pursue the matter further. No records of the Mobile Police Department's original investigation into the death could be located in its Municipal Archives, the autopsy report was apparently destroyed in a flood, and the Mobile coroner, who conducted the autopsy and also served as the pathologist at the Mobile Infirmary, could not recall anything about the investigation.

37. "Referral Vow was Refused by Physicians" *Mobile Register,* February 23, 1967, vertical files of the Mobile Register, Mobile Municipal Archives.

38. "Arrogance of HEW on Medicare Confirmed." *Mobile Register,* February 22, 1967, vertical files of the Mobile Register, Mobile Municipal Archives.

39. "Medicare, New Addition, Top '67 activities." *Mobile Register,* January 24, 1968, vertical files of the Mobile Register, Mobile Municipal Archives.

40. Rose, memorandum, 14.

41. Heffernan, "OCR Historical Record," 17.

42. Howard Bennett, interview by the author, June 21, 1995, tape recording.

43. *New Orleans States-Item,* November 25, 1966, 2.

44. 42 U.S.C. § 2000d-1 (1976). See discussion in Title VI of the Civil Rights Act 837–39.

45. See U.S. Commission on Civil Rights: The Federal Civil Rights Enforcement Effort—1974, part 4, To Extend Federal Financial Assistance 118–19; (1975)

and Civil Rights Issues in Health Care Delivery: A Consultation Sponsored by the United States Commission on Civil Rights, Washington, D.C.: U.S. Commission on Civil Rights, April 15–16, 1980, 850–82.

46. Committee on Public Relations, Indiana Medical Society, press release, November 1967, personal papers of Quentin Young.

47. Wilbur J. Cohen, memorandum to Henry Wills, the Attorney General, the Secretary of Labor, and Director, Bureau of the Budget, March 15, 1966, White House Central Files, LBJ Library; emphasis added.

48. Peter Libassi, memorandum to Harry McPherson, Special Counsel to the President, March 16, 1966, White House Central Files, LBJ Library.

49. U.S. Commission on Civil Rights, *HEW and Title VI* (Washington, D.C.: Government Printing Office, 1970), 10–11.

50. Jim Gaither, memorandum to Matt Nimetz, October 28, 1968, White House Central Files, LBJ Library.

51. Steve Polack, memorandum, to White House staff, October 17, 1968, White House Central Files, LBJ Library.

52. According to reports of recently released White House tapes, Nixon actively considered an idea put forward by speechwriter and later presidential candidate Patrick Buchanan to secretly divert 10 percent of the campaign money raised for Republicans to a third-party black candidate in order to undercut the Democratic nominee. Mike Feinsibler, "Nixon, Aides Secretly Planned to Finance Black Candidate," *Philadelphia Inquirer,* November 28, 1996, 1.

53. *Simkins v. Moses H. Cone Memorial Hospital,* 323 F.2d 959, 971 (1963).

54. An OCR staffer tells the story.

One day I went down to mail a letter. As I went to the corner to mail it, this guy tosses a bundle of newspapers off the delivery truck. The wire was still on them, but I notice the headline: "Panetta Resigns." . . . I walk into Panetta's office and . . . flash the headline at him. "Jesus! What the hell is this?" Anyway, it seems that someone had made an announcement in the Senate that he understood that Panetta had resigned, and that's where the headline had come from. Leon called the secretary to find out what was going on. It seems that the secretary had a call from the White House, asking to know what they knew about it. There had been no resignation, and the White House hadn't asked for one, but Panetta ended up writing one. (anonymous interview, July 17, 1995)

This account differs in a few minor details from Panetta's own. See Leon Panetta and Peter Gall, *Bring Us Together: The Nixon Team and the Civil Rights Retreat* (Philadelphia: Lippincott, 1971), 351–67.

55. Panetta and Gall, *Bring Us Together,* 368.

56. Richardson would latter serve as Nixon's attorney general and, in the dark endgame of the Watergate scandals, refuse to fire the special prosecutor investigating the incident and be fired himself in what became known as the Saturday Night Massacre. Potinger would become an attorney in the Civil Rights Division of the Justice Department after the Nixon administration stint in OCR and latter become

a best-selling author of murder mysteries. Panetta would return as President Clinton's chief of staff during his first term.

57. National Center for Health Statistics, *Health in the United States, 1994* (Hyattsville, Md.: Public Health Service, 1995), 229.

58. *Hospital Survey and Construction Act,* sec. 291c(e).

59. Rose, memorandum, 14.

60. Ibid., 15.

61. *Cook v. Ochsner.*

62. *Cook v. Ochsner,* 361.

63. The impact was watered down by concessions to the hospital industry in crafting the regulations and by delays in their enforcement. See Marilyn Rose, "The Federal Regulation of Services to the Poor under the Hill-Burton Act: Realities and Pitfalls," *Northwestern University Law Review* 70, no. 1 (1975): 168–201.

64. Peter Jacobson, telephone interview by the author, April 11, 1996.

65. Rose, memorandum, 18.

66. For contrasting views see, for example: Thomas Buchmeuller and Paul Feldstein, "Hospital Community Benefits Other than Charity Care: Implications for Tax Exemption Policy," *Hospital and Health Services Administration* 41 (1996):441, and Anthony Kovner, "The Hospital Community Benefit Standards Program and Health Reform," *Hospital and Health Services Administration* 39 (1994):143–58.

67. Peter Jacobson, telephone interview by the author, April 11, 1996.

68. Jacobson, interview.

69. Marilyn Rose, "Access for Minorities into Mainstream Hospital Care," *Clearing House Review,* June 1979, 83–86.

70. Institute of Medicine, *Health Care in a Context of Civil Rights* (Washington, D.C., 1981), appendix E, "Case Study: *Cook v. Ochsner,*" 174–84.

71. Alan Sager, "Urban Hospital Closings in the Face of Racial Change: A Statement on Hospital Financing Problems," in *Civil Rights Issues in Health Care Delivery* (Washington, D.C.: U.S. Commission on Civil Rights, 1980), 383–432.

72. Raymond A. Mohl, *Steel City: Urban and Ethnic Patterns in Gary, Indiana, 1906–1950* (New York: Holmes and Meier, 1986), 63.

73. Everett Johnson, interview by the author, June 10, 1996, tape recording.

74. Everett Johnson, Administrator, memorandum from to Steering Committee of Board of Directors et al., January 31, 1963, NAACP Legal Defense Fund files.

75. Minutes of the Board of Directors, Methodist Hospital of Gary, October 28, 1963, p. 3, NAACP Legal Defense Fund Pleading Files.

76. Ibid., March 18, 1964.

77. Minutes of the Executive Committee of the Board of Directors, Methodist Hospital of Gary, September 28, 1964, NAACP Legal Defense Fund Pleading Files.

78. *NAACP v. Wilmington Medical Center,* 426 F. Supp. 919 (D. Del. 1977).

79. Dewey E. Dodds, Director Office for Civil Rights, Region III, Letter of Findings to James Harding, President of the Wilmington Medical Center, July 5, 1977. Exhibit A Second Supplement to Court U.S. District Court. Delaware NAACP v. Wilmington Medical Center.

80. *NAACP v. Wilmington Medical Center Inc.* 491 F. Supp. 290 (D:Del 1980); aff'd 627 F.2d 1322 (3d Cir. 1981).

81. Norman L. Cannon, *The History of a Hospital Merger: The Wilmington Medical Center, 1965–1985* (Wilmington, Del.: Harpart House, 1987).

82. Ibid., 201.

83. Marilyn Rose, personal memo.

84. *Adams v. Richardson,* 356 F.Supp. 92, 95 (DC Cir. 1973); and *Women's Equity Action League v. Cavazos,* 906 F.2d 742 (DC Cir. 1990).

85. The basic framework was established in the Supreme Court decision in *Griggs v. Duke Power Co.,* 401 U.S. 424 (1971), considerably weakened in *Wards Cove Packing Co. v. Atonio,* 490 U.S. 641 (1989), and strengthened and clarified by the Civil Rights Restoration Act of 1991.

86. 45 C.F.R. Part 80.3(b)(2)(1993).

87. *Washington v. Davis,* 426 U.S. 224, 238–48 (1976). The case challenged the constitutionality (Fourteenth Amendment establishes that a state shall not "deny to any person within its jurisdiction the equal protection of the laws") of a police department qualifying test that excluded 57 percent of the black applicants but only 13 percent of the white. The Court concluded that the constitutional standard was purposeful discrimination.

88. J. C. McBride, "Title VI: The Impact/Intent Debate Enters the Municipal Services Arena," *St. John's Law Review* 44 (1980): 124–52; S. D. Watson, "Reinvigorating Title VI: Defending Health Care Discrimination—It Shouldn't Be So Easy," *Fordham Law Review* 58 (1990): 972–73.

89. *Guardians Association v. Civil Service Commission of New York,* 463 U.S. 582, 593–95 (1983) produced a muddled decision that said (1) the intent standard for the Fourteenth Amendment and Title VI are the same, but (2) agencies may develop impact standards that represent a less stringent test.

90. Watson, "Reinvigorating Title VI," 978.

91. *Terry v. Methodist Hospital of Gary,* Nos. H.-76–373 and H-77–154 (N.D. Ind.), consent decree June 8, 1979; *United States v. Bexar County Hospital District,* 484 F. Supp. 855 (W.D. Tex. 1980); *NAACP v. Wilmington Medical Center, Inc.* 491 F. Supp. 290 (D. Del. 1980), aff'd, 657 F.2d 1322 (3d Cir. 1981); *Bryan v. Koch,* 492 F. Supp. 212 (S.D.N.Y), aff'd, 627 F.2d 612 (2d Cir. 1980); and *Mussington v. St Luke's Roosevelt Hospital Center,* No. CIV.92–89618 (S.D.N.Y. filed Dec. 11, 1992) (complaint).

92. Marilyn P. Rose, "Can Hospital Relocations and Closures Be Stopped through the Legal System?" *Health Services Research* 18, no. 4 (1983): 551–74.

93. M. E. Lado, "Breaking the Barriers of Access to Health Care: A Discussion of the Role of Civil Rights Litigation and the Relationship between Burdens of Proof and the Experience of Denial," *Brooklyn Law Review* 60, no. 1 (1994): 262.

94. Indeed, in a book (Panetta and Gall, *Bring Us Together*) devoted to his brief, stormy tenure as the director of the Office for Civil Rights during the first year of the Nixon White House, Panetta makes no mention of health care.

95. R. J. Stewart, statement for U.S. Civil Rights Commission, "Civil Rights Issues in Health Care Delivery."

96. H. A. Foley, statement for "Civil Rights Issues in Health Care Delivery," 346–82.

97. Marilyn P. Rose, statement for "Civil Rights Issues in Health Care Delivery," 107.

98. K. Wing, "Title VI and Health Facilities: Forms without Substance," *Hastings Law Journal* 30 (September 1978): 162.

99. Jacobson, interview.

100. Sylvia Drew Ivie, telephone interview by the author, November 17, 1997.

101. Raymond Wolters, *Right Turn: William Bradford Reynolds, the Reagan Administration, and Civil Rights* (New Brunswick, N.J.: Transaction Publishers, 1996).

102. Jacobson, interview.

103. U.S. Congress, House Committee on Government Operations, Intergovernmental Relations and Human Resources Subcommittee, *Oversight of the Office for Civil Rights at the Department of Health and Human Services: Hearings before a Subcommittee of the Committee on Government Operations, House of Representatives,* Ninety-ninth Cong., 2d Sess., August 6–7, 1986 (Washington: Government Printing Office, 1986).

104. Office for Civil Rights, Health and Human Services Office for Civil Rights Strategic Plan, December 16, 1994, Washington, D.C. Unpublished document office for Civil Rights.

105. U.S. Commission on Civil Rights, *Funding Federal Civil Rights Enforcement* (Washington, D.C.: U.S. Commission on Civil Rights, June 1995).

106. U.S. Commission on Civil Rights, *Federal Title VI Enforcement to Ensure Nondiscrimination In Federally Assisted Programs* (Washington, D,C,: U.S. Commission on Civil Rights, June 1996).

107. Ibid., 221.

Chapter 6

1. HeathQuest, *Monmouth County Baseline Community Health Assessment.* (Lincroft, NJ: HeathQuest, 1996), 70.

2. Smith, Apt Associates, *Community Health Assessment for Broward County Florida* (Swarthmore, Penn: Smith, Apt Associates 1994), 119.

3. Smith, Apt Associates, *Bucks County Community Health Assessment Qualitative Profile* (Swarthmore, Penn: Smith, Apt Associates), 82–83.

4. Charles Johnson, MD. Interview by the author, June 24, 1996, tape recording.

5. Susan Moscow, "Do Race and Ethnicity Influence Perceptions of Health Care Practitioners?" paper presented to the Annual Meeting of the American Public Health Association, November 19, 1996.

6. See Avedis Donabedian, *Explorations in Quality Assessment and Monitoring,* vols. 1–3 (Ann Arbor: Health Administration Press, 1985).

7. John T. Foster, "Survey: What's Ahead for Negro Hospitals?" *Modern Hospital,* November 1967, 109.

8. W. Montague Cobb, "Factors Influencing the Fate of the Negro Hospital," *Journal of the National Medical Association* 59 (1967): 217–18.

9. Calvin Sampson, "Death of the Black Community Hospital: Fact or Fiction," editorial, *Journal of the National Medical Association* 66 (1974): 165.

10. Rice and Jones, *Public Policy,* 115–27.

11. Rob Levin, "Hughes Spalding Hospital Having Grand Opening for New Wing," *Atlanta Journal and Constitution,* July 1, 1984, cited in Wesley, "Struggle for Survival," Appendix III, 1.

12. Charles Johnson, interview.

13. Watts, interview, August 28, 1996.

14. Richard Douglas et al., "Representation of the Black Elderly in Detroit Metropolitan Nursing Homes," *Journal of the National Medical Association* 80(1988):283–88. The connection between these higher rates of nursing-home use and the history of black hospitals in Detroit was pointed out to me by Paul Cornely (personal communication, July 28, 1990). The gap between black and white use of nursing homes, long a source of commentary in the literature has closed, at least according to 1995 National Nursing Home Survey data. These issues will be dealt with in greater detail in chapter 8.

15. Robert Sigmond, interview by the author, tape recording, February 14, 1997.

16. This single-affiliation arrangement undercut the attractive patronage potential of the hospital for city politicians, and they began to lose interest in its operations (Paul Socolar, "The Closing of Philadelphia General Hospital," September 30, 1986 (Medical Committee for Human Rights Archives)). No longer able to play affiliation agreements with one school off against another, PGH began to be cannibalized by the Hospital of the University of Pennsylvania (Edward Sparer, "Medical School Accountability in the Public Hospital," Health Law Project Report, October 1974, Medical Committee for Human Rights Archives). After the passage of Medicare and Medicaid, other hospitals joined in, picking up care for the "better" PGH patients, which now included elderly and working class blacks. PGH was left with a shrinking population of "less desirable" patients. These patients included those with chronic alcohol and drug dependency, the indigent mentally ill, and those suffering from chronic problems related to sexually transmitted diseases, whom the voluntary hospitals wanted neither to deal with nor to mix with their regular patients. PGH completed its closure in 1977 with only a ripple of protest. There was little of the community passion that is typically unleashed by such events (Sigmond, interview).

17. Victor Rodwin et al., *Public Hospital Systems in New York and Paris* (New York: New York University Press, 1992), 66.

18. On the eve of the closing of the hospital's emergency department on September 15, 1980, community residents took over the administrative offices and began demonstrations outside. After the police erected barricades outside the hospital on the morning of September 20, a riot broke out, injuring at least nine persons, including four policemen ("Closing of City Hospital Raises Community Protest," *Hospitals,* October 16, 1980, 22–23).

19. "Judge Clears Hospital Closing in St. Louis," *Hospitals,* October 16, 1979, 20.

20. Kenneth Thorpe, "The Impact of Medicaid Reforms: Cook County and Parkland Memorial Hospitals," in *Managing Safety-Net Hospitals: Cases for Executive Development,* ed. Charles Brecker (Ann Arbor: Health Administration Press, 1993).

21. Andrew B. Bindman, Dennis Keane, and Nicole Lurie, "A Public Hospital Closes: The Impact on Patients' Access to Care and Health Status," *Journal of the American Medical Association* 264 (1990): 2899–2904.

22. Alan Sagar, *Urban Hospital Closings in the Face of Racial Change: A Statement on Hospital Financing* (Washington, D.C.: U.S. Commission on Civil Rights, 1980), 283–432.

23. David G. Whiteis, "Hospital and Community Characteristics in Closures of Urban Hospitals, 1980–87," *Public Health Reports* 107 (1992): 409–16. The percentage of black residents in a community overwhelmed other hospital operational and community characteristics including median household income in predicting closure ($p < .008$).

24. Falk, Klem, and Sinai, *Incidence of Illness,* 5.

25. National Center for Health Statistics, *Health, United States, 1995* (Hyattsville, Md.: National Center for Health Statistics, 1996) 190, data from the National Health Interview Survey.

26. See, for example, Karen Davis, "Equal Treatment and Unequal Benefits: The Medicare Program," *Milbank Quarterly* 53, no. 4 (1975): 449–88; and Martin Ruther and Alan Dobson, "Unequal Treatment and Unequal Benefits: A Reexamination of the Use of Medicare Services by Race, 1967–1976," *Health Care Financing Review* 2, no. 3 (1981): 55–83.

27. See for example, Ruther and Dobson, "Unequal Treatment"; and Charles Link, Stephen Long, and Russell Settle, "Access to Medical Care under Medicaid: Differentials by Race," *Journal of Health Policy Politics and Law* 7, no. 2 (1982): 345–65.

28. Mitchell F. Rice and Mylon Winn, "Black Heath Care and the American Health System: A Political Perspective," in *Health Politics and Policy,* ed. Theodor Litman and Leonard Robins (Albany, N.Y.: Delmar, 1991), 320–35; and Mitchell F. Rice and Mylon Winn, "Black Health Care in America: A Political Perspective," *Journal of the National Medical Association* 82 (1990): 429–36.

29. Robert J. Blendon et al., "Access to Medical Care for Black and White Americans: A Matter of Continuing Concern," *Journal of the American Medical Association* 261 (1989): 278–81; and Tracy A. Lieu, Paul W. Newacheck, and Margaret A. McManus, "Race, Ethnicity, and Access to Ambulatory Care among US Adolescents," *American Journal of Public Health* 83, no. 7 (1993): 960–65.

30. National Center for Health Statistics, *Health in the United States, 1995* (Hyattsville, Md.: National Center for Health Statistics, 1996); *Summary Report to Congress: Monitoring the Impact of Medicare Physician Payment Reform on Utilization and Access,* pub. no. 03357 (Baltimore: Health Care Financing Administration, 1994).

31. Ann Elixhauser, Robert Harris, and Rosanna Coffey, *Trends in Hospital Procedures Performed on Black Patients and White Patients, 1980–87,* Agency for Health Care Policy and Research Publications No. 94–0003, Provider Studies Research Note 20 (Rockville, Md: Public Health Service, 1994).

32. Kenneth C. Goldberg et al., "Racial and Community Factors Influencing Coronary Artery Bypass Graft Surgery Rates for All 1986 Medicare Patients," *Journal of the American Medical Association* 267 (1992): 1473–77; Jeff Whittle et al., "Racial Differences in Use of Invasive Cardiovascular Procedures in the Department of Veterans Affairs Medical System," *New England Journal of Medicine* 329 (1993): 621–27; and Earl S. Ford and Richard S. Cooper, "Racial/Ethnic Differences in Health Care Utilization of Cardiovascular Procedures: A Review of the Evidence," *Health Services Research* 30, no. 1 (1995), pt. 2, 237–52.

33. A. M. McBean and Marian Gornick, "Differences by Race in the Rates of Procedures Performed in Hospitals for Medicare Beneficiaries," *Health Care Financing Review* 15, no. 4 (1994): 77–90.

34. Bertram L. Kasiske et al., "The Effect of Race on Access and Outcome in Transplantation," *New England Journal of Medicine* 324 (1991): 302–7.

35. R. Horner, E. Oddone, and D. Matchar, "Theories Explaining Racial Differences in the Utilization of Diagnostic and Therapeutic Procedures for Cerebrovascular Disease," *Milbank Quarterly* 73, no. 3 (1995): 443–62.

36. William G. Weissert and Cynthia M. Cready, "Determinants of Hospital-to-Nursing Home Placement Delays: A Pilot Study," *Health Services Research* 23, no. 5 (1988): 619–48.

37. David Falcone and Robert Broyles, "Access to Long Term Care: Race as a Barrier," *Journal of Health Politics, Policy, and Law* 19, no. 3 (1994): 583–95.

38. McBean and Gornick, "Differences by Race."

39. Council on Ethical and Judicial Affairs, "Black-White Disparities in Health Care," *Journal of the American Medical Association* 263 (1990): 2344–46.

40. Whittle et al., "Racial Differences in Use."

41. National Center for Health Statistics, *Health in United States, 1996–97,* 115.

42. Gregory Pappas et al., "The Increasing Disparity in Mortality between Socioeconomic Groups in the United States, 1960 and 1986," *New England Journal of Medicine* 329 (1993): 103–9.

43. Richard Rogers, "Living and Dying in the USA: Socio-demographic Determinants of Death among Blacks and Whites," *Demography,* 29 (1992): 287–304.

44. See Barbara S. Starfield et al., "Race, Family Income, and Low Birthweight," *American Journal of Epidemiology* 134(1991):1167–74; and Joel C. Kleinman and Samuel S. Kessel, "Racial Differences in Low Birthweight," *New England Journal of Medicine* 317 (1987): 749–53.

45. For a thoughtful review of the stress and related hypotheses see Marsha Lillie-Blanton et al. "Racial Differences in Health: Not Just Black and White, but Shades of Gray," *Annual Review of Public Health* 17(1996):411–48.

46. Robert Flewelling, *National Household Survey on Drug Abuse: Race/Eth-*

nicity, Socioeconomic Status, and Drug Abuse, 1991 (Washington, D.C.: U.S. Department of Health and Human Services, 1993).

47. W. Montague Cobb, *Medical Care and the Plight of the Negro* (New York: National Association for the Advancement of Colored People, 1947), 7.

48. Smith, *Partners for Healthy Community,* 112.

49. Massey and Denton, *American Apartheid.*

50. The bulk of this section appeared previously in David B. Smith, "The Racial Segregation of Hospital Care Revisited: Medicare Discharge Patterns and Their Implications," *American Journal of Public Health* 88 (1998): 461–63 and is reprinted with permission of the American Public Health Association.

51. Dan Erman and John Gabel, "Multi-hospital Systems: Issues and Empirical Findings," *Health Affairs* 3 (1984): 50–64; Stanley Wohl, *The Medical Industrial Complex* (New York: Harmony, 1984).

52. I present data from two sources: (1) the Expanded Modified MEDPAR (Medicare Provider Analysis and Review) File for Fiscal Year 1993 and (2) the 1990 United State Census Summary, Tape File 1. The MEDPAR file (Health Care Financing Administration) contains records for 100 percent of all Medicare beneficiaries using hospital inpatient services. It includes 11,075,789 discharges from short-term acute and specialty hospitals in the United States in fiscal year 1993. The racial information on beneficiaries in the file is from Social Security enrollment records and subsequent enrollment surveys. This source provides more uniform and complete racial information than that collected through hospital claims data.

53. Massey and Denton, *American Apartheid;* Chung-Hao Li, Joshua G. Bagkas, and Joe T. Darden, "A Comparison of the U.S. Census Summary Tape Files 1a and 3a in Measuring Residential Segregation," *Journal of Economic Social Measures* 21 (1995): 145–55.

54. See Nicholas Lemann, *The Promised Land: The Great Black Migration and How It Changed America* (New York: Knopf 1991).

55. The linear regression model tested the independent effect of each of these five factors on the degree of hospital segregation in a metropolitan area. Specifically, the four measures included in the model were (1) LNPOP (natural log of SMSA total population), (2) HOSDEN (hospital density or the number of hospitals per 100,000 population), (3) RESSEG (index of dissimilarity for residential segregation), (4) INCSEG (index of dissimilarity of racial income differences), and (5) SOUTH (a dummy variable for location of the SMSA in this region).

56. Based on 1993–95 age adjusted rates see: National Center for Health Statistics, *Health in the United States 1996–97,* 109.

57. Katherine L. Kahn et al., "Health Care for Black and Poor Hospitalized Medicare Patients," *Journal of the American Medical Association* 271 (1994): 1169–74.

58. Lola Jean Kozak, "Under Reporting of Race in the National Hospital Discharge Survey," *Advance Data,* (1995): 265. DHHS publication PHS 95-1250.

59. Elixhauser, Harris, and Coffey, *Trends in Hospital Procedures.*

60. Eric Gibson and Jenny Culhane, "Effect of Previable Births on Philadel-

phia Infant Mortality Rates," paper presented to the Annual Meeting of the American Public Health Association, San Diego, November 1, 1995.

61. The May/June issue of *Health Affairs* 17, no. 3 (1998) is devoted to a series of articles that provide a useful review state-related Medicaid program initiatives. It is, however, admittedly difficult to interpret the regional and racial effects of these initiatives.

62. The ironies of "vertical integration" are generally attributed to Harry Golden, editor of the *Carolina Israelite* in Charlotte, North Carolina. See Harry Golden, "The Vertical Negro Plan," in *The Best of Harry Golden* (New York: World Publishing, 1967), 219–22). Golden once noted the evidence of progress toward "gradual integration" in a Charlotte emergency room that had three thermometers: one labeled "white," one "colored," and one "rectal." See John Egerton, *Speak Now Against the Day* (New York: Knopf, 1994), 546.

63. The maintenance of separate accommodations was prohibitively costly and inefficient for many practitioners. White physicians would simply schedule different office hours. Similarly, black barbers whose shops in some communities were patronized by whites during the day would serve black patrons during evening hours.

64. Benjamin Cone, letter to J. Spencer Love, May 31, 1956, Moses Cone Hospital Historical Collection.

65. Yoshi Morohashi, "The Health Care System of Japan," *Japan Hospitals* 14 (July 1995): 5.

66. See, for example, Karen E. Kun and Edward Muir, "Influences on State Legislators," *Public Health Reports* 112 (1997): 274–82; Tracy W. Smirnoff, "Drive-Through Deliveries: Indiscriminate Post partum Early Discharge Practices Presently Necessitate Legislation Mandating Minimum Hospital Stays," *Cleveland State Law Review* 44, no. 2 (1997): 321; and Laura Meckler, "Administration Warns against Pushing Medicare Mastectomies out the Door," Associated Press, February 12, 1997.

67. Uwe Reinhardt, quoted in *American Hospital Association News,* March 4, 1996, 3.

68. See William Barker, *Adding Life to Years* (Baltimore: Johns Hopkins University Press, 1987) for examples of the experimentation in the 1950s in the United States and the actual fruition of these efforts in Great Britain.

69. National Center for Health Statistics, *Health in United States, 1995.*

70. Burton Dunlop, *The Growth of Nursing Home Care* (Lexington Mass.: D.C. Heath, 1979).

71. Smith, *Partners for Healthy Community,* 106.

72. Interest and depreciation reimbursable costs typically exceed debt expenses during the first half of repayment (interest rather than principal, as in the case of a conventional home mortgage, accounts for the bulk of such payments), thus providing a short-term windfall. Some observers during the 1970s likened the behavior of some hospitals to a pyramid scheme, with new windfalls accumulated through more and more new construction. See, for example, the more or less tongue-and-cheek account of this process in George Ross Fisher, *The Hospital That Ate Chicago* (Philadelphia: Saunders Press, 1980).

73. Susan Chapman, R.N., interview by the author, tape recording, September 20, 1995.

74. Morohashi, "Health Care Japan."

75. Pinkston interview.

76. Charles Johnson, interview.

77. Watts, interview, August 28, 1996.

78. The current wave of concern at teaching hospitals is related to the competition from managed care and the need to upgrade services to assure the patient volumes necessary to assure continuing accreditation by the Accrediting Council for Graduate Medical Education. See observations related to an obstetric teaching program in chapter 8.

79. Lawrence Egbert and Ilene L. Rothman, "Relation between the Race and Economic Status of Patients and Who Performs Their Surgery," *New England Journal of Medicine* 297 (1977): 90–99.

80. Lawrence Egbert, letter to author, November 26, 1991.

Chapter 7

1. Bennett, interview.

2. See, for example, more general treatments by Howard Aldrich, *Organizations and Environments* (Englewood Cliffs, N.J.: Prentice-Hall, 1979); Carroll, "Organizational Ecology"; and Jeffrey Pfeffer and Gerald Salanik, *The External Control of Organizations: A Resource Dependent Perspective* (New York: Harper and Row, 1978); as well as efforts to apply such a framework to health care: Alexander, Kaluzny, and Middleton, "Organizational Growth"; and A. Kaluzny, issue ed., *Medical Care Review* 44, no. 2 (1987): 225–408.

3. Stephen Steinberg, *The Ethnic Myth: Race, Ethnicity, and Class in America* (Boston: Beacon Press, 1989), 195–96.

4. John G. Freymann, *The American Health Care System: Its Genesis and Trajectory* (Huntington, N.Y.: Krieger, 1980), chap. 3, cited in Barker, *Adding Life to Years.*

5. Sigmond, interview.

6. Colleen Johnson and Leslie Grant, *The Nursing Home in American Society* (Baltimore: Johns Hopkins University Press, 1985), 5.

7. Bruce Vladeck, *Unloving Care: The Nursing Home Tragedy* (New York: Basic Books, 1980), 30–70.

8. United States Congress, House of Representatives, Committee on Ways and Means, *Hearings on H.R. 4120, Economic Security Act,* 74th Cong., 1st sess., 1935, p. 438; William Thomas, *Nursing Homes and Public Policy* (Ithaca: Cornell University Press, 1969), 49.

9. National Center for Health Statistics, *Institutions for the Aged and Chronically Ill* (Washington, D.C.: Public Health Service, 1965), series 12, no. 1, p. 2.

10. Ibid., 4, 13.

11. Barker, *Adding Life to Years,* 199–200.

12. D. Littauer, F. Steinberg, and G. Gee, *A Chronic Disease Unit in a General*

Hospital: Analysis of Six Years Operating Experience (Chicago: American Hospital Association, 1963), 52, 54, quoted in Barker, *Adding Life to Years,* 112.

13. Health Care Financing Administration, Office of the Actuary: Data from the Office National Health Statistics, <http://www.hcfa.gov>, March 20, 1997.

14. National Center for Health Statistics, *Selected Operating and Financial Characteristics of Nursing Homes in the United States: 1973–74 National Nursing Home Survey,* series 13, no. 2. DHEW Publication No. (HRA) 76–1773 (1975), 10.

15. American Hospital Association, *Hospital Statistics 1995* (Chicago: American Hospital Association, 1996), 2.

16. David Smith, *Long-Term Care in Transition* (Ann Arbor, Mich.: Health Administration Press, 1981), 23; E. Cooros, "Rules Hurt Nursing Homes," *Rochester Democrat and Chronicle,* December 28, 1971.

17. Smith, *Long-Term Care,* 154.

18. Health Care Financing Administration, Summary HCFA-2082 Tables FY 1995, <http://www.hcfa.gov>, March 20, 1997.

19. Health Care Financing Administration, Office of the Actuary, Data from the Office of National Health Statistics, National Health Expenditures by Source of Funds, Calendar Year 1995, <http://www.hcfa.gov>, March 20, 1997.

20. Barker, *Adding Life to Years,* 119.

21. American College of Physicians, Health and Policy Committee, "Long Term Care of the Elderly," *Annals of Internal Medicine* 100 (1984): 760–63.

22. J. Holahan and J. Cohen, "Nursing Home Reimbursement: Implications for Cost Containment, Access, and Quality," *Milbank Quarterly* 665, no. 1 (1987): 112–36.

23. U.S. Commission on Civil Rights, *The Federal Civil Rights Enforcement Effort: One Year Later* (Washington, D.C.: Government Printing Office, 1971), 138, 140.

24. Rosemary Stevens, Chairperson of Institute of Medicine's Committee for a Study of Health Care of Racial/Ethnic Minorities and Handicapped Persons, interview by the author, June 1990.

25. Institute of Medicine, *Health Care in a Context of Civil Rights* (Washington, D.C.: National Academy Press, 1981), 7–8.

26. The Committee on the Cost of Medical Care in their reports in the early 1930s, the earliest systematic effort to study and make recommendations concerning the organization and financing of medical services, clearly envisioned such an integrated continuum of care. Most studies since then have advocated a similar approach. See: example, Barker, *Adding Life to Years.*

27. The avoidance of such risks is part of the widely shared assumptions built into efforts to protect frail, elderly patients. See, for example, Michael Schuster, Patricia DeMichele and Bruce Vignery, "Nursing Home Transfer and Discharge Protections: Rights Not Fully Recognized," *Clearing House Review* 26, no. 6 (1992): 619. There is much consistent anecdotal and some more rigorous evidence of the adverse risks accompanying the closure of a nursing home or long term-care unit. See, for example, John Warden, "Inquiry Ordered into Transfer of the Frail Elderly," *British Medical Journal* 316 (1998): 650; Susan Friedman et al., "Increase

Fall Rates in Nursing Home Residents After Relocation to a New Facility," *Journal of the American Geriatrics Society* 43, no. 11 (1995): 1237–42; Carol Robertson, Jill Warrington and John M. Eagles, "Relocation Mortality in Dementia: The Effects of a New Hospital," *International Journal of Geriatric Psychiatry* 6, no. 6 (1992): 51–76; Gregory B. Seathoff et al., "Mortality Among Elderly Patients Discharged from a State Hospital," *Hospital and Community Psychiatry* 43, no. 3 (1992): 280–82; and James A. Thorson, "Relocation of the Elderly: Some Implications from Research," *Gerontology Review* 1, no. 1 (1989): 28–36.

28. Vladeck, *Unloving Care,* 224–30.

29. Barker, *Adding Life to Years.*

30. Health Care Financing Administration, Office of the Actuary, Data from the Office of National Health Statistics, <www.hcfa.gov/news//n970127.htm>, March 20, 1997.

31. See, for example, "Planning to Be Poor: With a Little Help, the Nursing Home Won't Get Your Savings—Your Kids Will," *Newsweek,* November 30, 1992, 66–67; and Terry A. Donner, "Medicaid Estate Planning: Still Not Resolved," *Nursing Homes* 46, no. 10 (1997): 21–24.

32. Lee Labeck, M. Shaffer, and Sharon Shaffer, *Assessing the Feasibility of Developing and Marketing Long Term Care Insurance in Pennsylvania* (Harrisburg, Penn.: Department of Insurance, 1988), vi.

33. See for example, John Wennberg, *A Small Area Approach to the Analysis of Health System Performance* (Rockville, Md.: U.S. Department of Health and Human Services, 1980); *The Dartmouth Health Atlas* (Chicago: American Hospital Publishing, 1998); and David Smith and Joel Telles, *A Population-Based Analysis of the Effect of Disproportionate Share on Patterns of Hospital Care in a Metropolitan Area* (Philadelphia: Delaware Valley Health Education and Research Foundation, 1991).

34. Prospective Payment Assessment Commission, *Report and Recommendations to Congress, March 1, 1997* (Washington, D.C.: Prospective Payment Assessment Commission, 1997), 30.

35. Summary HCFA-2082 Tables Fiscal Year 1995.

36. Margaret K. Bishop, "Commercial Nursing and Boarding Homes in Philadelphia," *Social Security Bulletin,* June 1946, 16–18.

37. Pennsylvania Economy League, *Caring for Philadelphia's Needy Aged,* Report No. 350, (Philadelphia, 1968).

38. Ibid.

39. "Abandoning the Helpless," editorial, *Philadelphia Bulletin,* March 13, 1978, 2.

40. Ibid., quoting Seymour Rosenthal, report of the Temple University Center for Social Policy and Community Development.

41. "Goode Orders Crackdown on Boarding Homes," *Philadelphia Bulletin,* March 4, 1980.

42. Ann Torregrossa, interview by the author, tape recording, March 24, 1997.

43. David Smith and Robert Pickard, "Evaluation of the Impact of Medicare

and Medicaid Prospective Payment on Utilization in Philadelphia Area Hospitals," *Health Services Research* 21, no. 4 (1986): 529–46.

44. Torregrossa interview.

45. Torregrossa interview.

46. Torregrossa interview.

47. See Gilbert M. Gaul, "Nursing-Home Doors Slam Shut on the City's Poor," *Inquirer,* November 29, 1987, A1; "Racial Segregation Is Seen in Phila. Nursing Homes," *Inquirer,* November 30, 1987, A1; and "The Elderly Poor vs. the Elderly Middle Class," *Inquirer,* December 11, 1987, B16.

48. Torregrossa interview.

49. These tables are updated from David Smith, "Racial Integration of Health Facilities," *Journal of Health Policy, Politics, and Law* 18, no. 4 (1993): 851–69 and are reprinted with permission of Duke University Press.

50. A significantly higher proportion of black elderly Medicare enrollees living in the community have functional impairments: Candace L. Macken, "A Profile of Functionally Impaired Elderly Persons Living in the Community," *Health Care Financing Review* 7, no. 4 (1986): 33–49. While the racial gap in life expectancy at birth narrowed after the passage of Medicare and Medicaid, it widened for life expectancy at 65: Kenneth Manton, Clifford Patrick, and Katrina Johnson. "Health Differentials between Blacks and Whites: Recent Trends in Mortality and Morbidity," *Health Policies and Black Americans,* ed. David Willis, (New Brunswick, N.J.: Transaction, 1989), 129–99.

51. *Pennsylvania Bulletin* 19, no. 38 (September 23, 1989): 4116–18.

52. *Taylor v. White,* No. 90–3307 (E.D. Pa., amended complaint filed Aug. 15, 1990).

53. Torregrossa interview.

54. *Linton v. Commissioner of Health & Envt.,* 973 F.2d 1311, 1318 n. 12 (6th Circ. 1992).

55. RFP No. 5–96, *Commonwealth of Pennsylvania Request for Proposals for a Mandatory Medical Assistance Managed Care Program for Bucks, Chester, Delaware, Montgomery, and Philadelphia Counties,* 59.

56. Pennsylvania Department of Public Welfare, MA/LTC Participation Review, August 8, 1997, 5, 7.

57. The Department of Welfare is attempting to expand this obligation on the part of the Health Choices plans to ninety days.

58. Donald Snook, interview by author, tape recording, April 4, 1997.

59. Ibid.

60. Ibid.

61. Jonathan Rabinovitz, "Connecticut Pulls Back from a Managed Care Plan for the Elderly," *New York Times,* December 27, 1997, B1, B4.

Chapter 8

1. *Simkins v. Cone,* 970 n. 23.

2. National Center for Health Statistics, *Health in United States, 1996–1997,* 102, 103.

3. For a review of studies attempting to adjust for risk, income and educational differences in birth outcomes see Marsha Lillie-Blanton et al., "Racial Differences in Health," 416–19. Except for populations in the armed forces and thus provided uniform access to health care disparities persist.

4. See Jonathan B. Kotch et al., *A Pound of Prevention: The Case for Universal Maternity Care in the U.S.* (Washington, D.C.: American Public Health Association, 1992).

5. National Center for Health Statistics, *Health in United States, 1996–1997,* 106, 250.

6. Confidential interview by the author, tape recording, June 24, 1992.

7. David Smith, "Lower Merion Township Community Health Assessment," October 1992, 77. National physician population ratios are from National Center for Health Statistics, and local physician population ratios are derived from local physician listings, adjusting for multisite practices.

8. Hospital birth statistics were extracted from hospital discharge files obtained from the Pennsylvania Health Care Cost Containment Council for calendar year 1992.

9. The birth segregation index was calculated from data obtained from the Pennsylvania Health Care Cost Containment Council. The overall hospital segregation index was calculated from the Heath Care Financing Administration MEDPAR files, described in more detail in chapter 6. The residential segregation index was computed from 1990 census data.

10. National Center for Health Statistics, *Health in United States, 1995,* 194 (data from the National Ambulatory Medical Care Survey and the National Hospital Ambulatory Care Survey for 1993).

11. Anthony P. Polednak, "Black-White Differences in Infant Mortality in Thirty-eight Standard Metropolitan Statistical Areas," *American Journal of Public Health* 81, no. 11 (1991): 1480–82.

12. Smith, *Partners for Healthy Community,* 112.

13. Smith, Apt Associates, *Bucks County Community Health Assessment.*

14. Ibid., 95.

15. Ibid., 97–98.

16. Ibid., 98.

17. Ibid., 96.

18. Ibid.

19. Ibid, 97.

20. These were focus groups conducted between 1994 and 1996 for the Department of Obstetrics and Gynecology, Temple University Medical School, Temple University Hospital, Germantown and Chestnut Hill Hospitals, and for a coalition of hospitals and other services providers in neighboring Bucks County.

21. The author participated as the external evaluator of the Temple Infant and Parents Support and Services Program developed by the Department of Obstetrics and Gynecology at Temple University with the support of the William Penn Foundation between 1991 and 1994. The comments were extracted from taped interviews with staff.

22. Smith, Apt Associates, *Buck County Community Health Assessment,* 41, 58.

23. Roy Penchansky and Daniel Fox, "Frequency of Referral and Patient Characteristics in Group Practice," *Medical Care* 8, no. 5 (1970): 368–85.

24. An account of the integration of the facilities owned by state medical societies appears in chapter 5. See *United States v. Medical Society of South Carolina.*

25. Medical University of South Carolina, "Policy II07, Management of Drug Abuse during Pregnancy," Charleston, October 1989.

26. Ibid.

27. Ken Wittenmore, interview by the author, tape recording, October 30, 1997.

28. *Ferguson et al. v. City of Charleston, South Carolina,* C/A No. 2:93–2624–2 Corrected Copy Plaintiffs Memorandum in Support of Their Partial Cross-Motion for Summary Judgement and in Opposition to Defendents Motion for Summary Judgement (October 1995), 25–26.

29. *Ferguson v. City of Charleston.*

30. Edgar Horger, Shirley Brown, and Charles Condon, "Cocaine in Pregnancy: Confronting the Problem," *Journal of the South Carolina Medical Association* 86, no. 10 (1990): 527–31.

31. Linda G. Tribble et al., "Analysis of a Hospital Maternal Cocaine Testing Policy: Its Association with Prenatal Care Utilization Patterns." Unpublished abstract, (Exhibit 4 in *Ferguson v. City of Charleston* Defendents Memorandum in support of Summary Judgment).

32. David Annibale et al., "Re: Analysis of Hospital Cocaine Testing Policy: Its Association with Prenatal Utilization Patterns (Tribble et al.)," memorandum, May 17, 1994.

33. Philip H. Jos, Mary Faith Marshall, and Martin Perlmutter, "The Charleston Policy on Cocaine Use during Pregnancy: A Cautionary Tale," *Journal of Law, Medicine, and Ethics* 23 (1995): 120–28.

34. This section was written in conjunction with the local evaluation of Philadelphia's Health Start Initiative. It involved in-depth interviews with twelve key early participants in the development of that program. About half of this group represented service providers and the other half neighborhood leaders and organizers.

35. Huntley Collins, "From Healthy Start, Mixed Results," *Philadelphia Inquirer,* December 23, 1997, A1.

36. E. Digby Baltzell, *Puritan Boston and Quaker Philadelphia: Two Protestant Ethics and the Spirit of Class Authority and Leadership* (New York: Free Press, 1979).

37. Pennsylvania Department of Health, *Need Index for Maternal and Infant Health Services* (Harrisburg: Pennsylvania Department of Health, 1993).

38. Greenberg, *Crusaders in the Courts,* 341.

39. R. Gold et al., *Blessed Events and the Bottom Line: Financing Maternity Care in the United States* (New York: Allan Guttmacher Institute, 1987).

40. D. Hughes et al., *The Health of America's Children: Maternal and Child Health Data Book* (Washington, D.C.: Children's Defense Fund, 1988).

41. See, for example, Institute of Medicine, Committee to Study the Prevention

of Low Birth Weight, Division of Health Promotion and Disease Prevention, *Preventing Low Birth Weight* (Washington, D.C.: National Academy Press, 1985); Gold et al., *Blessed Events.*

42. Sandra Tannenbaum, "Medicaid Eligibility Policy in the 1980's: Medical Utilitarianism and the Deserving Poor," *Journal of Health Policy, Politics and the Law* 30, no. 4 (1995): 933–34.

43. See, for example, J. Haas et al., "The Effect of Providing Health Coverage to Poor Uninsured Pregnant Women in Massachusetts," *Journal of the American Medical Association* 269 (1993): 87–91; G. Kenney, "The Medicaid Expansions and Birth Outcomes: A Descriptive Analysis," Working Paper 6217–07, Washington, D.C., Urban Institute, 1994; P. Braverman et al., "Access to Prenatal Care following Major Medicaid Eligibility Expansions," *Journal of the American Medical Association* 269 (1993): 1285–89; and L. Dubay et al., "Local Responses to Expanded Medicaid Coverage for Pregnant Women," *Milbank Quarterly* 73, no. 4 (1995): 535–63.

44. *Philadelphia Inquirer,* September 28, 1995, A10.

45. Robert Pear, "Bush Plan to Fight Infant Deaths Would Use Money Going to Poor," *New York Times,* February 6, 1991, A1.

46. Robert Pear, "19 Cities Listed for Aid to Cut Infant Mortality," *New York Times,* March 7, 1991, A12.

47. Ibid.

48. Ibid.

49. N. Goldfarb et. al., "Impact of Mandatory Medicaid Case Management Program on Prenatal Care and Birth Outcomes: A Retrospective Analysis," *Medical Care* 29, no. 1 (1991): 64–71.

50. General Accounting Office, *HealthPASS: An Evaluation of a Managed Care Program for Certain Philadelphia Recipients,* GAO/IIRD-93–67 (Washington, D.C.: U.S. General Accounting Office, May 1993).

51. Philadelphia Department of Health, *Healthy Start Plan,* 1992, 55–76.

52. D. Strobino et al., "A Strategic Framework for Infant Morality Reduction: Implications for Healthy Start," *Milbank Quarterly* 73, no. 4 (1995): 507–33.

53. See Arthur T. Himmelman, *Final Report on the Healthy Start Initiative,* unpublished report, October 1996. The report describes the project as a "collaborative betterment" as opposed to a "collaborative empowerment" approach driven by a large institution (the Health Department) seeking collaborative community partners but pushed and pulled by the partners arguing for more of an empowerment approach.

54. L. Schorr, *Within Our Reach: Breaking the Cycle of Disadvantage* (New York: Anchor, 1988).

55. James P. Robinson and Lawrence P. Casalino, "Vertical Integration and Organizational Networks in Health Care," *Health Affairs* 15, no. 1 (1996): 7–22.

56. Collins, "From Healthy Start," A1, A12.

57. From "Healthy Start, Mixed Results," *Philadelphia Inquirer* December 23, 1997, A12.

Chapter 9

1. David Falcone and Robert Broyles, "Access to Long Term Care: Race as a Barrier," *Journal of Health Politics, Policy and Law* 19, no. 3 (1994): 593.

2. Stevens, *Sickness and Wealth,* 361.

3. Marianne Engleman Laddo, interview by author, tape recording, February 15, 1995.

4. For a description of this earlier period see W. Montague Cobb, "Medical Deans Static," editorial, *Journal of the National Medical Association* 43 (1951): 57–58. For the current status see Jordan Cohen, "Finishing the Bridge to Diversity," *Academic Medicine* 72, no. 2 (1997): 103.

5. Howard Zinn, *You Can't Be Neutral on a Moving Train* (Boston: Beacon Press 1995), 92.

6. E. H. Beardsley, "Goodbye to Jim Crow: The Desegregation of Southern Hospitals, 1945–1970," *Bulletin of the History of Medicine* 60 (1986): 386.

7. African American Focus Group, *Bucks County Community Health Assessment: Qualitative Profile,* November 21, 1994, 83.

8. M. Meltsner, "Equality and Health," *Pennsylvania Law Review* 115, no. 1 (1966): 38.

9. U.S. Commission on Civil Rights, *Funding Civil Rights Enforcement.*

10. Jeremy Rabkin, "The Office for Civil Rights," in *The Politics of Regulation,* ed. James Q. Wilson (New York: Basic Books, 1980), 304.

11. U.S. Commission on Civil Rights, *To Know or Not to Know: Collection and Use of Racial and Ethnic Data in Federal Assistance Programs* (Washington, D.C.: Government Printing Office, 1973).

12. *Madison-Hughes v. Shalala,* No. 3–93–0046 (M.D. Tenn. filed January 19, 1993).

13. G. Bonnyman et al., Memorandum to Individuals and Organizations Concerned about Civil Rights, December 20, 1994, correspondence of author.

14. G. Orfield and C. Ashkinaze, *The Closing Door: Conservative Policy and Black Opportunity* (Chicago: University of Chicago Press, 1991).

15. H. Jack Geiger, "Race and Health Care—an American Dilemma," editorial, *New England Journal of Medicine* 336 (1996): 816. The section is extracted from a paper previously published, David Smith, "Addressing Racial Inequities in Health Care: Civil Rights Monitoring and Report Cards," *Journal of Health Policy, Politics, and Law* 23, no. 1 (1998): 75–105 and is reprinted with permission of Duke University Press.

16. Geiger, "Race and Health Care," 816.

17. These distinctions in approaches to assessment were first clearly codified by Avedis Donabedian. See Avedis Donabedian, *The Definition of Quality and Approaches to Its Assessment* (Ann Arbor: Health Administration Press, 1980).

18. Robert E. Hurley, "The Purchaser Driven Reformation in Health Care: Alternative Approaches to Leveling our Cathedrals," *Frontiers of Health Services Management* 9, no. 4 (1993): 5–35.

19. Office of Management and Budget, "Revisions to Standards," 58789.

20. Research Triangle Institute, *Design of a Survey to Monitor Consumer's Access to Care, Use of Services, Health Outcomes, and Patient Satisfaction: Final Report* (Rockville, Md: Agency for Health Policy and Research, DHHS, 1995).

21. Joint Commission on Accreditation of Health Care Organizations *National Library of Healthcare Indicators: Health Plan and Network Edition* (Oakbrook Terrace, Ill: JCAHO, 1997).

22. See Alicia H. Munnell et al., "Mortgage Lending in Boston: Interpreting the Data," working paper (Federal Reserve Bank of Boston, 1992), and William Hunter and Mary Beth Walker, "The Cultural Affinity Hypothesis and Mortgage Lending Decisions," working paper (Federal Reserve Bank of Boston, July 1995).

23. National Community Reinvestment Coalition, "1994 Home Mortgage Shows Improvement," *NCRC Reinvestment Compendium* 2, no. 3 (1996): 9.

24. Marsha L. Gold et al., "Behind the Curve: A Critical Assessment of How Little is Known about Arrangements between Managed Care Plans and Physicians," *Medical Care Research and Review* 52, no. 3 (1995): 307–41.

25. Ibid.

26. Roy Penchansky and Daniel Fox, "Frequency and Patient Characteristics in Group Practice," *Medical Care* 8, no. 5 (1970): 368–85.

27. Smith, Apt Associates, *Community Health Assessment for Broward County, Florida,* Teen Focus Group, December 1994, 147.

28. P.L.105–33, 105th Cong. 1st. sess.

29. The Sentencing Project, *Intended and Unintended Consequences: State Racial Disparities in Imprisonment* (Washington, D.C.: The Sentencing Project, 1997).

30. Rodrick Wallace and Deborah Wallace, "The Coming Plagues."

31. Solomon R. Benatar, "Health Care Reform in the New South Africa," *New England Journal of Medicine* 336, no. 12 (1997): 891.

32. Tim Smith, "A Nation Examines Its Conscience," *America,* November 8, 1997, 22–26.

Index

373

386   Index